VASCULAR SURGICAL TECHNIQUES

VASCULAR SURGICAL TECHNIQUES

An Atlas

Second Edition

Edited by

ROGER M. GREENHALGH MA, MD, MChir, FRCS

Professor of Surgery, Charing Cross and Westminster Medical School, London, UK.

W. B. Saunders Company

London · Philadelphia · Toronto · Sydney · Tokyo

W.B. Saunders   24–28 Oval Road
Baillière Tindall   London NW1 7DX, UK

The Curtis Center
Independence Square West
Philadelphia, PA 19106–3399, USA

1 Goldthorne Avenue
Toronto, Ontario M8Z 5T9, Canada

Harcourt Brace Jovanovich Group (Australia) Pty Limited
32–52 Smidmore Street, Marrickville,
NSW 2204, Australia

Harcourt Brace Jovanovich Group Japan Inc
Ichibancho Central Building, 22–1 Ichibancho
Chiyoda-ku, Tokyo 102, Japan

British Library Cataloguing in Publication Data

Greenhalgh, Roger M. (Roger Malcolm)
   Vascular surgical techniques: an altas 2nd edition
   1. Blood vessels — Surgery
   617'.43   RD598.5
ISBN 0702013773

Typeset by Lasertext Ltd, Stretford, Manchester
Printed and bound in Great Britain by
Mackays of Chatham PLC, Letchworth, Herts.

CONTENTS

Contributors

George Andros, MD
Vascular Laboratory, Saint Joseph Medical Center, Burbank, California, USA

Enrico Ascer, MD
Associate Professor of Surgery, Albert Einstein College of Medicine, New York, USA;
Vascular Surgeon in Charge, North Central Bronx Hospital, New York, USA

Roger N Baird, ChM, FRCS
Consultant Surgeon, The Royal Infirmary, Bristol, UK

Aires A B Barros D'Sa, MD, FRCS, FRCS (Ed)
Consultant Vascular Surgeon, Vascular Surgical Unit, Royal Victoria Hospital, Belfast, UK

Y Bensaïd
Service de Chirurgie Vasculaire, Groupe Hospitalier Pitié-Salpétrière, Paris, France

John J Bergan, MD
Clinical Professor of Surgery, University of California, San Diego, California, USA;
Magerstadt Professor Emeritus of Surgery, Northwestern University Medical School, Chicago, Illinois, USA

Sven-Erik Bergentz, MD
Department of Surgery, Lund University, Malmö General Hospital, Malmö, Sweden

Giorgio M Biasi, MD
Professor, Institute of General and Cardiovascular Surgery, University of Milan, Milan, Italy

Martin Birnstingl, MS, FRCS
Consultant Surgeon, St Bartholomew's Hospital, London, UK

N L Browse, MD, FRCS
Professor of Surgery, Department of Surgery, St. Thomas' Hospital, London, UK

K G Burnand, MS, FRCS
Assistant Director, Department of Surgery, St. Thomas' Hospital, London, UK

Benjamin B Chang, MD, FACS
Associate Professor of Surgery, Albany Medical College, Albany, New York, USA

Albert K Chin, MD
Cardiovascular Research Staff, Sequoia Hospital, Redwood City, California, USA

F B Cockett, MS, FRCS
Consulting Surgeon, St. Thomas' Hospital, London, UK

M Colonna, MD
Department of Vascular Surgery, University Hospital of Rome, Rome, Italy

R Courbier
Professeur Agrégé à la Faculte de Medecine et Chef du Service de Chirurgie Cardio Vasculaire, Hôpital Saint Joseph, Marseille, France

Herbert Dardik, MD, FACS
Chief, General and Vascular Surgery, Englewood Hospital, Englewood, New Jersey, USA;
Clinical Associate Professor of Surgery, New Jersey Medical School, Newark, New Jersey, USA

Michael E DeBakey, MD
Olga Keith Wiess Professor of Surgery and Chairman, Cora and Webb Mading Department of Surgery, and Chancellor, Baylor College of Medicine, Houston, Texas, USA

Ralph G DePalma, MD
Chairman, Department of Surgery, George Washington University Medical Center, Washington DC, USA

Alexander C De Vries, MD
St. Antonius Hospital, Nieuwegein, The Netherlands

Do-Dai-Do
Medical Department of the University of Berne, Berne, Switzerland

Leopoldo B Dulawa, MD
Vascular Laboratory, Saint Joseph Medical Center, Burbank, California, USA

William K Ehrenfeld, MD
Professor of Surgery, University of California, San Fransisco, California, USA

Bert C Eikelboom, MD, PhD
St. Antonius Hospital, Nieuwegein, The Netherlands

Harold Ellis, CBE, DM, MCh, FRCS
Professor of Surgery, Westminster Hospital, London

V Faraglia, MD
Department of Vascular Surgery, University Hospital of Rome, Rome, Italy

James C Finn, MD
Stanford University Medical Center, Stanford, California, USA

P Fiorani, MD
Professor of Vascular Surgery, University Hospital of Rome, Rome, Italy

Thomas J Fogarty, MD, FACS
Chief, Cardiovascular Section, Sequoia Hospital, Redwood City, California, USA

Roger M Greenhalgh, MA, MD, MChir, FRCS
Professor of Surgery, Charing Cross and Westminster Medical School, London, UK

Lazar J Greenfield, MD
Professor and Chairman, Department of Surgery, University of Michigan, Ann Arbor, Michigan, USA

Sushil K Gupta, MD
Associate Professor of Surgery and Associate Chief of Vascular Surgery, Albert Einstein College of Medicine and Montefiore Medical Center, New York, USA

P L Harris, MD FRCS
Consultant in Vascular Surgery, Broadgreen Hospital,
Liverpool, UK;
Lecturer in Clinical Surgery, University of Liverpool,
Liverpool, UK

Robert W Harris, MD
Vascular Laboratory, Saint Joseph Medical Center,
Burbank, California, USA

Larry H Hollier, MD, FACS, FACC
Chairman, Department of Surgery, Ochsner Clinic, New
Orleans, Louisiana, USA

Crawford W Jamieson, MS, FRCS
Consultant Surgeon, St. Thomas's Hospital, London, UK;
Honorary Consultant Surgeon, Hammersmith Hospital
and Royal Postgraduate Medical School, London, UK

J M Jausseran
Assistant du Service de Chirurgie Cardio Vasculaire,
Hôpital Saint Joseph, Marseille, France

Jeffrey L Kaufman, MD, FACS
Associate Professor of Surgery, Albany Medical College
and Veterans Administration Medical Center, Albany, New
York, USA

E Kieffer
Service de Chirurgie Vasculaire, Groupe Hospitalier Pitié-
Salpétrière, Paris, France

G Kretschmer, MD
1st Clinic of Surgery, University of Vienna, Vienna, Austria

Rodney J Lane, MS, FRCS, FRCS(Ed), DDU, FRACS
Visiting Vascular Surgeon, The Royal North Shore Hospital,
St. Leonard's, New South Wales, Australia;
Visiting Vascular Surgeon, North Harbour Private Hospital,
Harbord, New South Wales, Australia

Robert P Leather, MD, FACS
Professor of Surgery, Albany Medical College, Albany,
New York, USA

F Mahler
Medical Department of the University of Berne, Berne,
Switzerland

John A Mannick, MD
Moseley Professor of Surgery, Harvard Medical School;
Surgeon-in-Chief, Brigham and Women's Hospital, Boston,
Massachusetts, USA

Averil O. Mansfield, ChM, FRCS
Consultant Surgeon, St. Mary's Hospital, London;
Honorary Senior Lecturer in Vascular Surgery, Royal
Postgraduate Medical School, London, UK

Charles N McCollum, MD, FRCS
Reader in Surgery, Charing Cross and Westminster
Medical School, London, UK;
Consultant Surgeon, Charing Cross Hospital, London, UK

James McIvor, MBChB, FRCR, FFR, FDSRCS
Consultant Radiologist, Charing Cross Hospital, London,
UK;
Senior Lecturer (Radiology), Institute of Dental Surgery,
London, UK

Sergio Miani, MD
Professor, Institute of General and Cardiovascular Surgery,
University of Milan, Milan, Italy

Justin H Miller, MBBS, FRCS, FRACS, FACS
Royal Adelaide Hospital and Repatriation General Hospital,
Adelaide, South Australia

Hans O Myhre, MD, PhD
Professor and Chairman, Department of Surgery,
Trondheim University Clinic, Trondheim, Norway

B Nachbur
Department of Thoracic and Cardiovascular Surgery,
University of Berne, Berne, Switzerland

J Natali
Service de Chirurgie Vasculaire, Groupe Hospitalier Pitié-
Salpétrière, Paris, France

B Niederle, MD
1st Clinic of Surgery, University of Vienna, Vienna, Austria

Robert W Oblath, MD
Vascular Laboratory, Saint Joseph Medical Center,
Burbank, California, USA

Michael J Olding, MD
Department of Surgery, George Washington University
Medical Center, Washington DC, USA

Malcolm O Perry, MD
Department of Surgery, Division of Vascular Surgery,
Vanderbilt University School of Medicine, Nashville,
Tennessee, USA

C Petitjean
Service de Chirurgie Vasculaire, Group Hospitalier Pitié-
Salpètrière, Paris, France

Peter G Qvarfordt, MD
Vascular Research Fellow, University of California, San
Francisco, California, USA

M Kathleen Reilly, PhD, MD
Department of Surgery, Division of Vascular Surgery,
Vanderbilt University School of Medicine, Nashville,
Tennessee, USA

K W Reynolds, MS, FRCS
Consultant Surgeon, Gastrointestinal Unit, Charing Cross
Hospital Medical School, London, UK

Norman M Rich, MD, FACS
Professor and Chairman, Department of Surgery, and
Chief, Division of Vascular Surgery F Edward Herbert School
of Medicine, Uniformed Services University of the Health
Sciences, Bethesda, Maryland, USA;
Co-Director, Vascular Fellowship Program, Walter Reed
Army Medical Center

John V Robbs, ChM(CT), FRCS (Ed)
Chief, Vascular Service and Head, Division of Surgery,
University of Natal Medical School, Durban, South Africa

Kingsley Robinson, MS, FRCS(Ed), FRCS(Eng)
Consultant Surgeon, Westminster Hospital, London;
Director, Limb-Surgery Unit and Consultant Surgeon,
Queen Mary's Hospital, Roehampton

Sidney S Rose, MB ChB, FRCS
Consulting Surgeon, University Hospital of South
Manchester, Withington Hospital, Manchester, UK

John P Royle, MBBS, FRCS(Ed), FRCS, FRACS, FACS
Director of Vascular Surgery, Surgery Unit, Austin
Hospital, Heidelberg, Australia;
Senior Associate, University of Melbourne, Australia;
Consultant Vascular Surgeon, Fairfield Hospital,
Melbourne, Australia

Ola D Saether
Senior Registrar, Department of Surgery, Trondheim University Clinic, Trondheim, Norway

Sergio X Salles-Cunha, PhD
Vascular Laboratory, Saint Joseph Medical Center, Burbank, California, USA

Wilhelm Sandmann
Department of Vascular Surgery and Kidney Transplantation, Chirurgische Universitätsklinik Düsseldorf, Düsseldorf, Federal Republic of Germany

E Schneider
Division of Angiology, Medical Department of the University of Zürich, Zürich, Switzerland

Dhiraj M Shah, MD, FACS
Associate Professor of Surgery, Albany Medical College and Veterans Administration Center, Albany, New York, USA

F Speziale, MD
Department of Vascular Surgery, University Hospital of Rome, Rome, Italy

Ronald J Stoney, MD
Professor of Surgery, University of California, San Francisco, California, USA

M Taurino, MD
Department of Vascular Surgery, University Hospital of Rome, Rome, Italy

Peter R Taylor, MA, FRCS
Senior Clinical Vascular Fellow, St. Mary's Hospital, London, UK

N A Theodorou, FRCS
Senior Surgical Registrar, Department of Surgery, Charing Cross Hospital Medical School, London, UK

Jesse E Thompson, MD, FACS
Attending Surgeon, Baylor University Medical Center, Dallas, Texas, USA;
Clinical Professor of Surgery, University of Texas, Southwestern Medical School, Dallas, Texas, USA

Hero Van Urk, MD
Chief, Vascular Surgery, University Hospital, Erasmus University, Rotterdam, The Netherlands

Frank J Veith, MD
Professor of Surgery and Chief of Vascular Surgical Services, Albert Einstein College of Medicine and Montefiore Medical Center, New York, USA

O Wagner, MD
Professor of Surgery, University of Vienna, Vienna, Austria

Kurt R Wengerter, MD
Assistant Professor of Surgery and Assistant Attending Vascular Surgeon, Albert Einstein College of Medicine and Montefiore Medical Center, New York, USA

Anthony D Whittemore, MD
Assistant Professor of Surgery, Harvard Medical School; Surgeon, Brigham and Women's Hospital, Boston, Massachusetts, USA

John H N Wolfe, MS, FRCS
Consultant Vascular Surgeon and Honorary Senior Lecturer, St. Mary's Hospital Medical School, London, UK; Consultant Vascular Surgeon and Honorary Senior Lecturer, Royal Postgraduate Medical School, Hammersmith Hospital, London, UK

M Wunderlich, MD
1st Clinic of Surgery, University of Vienna, Vienna, Austria

James S T Yao, MD, PhD
Professor of Surgery and Director, Blood Flow Laboratory, Northwestern University Medical School, Chicago, Illinois, USA

Dedication

I wish to dedicate this Atlas to Professor G. W. Taylor, Emeritus Professor of Surgery at St. Bartholomew's Hospital – London, my first teacher of operative technique. Gerry Taylor achieved excellent technical results by never failing to be well read and prepared for each procedure, always performed with natural flair.

PREFACE

The aim of the second edition remains to describe operations which are currently performed by the most eminent vascular surgeons from around the world. During the five years since the first edition, the practice of vascular surgery has continued to evolve and many of these exciting developments are reflected in the contents of this edition.

All of the chapters retained from the last edition have been fully reconsidered, re-edited and in some cases rewritten by the original or new authors so they are completely up-to-date. There are also additional chapters by distinguished authors to reflect and highlight important techniques of the moment. In the Basic Principles section a chapter has been added on *Intra-operative Proof of Patency*. During recent years vascular surgeons have taken even greater care to prove patency on the operating table and indeed to design the intended procedure before surgery with greater precision. This chapter illustrates how these techniques can achieve optimal reconstruction results. Infected grafts are the bane of the vascular surgeon's life. Correct management frequently requires courage, timely intervention and an informed appreciation of the extent of graft excision. There is a new section devoted to vascular trauma as we continue to live in troubled times. The chapters from South Africa and Belfast reflect tremendous experience in the management of violent wounds. Dr. Malcolm Perry has had a life interest in vascular trauma and had experience of a number of distinguished casualties when he worked in Dallas before moving on to take his expertise to other centres. The chapters on carotid surgery by Jesse E. Thompson of Dallas and on aortic bifurcation grafting by Michael E. DeBakey of Houston, greatly strengthen this edition.

During the last five years, the advance of vascular surgery has been marked by increasingly important contributions from the continent of Europe and we have seen the foundation of the European Society for Vascular Surgery in 1987. Significantly, this edition contains many contributions from authors in the continent of Europe, not only from France and Italy as before but now from Scandinavia, Holland, Germany, Austria and Switzerland where there has been a notable upsurge of enthusiasm in vascular surgery.

The standard embolectomy technique for acute ischaemia as described in this edition by Hans Myhre, is challenged as the optimal technique for all situations by Bernard Nachbur who describes his preferred technique of initial lysis and catheter clot removal which he employs in many cases.

Few operative procedures have disappeared since 1984 but extracranial/intracranial bypass suffered severe criticism and has been excluded from this edition. The *in situ* vein bypass of Karmody and Leather was becoming established when these authors described their method in the first edition. I greatly regret the premature death of Alistair Karmody who, in partnership with Bob Leather, taught so many of us this excellent operation. Their method remains and has gathered momentum to the extent that vein utilization for femoropopliteal and femorotibial bypass has increased to over 90% in the best centres. This has lead to a great reduction in the use of prosthetic bypass below the knee and the chapters on these subjects have been thoroughly revised. The harvesting of arm vein described again is, if anything, even more vital five years later because of this increasing disenchantment with prosthetic material for distal sites.

Whilst percutaneous transluminal angioplasty has certainly found its role in the management of vascular surgical patients there are yet more recent intra-arterial techniques available. The name of Thomas Fogarty has always been associated with innovation and he has authored two excellent chapters which show advances in this field, notably the description of the atherectomy device.

A new section on amputations has been included in this edition as the Editor is reluctantly accepting that some legs cannot be saved and are best amputated. Nevertheless, only a small percentage of critically ischaemic limbs should come to major amputation and it is important to relate the level of amputation to the best available prosthesis. If a forefoot amputation is not possible many believe that the next best option for rapid mobility is a below-knee amputation. The long posterior flap (Burgess procedure) is favoured by many but Kingsley Robinson has shown us that the skew flap amputation can be performed in circumstances where the long posterior flap is not possible and only this technique can preserve the knee joint in some patients. Above this level few surgeons see the place for any amputation other than at mid-thigh, with good myoplastic flaps, if the patient is to be mobilised. The prosthesis for a patient having a through-knee amputation is very cumbersome and this procedure virtually disappeared for some years. It has been reintroduced for the very sick patient requiring an amputation who is not expected to walk again. This amputation is ideal for this situation; it is a totally soft tissue procedure finishing with a tiny scar. This re-emergence is welcomed.

Finally, the management of varicose veins has changed little, but the management of venous ulceration and venous insufficiency of the lower limb is still evolving. Chapters are included on venous reconstructive surgery and techniques to improve the competence of deep valves, deep venous thrombectomy and placement of the Kimray-Greenfield inferior vena caval filter to prevent pulmonary embolism. It is clear that practices concerning deep venous surgery are greatly divergent in different parts of the world. For example, on the continent of Europe many deep venous thrombectomies are performed whereas in the United Kingdom this seldom occurs. In the United States and Australia deep vein reconstructions are being performed but there is less enthusiasm elsewhere.

What has emerged is that there is a range of possibilities and a variety of known pathologies which can lead to venous insufficiency in the lower limb and ulceration. Venous assessments, not only ascending and descending venography, are required to investigate these limbs. Even more important is the advent of venous non-invasive testing which is still not being applied the world over. Venous pressure testing and prediction tests are emerging. It appears that venous insufficiency can be improved very easily in a large number of patients by simple ligation of superficial veins and ligation of perforating veins. It is extremely important that the techniques seen in this Atlas in the section on deep venous surgery should be applied to the limb requiring that procedure. We shall certainly see advances in this field over the next five years.

I should like to thank all of the authors for their excellent contributions. Their ability to produce these detailed descriptions in their busy lives is greatly appreciated by me as it certainly will by all those who read this volume. The contributors are the leading experts in the field whom we visit to learn and improve our techniques and it is appropriate that their unique technical expertise should be recorded in these pages. I am extremely happy that Sean Duggan has commissioned this second edition as he did the first. It has been a great pleasure to work with him once again.

Roger M. Greenhalgh

Operation planning

Roger M. Greenhalgh   MA, MD, MChir, FRCS

Professor of Surgery, Charing Cross and Westminster Medical School, London, UK

Introduction

All operative procedures require careful planning and this is especially important for arterial reconstructive surgery. The desired result cannot be achieved if patient selection is poor. Learning how to choose the right procedure for the right patient takes at least as much experience as learning how to do the vascular surgical techniques and both should form an integral part of training for vascular surgeons. The indications for the individual procedures are mentioned at the beginning of the later chapters but are only given in outline, as this really is a separate subject.

Preoperative assessment, non-invasive testing and angiography are essential stages in accurate patient selection for a procedure and these are outlined here. This is followed by a note on anaesthetic aspects and monitoring during the operative procedure, followed by some haematological considerations.

Preoperative assessment

A very careful history of the patient must initially be taken. It is vital to relate the patient's complaint to age, occupation and way of life before deciding what is the best treatment.

Almost all patients with severe arterial disease have been heavy smokers for many years. Patients at risk of stroke or suffering from ischaemic rest pain or imminent gangrene should be offered any possible operative procedure immediately. If the situation is not so urgent, the surgeon must decide whether to ask the patient to stop smoking before the operation is carried out.

The cardiac status needs to be thoroughly assessed. Approximately half of the patients presenting with the symptoms of peripheral arterial disease have already had a myocardial infarction in the past as demonstrated by resting electrocardiographic abnormality and a greater proportion have exercise ECG changes. Those centres with the facility should always perform ventricular ejection fractions on their patients to assess the cardiac status before embarking upon arterial reconstruction in the extremities. Centres without this facility can still rely to a great extent on careful history taking and examination of cardiac function to establish which patients are at high risk of cardiac failure. Often, such as for impending gangrene or stroke, there is no alternative but to perform a reconstruction.

Approximately 10% of patients with peripheral arterial disease are diabetic and just as it is important to work closely with a cardiologist for cardiac problems, it is equally important to work hand in hand with an endocrine physician when dealing with diabetic patients. Each endocrine specialist has his own way of managing the problem. There is increasing use of a constant infusion of insulin over the perioperative period. It is claimed that this facilitates easier moment-to-moment control of diabetes mellitus. Of course, the most important rule is that the blood glucose level should never be allowed to fall; a slight rise is preferable but the expert will aim at perfect control of the blood glucose level over the whole perioperative period.

If patients are taking warfarin or a similar oral anticoagulant drug this should be stopped and the prothrombin time should become normal before surgery. If it is thought that a prosthetic graft is going to be used in a low flow situation, an antithrombotic regimen may be instituted 48 h before surgery. Aspirin 300 mg daily with dipyridamole 75 mg three times daily is found to be an acceptable dosage in most centres.

A complete physical examination should be undertaken for all patients. The chest must, of course, be examined most carefully in those patients who are to undergo general anaesthesia. All of the pulses are felt and a careful examination is made for aneurysmal disease over the aorta, femoral and popliteal regions. It is important to listen for bruit over diseased arteries, particularly in the neck.

Two of the most important special investigations that are performed are for detection of diabetes mellitus and renal disease. Examination of the urine and measurement of blood sugar and plasma creatinine levels is essential and any abnormalities discovered require further investigation.

Non-invasive testing

Until recently it was felt that a thorough clinical examination and an angiogram were all that were required for correct patient selection. Increasingly, the place of non-invasive tests has become established. These now have a firm place in the investigation of carotid artery disease and disease of the arteries supplying the lower limbs. Ideally the carotid vessel should be investigated whenever the arterial tree is to be operated upon at another site. It is mandatory to evaluate the carotids in patients who have a carotid bruit. Oculoplethysmography (OPG) and carotid phonangiography have been used to assess the carotid vessels by an indirect method. The Kartschner and McRae OPG system compares the transit time to the eyeballs and the transit times to the ears. The Gee OPG works on a completely different principle and measures pressure in the orbit.

The indirect methods are now largely superceded by imaging methods. The first generation imaging systems incorporated pulsed gated Doppler imaging methods. These have given way to the duplex scanner which now has a colour coding facility. The duplex scanner combines B-mode ultrasound with Doppler velocity profile. This scanner has been shown to have a 98% correlation with conventional angiography. Digital subraction angiography also provides valuable additional anatomical information about the carotid vessels but this is strictly invasive because the contrast material is injected into a vein. This technique also has approximately 98% correlation with conventional angiography, and when combined with duplex scanning, a 99% correlation. The main concern about conventional angiography is that it carries a small but definite morbidity risk. This suggests that its use is only justified in patients with symptomatic carotid arterial disease, whereas the non-invasive tests mentioned here have no morbidity and provide an extremely convenient method of assessment of the carotid vessels before arterial reconstruction at another site is undertaken.

Non-invasive tests are equally valuable in assessing the arteries supplying the lower limbs. The simplest test involves the use of a Doppler probe with a blood pressure cuff. This enables the ultrasonic systolic pressure to be recorded at a particular segment. If the cuff is placed around the ankle, calf and upper thigh, segmental pressures can be measured on both legs and this can give vital information to be considered alongside an arteriogram. Where all pulses are present, and the Doppler systolic pressure in the ankle is normal compared to that in the arm, it is important to perform an exercise test to ensure that pressure is maintained after exercise (Laing and Greenhalgh, 1980). The waveforms of the velocity profiles on different points along the leg can also give vital information on the site and severity of disease.

An example of where these tests are of a special value is before performance of a femorofemoral cross-over graft. For this procedure it is not enough just to look at the arteriogram; it is absolutely essential to know that the donor iliac segment is normal and that it is a suitable source of blood supply for the opposite limb. A combination of waveform analysis, segmental pressure measurement and exercise testing can be most helpful here.

Angiography

The perfemoral Seldinger technique is the most commonly used method of arteriography today. With this approach it is possible to pass catheters to almost all parts of the arterial tree, provided that there are no arterial occlusions or very tight stenoses. If the iliac system above or the aorta is occluded it may be necessary to approach the arterial tree from another route. The transaxillary approach gives the same degree of flexibility as the femoral approach but this requires proper training to avoid damage to the nearby brachial plexus. The advantage of this approach is the ability to perform selective arterial catherization, e.g. of the carotid subclavian, vertebral, renal or visceral vessels. These techniques do not require general anaesthesia but the patient is frequently slightly sedated.

Translumbar aortography requires general anaesthesia but can be performed as an outpatient procedure. It is difficult though to take films in more than one plane and this is essential, at, for example, the origin of the profunda femoris artery which arises from behind the main vessel.

Anaesthetic options and monitoring

Most of the contributors to this book draw attention to the great value of the expertise of the anaesthetist who has experience with vascular surgical patients. Either a general anaesthetic or a light anaesthetic with continuous epidural can be used. It is essential to assess pulmonary function properly before embarking upon a procedure and to decide on the most appropriate form of anaesthesia. In some circumstances it is possible to provide a local block or even local infiltration to perform simple procedures as, for example, in the groin. The monitoring system which is used for continuous assessment of the patient during the operative procedure is designed for the benefit of the anaesthetist and the surgeon. A radial intra-arterial catheter should be passed so that continuous monitoring of the systolic and diastolic pressures is possible throughout the procedure. A central venous pressure line and ECG monitor are essential for every arterial operation. A number of venous lines is required – up to four if rapid transfusion is envisaged as, for example, when operating upon thoracoabdominal aneurysms. The insertion of a Swan-Ganz catheter is more controversial, but this is being used increasingly. Ideally, the catheter is inserted a day or so before the operation so that the optimal capillary wedge pressure for maximal cardiac output can be determined and this knowledge is used during surgery.

During the operation it is vital to estimate blood gases at least every 30 min so an anaesthetic is chosen that does not depress the myocardium. For muscle relaxation, muscle relaxant drugs are used. A urinary catheter is passed so that the hourly urine output can be monitored. When the surgeon clamps a major blood vessel he should work with the anaesthetist, observe the monitoring system and, if necessary, perform the clamping and unclamping very slowly. The use of heparin is very controversial. Most surgeons performing arterial bypass use approximately 5000 i.u. of heparin intravenously before cross-clamping. A wait of approximately 3 min before applying the clamps is generally recommended to allow the heparin to circulate. For emergency abdominal aneurysms and for all thoracoabdominal aneurysm replacements the use of heparin is not advisable.

Haematological considerations

It is necessary to work closely with the haematology department. Adequate whole blood needs to be cross-matched before the operation, and if excessive blood loss is anticipated, albumin and fresh frozen plasma should be at hand. For major procedures such as thoracoabdominal aneurysms, 10–16 u of platelets should be available so that these can be infused the moment the blood flow is restored to the graft. For major transfusions it is wise to alternate 1 u of frozen plasma to every 2 u of whole blood.

The planning of venous procedures is just as important as the planning of arterial ones. Varicose veins are assessed and marked following clinical examination and the the use of the Doppler probe can be valuable to determine whether there is any incompetence at a particular site. When considering surgery of the deep venous system, it is important to perform ascending and descending venograms.

Reference

Laing, S. P. and Greenhalgh, R. M. (1980). Standard exercise test to assess peripheral arterial disease. *British Medical Journal* **280**, 13.

Techniques of anastomosis

Roger M. Greenhalgh MA, MD, MChir, FRCS

Professor of Surgery, Charing Cross and Westminster Medical School, London, UK

Introduction

The various techniques of anastomosis, or joining of blood vessels, fall into two main types: end-to-end anastomosis and end-to-side anastomosis. Various graft materials are preferred for bypass in different parts of the body and these are described in detail in subsequent chapters. For replacement of large vessels such as the aorta, Dacron has become the material of choice. Essentially, Dacron prostheses are of two main types, woven and knitted. The woven variety has the advantages that it does not require any preclotting of the Dacron and it does not leak blood. Its disadvantage is that it is rather stiff and when cut it frays. It is advisable to cut woven Dacron with an electric diathermy needle so that the ends are sealed, but this can be quite a tricky procedure compared with the precise cutting of a knitted Dacron graft which can be performed with scissors. The great advantage of knitted Dacron is that it can be shaped exactly as required but must be preclotted. Preclotting can be achieved by taking approximately 100 ml of blood from a nearby vein such as the vena cava and syringing it down through the graft so that the blood pours through the holes. The blood is then caught in a dish and syringed through the graft again and again with some pressure until the interstices become blocked by the clotting blood. The blood is then squeezed out of the Dacron which should be leak-proof and it is ready for anastomosis. To dispense with or minimize preclotting, collagen impregnation and albumen coating of Dacron has recently been introduced. An externally supported Dacron graft has gained much favour and may prove ideal in sites where it is important that the graft should not be squashed, such as for axillofemoral bypass.

Dacron is perphaps the material of choice for the replacement or bypass of arteries ranging in size from the aorta to the common femoral artery. Expanded polytetrafluoroethylene (PTFE) is mainly used in long straight tubes for the replacement of smaller arteries than is ideal for Dacron. However, a bifurcated graft of PTFE is now available to replace or bypass the aortic bifurcation; it does not require preclotting and is easy to work. Patients who are expected to have a PTFE graft should begin aspirin and dipyridamole 48 h before surgery to minimize postoperative graft thrombosis. It is an excellent graft material for femorofemoral cross-over, axillobifemoral bypass and bypass of the femoral artery in the thigh.

Human umbilical vein does not require preclotting and remains an alternative to autologous vein for bypass from the groin to below the knee. It is also advisable to give aspirin and dipyridamole 48 h before the insertion of this graft as this is thought to reduce the risk of graft thrombosis.

Antibiotics and suture materials

When a prosthetic graft material is to be used it is advisable to commence prophylactic antibiotics either the day before surgery or at the time of the premedication 1 h before the operation. Some surgeons prefer to begin a day early, but virtually all would agree that it is essential to have satisfactory antibiotic levels in the blood at the time the graft material is implanted. The most threatening organism is *Staphylococcus aureus* and flucloxacillin is effective against this, but if this is used on its own there is a small risk of infection of the graft from Gram-negative organisms and it is, therefore, wise to combine ampicillin with flucloxacillin. Some prefer to use a cephalosporin prophylactic antibiotic which has antistaphylococcal ability as well as providing cover for the Gram-negative organisms.

Fashions have changed for the choice of suture for vascular anastomosis. Only recently silk was in common usage but it is now used very rarely. It fragments after some time, but those who use it maintain that the strength of the anastomosis is in the healing of the graft to the vessel. Mersilene handles like silk; it is a braided material made of Dacron and so, in many respects, is ideal for anastomosing a Dacron graft to a large vessel. It has the advantages that is does not slip and it is easy to use. Polypropylene is a slippery monofilament suture which is without doubt the most commonly used suture material for vascular anastomoses. Using a double-ended atraumatic needle of polypropylene, great flexibility of anastomotic technique is achieved. A disadvantage of this material, however, is that when it is tied it slips and it is wise to place up to six knots to guarantee a secure anastomosis. The slippery quality of polypropylene can however be used to advantage; sutures can be left long and the graft slid down along their length before tying.

Lighting and magnification

It is essential to perform any anastomosis in good light. Not every operating room has an excellent lighting system and the best can be adjusted by the surgeon himself. The types which have sterile handles are the easiest to use, and at least two and preferably four lights, which can all be adjusted by the surgeon, are ideal. Few vascular surgeons have this facility. The absolute minimum is two good lights, but, all too frequently, it is not possible for the surgeon to adjust them himself. In such instances an alternative is for the surgeon to wear a fibre optic headlight. The best variety have a sterile adjuster so that once again the surgeon can direct the light exactly where it is required.

It takes time to adjust to any form of magnification but × 2.5 magnification with a simple loupe is easy to use. The focal length is usually about 50 cm but this can be varied according to the particular circumstances. For anastomoses to vessels of 2 or 3 mm diameter such as tibial vessels, this degree of magnification is essential. For smaller vessels of 1–2 mm diameter an operating microscope is required and a triploscope is ideal. This has a split beam, enabling the surgeon and assistant and a television camera to view to the same work through one prism. Microvascular anastomoses require special training in a laboratory and should not be attempted in theatre by the novice surgeon.

All vascular anastomoses are either end-to-end or end-to-side. The different techniques described here are variations of end-to-end and end-to-side techniques. *It is a vital principle of all anastomoses, whether end-to-end or end-to-side, that the edges should always be everted. In this way the intima of the artery and lining of the graft material are brought into apposition.*

Techniques

End-to-end anastomosis of a graft to a large vessel

1

For an end-to-end anastomosis of large vessels (such as the aorta) it is convenient to use a polypropylene suture and place the first four or five sutures before pulling down the graft. This facilitates careful placement of the sutures in the back row. It is much easier to do this rather than to place anchoring stitches which make the subsequent adjacent suturing more difficult. It is important to take a deep bite of the posterior wall in the artery and pull it up into a ridge. It is not necessary to cut the vessel right across. Rather it can be cut approximately half-way to two-thirds across and opened like the leaves of a book. The posterior sutures are then placed long as shown.

2

After the graft is pulled down the suturing is continued to the mid-point, the polypropylene sutures being pulled tight in opposite directions as suturing proceeds to avoid slippage. Slippage will lead to leakage around the back of the anastomosis which is difficult to correct subsequently.

3 & 4

The suturing is continued over and over until the sutures meet. Frequently, it does not matter if the needle passes from the Dacron to the artery or from the artery to the Dacron. Whichever is the more comfortable should be performed. However, if it is anticipated that passing the needle from aorta to Dacron will dissect atheroma it is then essential to pass the needle in the conventional method from Dacron to aorta at all times.

3

4

End-to-end anastomoses of smaller vessels

5

Wherever smaller vessels are to be anastomosed end-to-end, the vessel should be cut obliquely as shown. This will increase the length of the suture line thus reducing tension and will minimize the risk of stenosis.

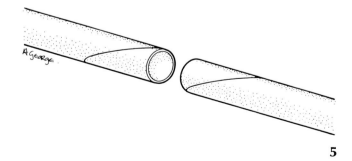

5

6

Two double-ended polypropylene sutures are passed through the opposing cut ends of the vessels.

6

7 & 8

One end is tied and the other is held with rubber-shod mosquito forceps. One end of the tied suture is used to sew over and over towards the other corner, while the other is held as a stay suture with rubber-shod mosquito forceps. On completion of one side, the vessel is rotated as shown.

The other side is sewn over and over between the held suture ends. At the end of the procedure the polypropylene sutures are cut long to avoid slippage.

7

8

End-to-side anastomosis

9

This illustration shows a conventional method of anastomosis of a Dacron limb to the side of the common femoral artery. The arteriotomy is cut to match the length of the obliquely cut Dacron tube and sutures are passed through each apex and tied and held with rubber mosquito forceps.

9

10

Suturing progresses forwards from the heel and backwards from the toe. Again, most surgeons sew from Dacron to artery to avoid freeing atheroma from the artery wall, but in some instances this is not essential. The disadvantage of this technique is that the toe end can pull away from the apex and once the sutures are pulled down it is difficult to place the adjacent sutures, particularly at the heel end. This technique is perfectly satisfactory when performed on the common femoral artery but when the Dacron is angled into the origin of the profunda artery this recipient vessel can be very thin and the Dacron frequently pulls away from the apex causing tearing of the vessel.

10

Alternative end-to-side method with eccentric stitch

11

The illustration shows autologous reverse vein with carefully placed dots along its length so that twisting is avoided when it is tunnelled. In this illustration the first double-ended suture is placed at the heel of the anastomosis as before but the second is placed eccentrically rather than at the apex. The suturing progresses as before, forwards from the heel suture and backwards from the eccentric stitch. The other eccentric stitch is continued forwards around the toe of the graft to meet the other suture. This minimizes the risk of the graft tearing from the apex.

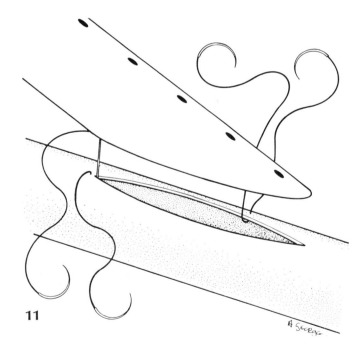

11

Alternative end-to-side anastomoses using a loose stitch at the heel end

12 & 13

This method is commonly used for anatomosing the end of expanded PTFE to the side of the popliteal artery. It is very convenient, especially for the more experienced vascular surgeon, to place the sutures at the heel end of the graft and leave them long as shown. When the first suture is pulled down and tied as described above, it can be quite difficult to place sutures on either side. This method shown here makes the rest of the anastomosis very easy. It is essential that the sutures be placed without any crossing and it is also vital to use polypropylene because of its slippery quality.

The rest of the anastomosis is either with one double-ended polypropylene suture carried around the toe of the anastomosis to meet the other suture or else a second double-ended suture can be adopted and tied in the eccentric position as shown. With practice a single double-ended polypropylene suture is the fastest way of anastomosis and is technically satisfactory.

12

13

14

14

In *Illustration 12* a long suture is sewn over and over so that on one side the sewing is from graft to artery and from the other side it is from artery to graft. Some surgeons prefer to avoid this and instead insert the first suture as a mattress stitch so that it then becomes possible to complete the anastomosis by sewing with both needles from graft to artery. This is more like the conventional approach and will pin the atheroma to the artery wall. However, the disadvantage is that it leads to many 'backhand' sutures and this prolongs the anastomosis. If the surgeon is prepared to turn so that he always sews 'forehand' and does not mind whether he sews from graft to artery or artery to graft the whole procedure can be completed much more easily, but this is not possible if there is any risk of dissecting the diseased artery wall.

End-to-side anastomoses in a small vessel using interrupted sutures

15

The example shown is the umbilical vein with its Dacron sheath being anastomosed to a small vessel. The heel of the graft is sewn in the usual way. It is essential to pick up the whole thickness of the graft material including the intima and the Dacron mesh with each stitch. For the toe end of the graft it may be preferable to use interrupted stitches so that they can be placed accurately before being tied. It is a very useful technique and provides an alternative method of ensuring accurate placement of the sutures in this vital part of the anastomosis.

15

16 & 17

On completion of the anastomosis the interrupted sutures are tied, held long and then cut one by one.

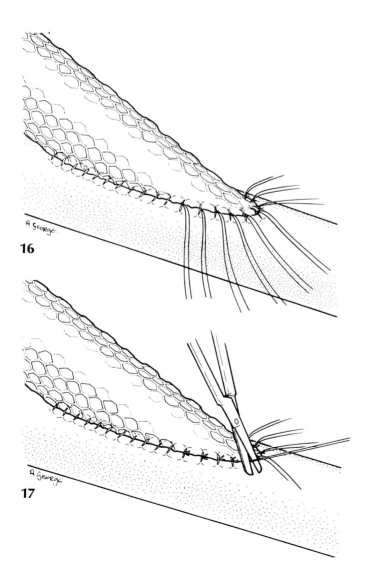

16

17

Confirming patency

Patency must be assessed before the wound is closed. Each surgeon has his own method of doing this and the subject cannot be dealt with in any detail here. The most conventional test, however, is to perform an on-table operative arteriogram. This will demonstrate the anatomy of the anastomoses and if nothing else it is a very useful teaching manoeuvre. Many anastomoses which were thought to be satisfactory are discovered by this method to be unsatisfactory. Such quality control leads to improved surgery.

The electromagnetic flow probe provides physiological data and is very much quicker than the operative arteriogram. The flow probe is placed around the graft and the volume flow per minute is measured. Additionally, a waveform of the flow is printed out for a permanent record.

Another method of checking an anastomosis is by direct pressure readings above the inflow and below the outflow. The needle can be connected to a thin polythene catheter which the anaesthetist attaches to a three-way tap to which the radial line is attached for monitoring. This technique is in its infancy and is probably best used in conjunction with flow readings.

Duplex scanning is now used in the operating room. A sterile Doppler probe may be used to image the vessel and assess the velocity of the blood flow in it.

Digital subraction angiography is also of tremendous value. It enables operative arteriography to be performed much more easily and can play back the result in order to minimize the problem of the timing of taking the film.

Wound closure

Clearly, meticulous aseptic technique is vital whenever prosthetic material is introduced into the body because if any infection is present the graft will be rejected. Wound infection can be minimized by closing the wound very carefully in several layers and it can be helpful to mop the wound edges with an aqueous solution of chlorhexidine. Before the final placement of the skin sutures a spray of povidone-iodine is given. Groin wounds are the most difficult and a subcuticular polypropylene suture fixed in place with beads is an ideal method of closure. This suture is removed after 7 days and leaves a good cosmetic result.

Intraoperative proof of patency

Bert C. Eikelboom MD, PhD
Alexander C. de Vries MD
St Antonius Hospital, Nieuwegein, The Netherlands

Introduction

Technical errors during vascular reconstructive surgery should be detected intraoperatively because they are partly responsible for the failure of these procedures. Graft failure of up to 18% within 1 month of femorocrural bypass surgery, and complications like stroke and restenosis after carotid endarterectomy, are to some degree caused by technical inaccuracies such as intimal flaps, anastomotic and endarterectomy suture line strictures, and intraluminal thrombi.

Intraoperative detection of these imperfections will enhance quality and patency in vascular surgery. The two most common and readily available techniques — angiography and Doppler flow assessment — will be described in detail. Other techniques, such as vascular endoscopy, outflow resistance measurement, as well as the more sophisticated forms of ultrasound assessment (e.g. spectral analysis and duplex scanning), will be discussed briefly.

Angiography

Intraoperative angiography is considered to be the best form of intraoperative assessment, especially in lower limb bypass surgery. In general, we prefer to use Doppler ultrasound, as described in the next section, because we find it a less time-consuming screening technique before angiography. We perform prebypass intraoperative angiography if more information is required regarding the outflow tract.

1, 2 & 3

The foot lies at an angle of 45° and the plate is placed flat on the table so that the angiogram is effectively shot obliquely through the leg. Depending on the type of bypass surgery, slightly different access routes are utilized. For the most common – angiography of autologous reversed saphenous vein bypass – we prefer to perform the proximal anastomosis first, allowing arterial blood pressure to straighten the graft and thus avoid kinking and rotation. In this way graft inflow can also be checked. After completion of the distal anastomosis, angiography is performed as shown, via a proximal side branch of the vein in the functioning graft.

1

2

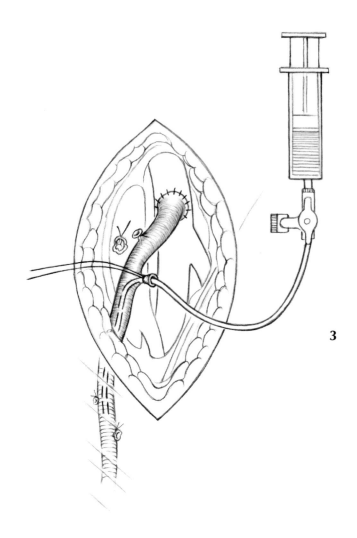

3

4

Alternatively, a vein bypass can be punctured using a standard infusion needle system (venflon 1.4 mm o.d.) as advocated for synthetic graft assessment. *In situ* bypass can be assessed in exactly the same way as reverse vein, but Doppler techniques are our preferred procedures.

Even in experienced hands, erroneous anastomosis to the venous system is possible on occasions and a distal bypass outflow angiogram will alert the surgeon to this mistake. Sometimes, the distal anastomosis is performed first to allow better exposure. The angiogram is then performed before the upper anastomosis is completed.

Following distal outflow angiography, flushing with heparinized saline is advised. If necessary, additional X-rays are performed of the foot region or the graft itself.

4

5

5

In the previous illustration an externally supported PTFE bypass is cannulated with a simple butterfly needle. Alternatively, as is shown here, at the end of both anastomoses a bypass (vein or prosthesis) can be occluded and a distal silastic catheter can be passed towards the lower anastomosis to allow good contrast delineation of the critical run-off area.

Doppler flow assessment

6

The Doppler system is a valuable tool for screening technical difficulties during vascular reconstructive surgery. We use this system in the most simple form, which comprises sterilizable probes connected to the basic apparatus which remains outside the operative field. Only audible processing is used. The apparatus remains on standby during all vascular surgery. It is less time-consuming and there are no disadvantages. It is used before or in some instances instead of angiography.

6

7

7

During surgery the functioning graft or reconstructed area is checked. The probe is placed near to the vessel to be assessed, preferably at an angle of 60°. Conduction of ultrasound is easily achieved by placing both the probe and the vessel under heparin saline solution in a vertebral-truncus thyrocervical transposition, as shown. In this way audible signals are processed. These sounds are easily recognized, even by untrained ears. A 'good' signal is characterized by an uninterrupted flow with three components, i.e. a triphasic pattern. A 'poor' signal consists of so-called 'damped' signals of short systolic peaks of low frequency with intermissions without any recognizable flow. The haemodynamic equivalent of this is a stepwise, slow flow through the assessed vessel. The traces are shown from a directional Doppler trace but the ear can tell the difference. Stenoses are recognized by frequency shifts, while at the site of anastomoses some turbulence must be accepted. For *in situ* bypass surgery, it can be used to locate side branches as previously described (Greenhalgh *et al.*, 1985).

Miscellaneous techniques

Spectrum analysis of directional Doppler ultrasound

Doppler-derived signals can be interpreted more accurately by means of computer processing, i.e. spectral analysis. The spectrum is then visualized and can be further analysed by means of indexes. These analyses require meticulously obtained samples and are therefore not always ideal for intraoperative use. Moreover, the indexes obtained are not easily interpreted.

Duplex scanning

Duplex scanning combines Doppler with B-mode ultrasound. This image allows visualization of reconstructed areas (Flanigan, 1985). The apparatus is expensive and requires its operators to be highly trained. The scan heads used are large in comparison to the operative site to be analysed. They are not sterilized but covered by plastic bags. The instrument itself needs constant operation and adjustment, which means that a technician and a skilled surgeon skilled in the use of ultrasound are required in the operating theatre. On the other hand, it offers all ultrasound possibilities, which makes this system the most versatile for the trained operator. When this system is operational, it offers the best information possible, especially for carotid surgery.

Vascular endoscopy

Vascular endoscopy requires the availability of special instruments and demands expert skills. It can only be used before completion of the reconstruction and has a limited indication.

Outflow resistance measurement

This technique offers outflow resistance measurements (Ascer and Veith, 1985). The value of this parameter is limited and the system is not yet commercially available.

Flow measurement

Electromagnetic flow measurement has been largely abandoned owing to technical problems (difficult probe fit) and because results have been of limited value. In the future, it will probably be replaced by Doppler-derived volume flow measurement which offers greater technical simplicity.

Summary

Doppler ultrasound, where simple audible processing is satisfactory for intraoperative use, offers a valuable tool in vascular reconstructive surgery. It is less time-consuming and requires little experience. It is advocated for screening and technical inaccuracies. We prefer its use before angiography, especially in peripheral bypass surgery. Of the other techniques mentioned, duplex scanning is the most promising. It offers all ultrasound-derived possibilities, including true visualization. However, its complexity makes its use in intraoperative application limited as yet.

References

Ascer, E. and Veith, F. J. (1985). Outflow resistance measurements in infrainguinal bypass operations by injecting saline and measuring the integral of pressure. In *Diagnostic Techniques and Assessment Procedures in Vascular Surgery*. Greenhalgh, R. M., ed. London and Orlando: Grune and Stratton.

Flanigan, D. P. (1985). Peroperative Doppler testing and imaging in patients with lower limb ischaemia. In *Diagnostic Techniques and Assessment Procedures in Vascular Surgery*. Greenhalgh, R. M., ed. London and Orlando: Grune and Stratton.

Greenhalgh, R. M., Heather, B. P., Green, I. L. and McCollum, C. N. (1985). Intra-operative detection of arteriovenous fistulae after *in situ* vein bypass. In *Diagnostic Techniques and Assessment Procedures in Vascular Surgery*. Greenhalgh, R. M., ed. London and Orlando: Grune and Stratton.

Loeprecht, H., Weber, H., and Monnig, J. (1985). Vascular endoscopy. In *Diagnostic Techniques and Assessment Procedures in Vascular Surgery*. Greenhalgh, R. M., ed. London and Orlando: Grune and Stratton.

Management of aortic graft infection

Larry H. Hollier MD, FACS, FACC
Chairman, Department of Surgery, Ochsner Clinic, New Orleans, Louisiana, USA

Introduction

Aortic graft infection is a complication that is universally dreaded by vascular surgeons since it often represents not only a breakdown in surgical technique but also a potentially lethal problem. The natural history of aortic graft infection can vary from a chronic draining fistula to acute arterial wall necrosis with false aneurysm, sepsis, or exsanguinating haemorrhage. Obviously, the management of graft infection is influenced by multiple factors, the most prominent of which are time of offset in relation to surgery, site of infection, extent of infection, location of the graft, aortoenteric fistula, and run-off vessels.

In general, aortic graft infections that occur shortly after surgery should be considered as diffuse infections that will involve the entire graft, since true tissue incorporation and obliteration of perigraft spaces have not yet occurred. These almost invariably require removal of the entire graft. Infections occurring months or years after graft implantation, however, will often be found to be localized to a specific segment of the graft which may allow extra-anatomic revascularization with salvage of most of the previous graft and excision of only the area infected. This technical discussion relates to this aspect of segmental excision of graft infection with preservation of the uninfected graft segments.

Evaluation

Although the literature is replete with multiple modalities used for identifying graft infection, we find only a few tests of significant value.

The physical examination

The presence of a draining sinus in the groin in a patient who has a previous aortofemoral graft should be sufficient evidence to make the diagnosis of graft infection. The only question to be answered subsequently relates to the extent of the infection. In this situation, performance of a sinugram with thin barium or Hypaque is often sufficient to delineate any proximal extension of the infection. A more subtle side of intra-abdominal graft infection is unilateral lower extremity osteoarthropathy with joint swelling and clubbing of the toes that are indicative of bowel erosion by one limb of an aortic bifurcation graft.

Computerized tomography

Computerized tomography (CT scan) is a valuable tool in the evaluation of patients with suspected aortic graft infection and particularly in the evaluation of upper gastrointestinal bleeding in a patient with previous placement of an aortic graft. A CT scan may uncommonly show inflammatory changes and fluid around an aortic graft, though these do not necessarily indicate graft infection. However, perigraft air that is present more than 3 months after aortic graft placement should be considered diagnostic of graft infection. Although one cannot definitively make a diagnosis of aortoenteric fistula on a CT scan, the presence of a continuous and uninterrupted fat line separating the graft line from the overlying bowel is presumptive of there being no aortoenteric fistula if the CT sections are taken at 0.5-cm intervals.

Endoscopy

Upper gastrointestinal endoscopy should be performed routinely in patients with a prior aortic graft who present with gastrointestinal bleeding. Attempts should be specifically made to examine the entire duodenum since graft erosion commonly occurs in the third or fourth portion of the duodenum. While endoscopy may be helpful if a graft is visualized through the distal duodenal wall, failure to identify a bleeding point does not necessarily exclude the possibility of aortoenteric fistula. Additionally, identification of other bleeding sites, such as gastric erosion or duodenal ulcer, likewise does not exclude aortoenteric fistula but does mandate the need for further evaluation.

Purified white cell scan

Indium-labelled purified white cells may be injected intravenously and used for identification of indolent graft infection. Although this can occasionally provide some false-positive or false-negative findings, if the scan does show a 'hot spot' along the course of the graft or one of its limbs, it may be helpful in localizing and identifying the extent of infection.

Angiography

Angiography is generally not useful in determining the presence of graft infection or aortoenteric fistula. None the less, we routinely recommend angiography in patients with graft infection, primarily for full delineation of the status of run-off vessels. We believe that this allows better planning for operative intervention for removal of the graft, assessment of collaterals, and revascularization of the lower extremities.

Management

1a, b & c

Unilateral groin infection

Under general anaesthesia, the draining site in the groin is carefully sealed with an occlusive dressing and the abdomen and lower extremity is wrapped with povidone-iodine solution and draped in a sterile fashion. A vertical transabdominal incision is made and the peritoneum over the aortic graft bifurcation is incised transversely. The graft limb to the involved side is dissected proximally just beyond the bifurcation of the graft. Good incorporation of surrounding tissues suggests that the graft in this area is free of infection. Even though some perigraft fluid may be present, if the perigraft space does not obviously connect to the groin and if the perigraft fluid is free of bacteria (as evidenced by Gram stain), we would proceed with proximal graft preservation and distal revascularization through the obturator canal. The involved limb is doubly clamped, transected and oversewn distally. That end of the graft is then pushed distally and the peritoneum overlying it is closed to the retroperitoneal space with running sutures of 3/0 prolene to separate the distal graft limb completely from the proximal graft. An 8-mm thin-wall ringed GoreTex graft is then sutured end-to-end to the proximal stump of the bifurcation graft and a separate retroperitoneal tunnel is made down to the obturator foramen. A vertical incision is then made distally on the medial thigh and the popliteal artery at this level is exposed and isolated. Using a long metal tunneller, the GoreTex graft is passed through the obturator foramen to lie in the space posterior to the pectineus, abductor longus and abductor brevis, and anterior to the abductor magnus. The graft is then anastomosed to the popliteal artery above the knee and flow is restored through the graft (b).

The abdominal incision and medial thigh incisions are then closed in standard fashion and sterile dressings are applied. The patient is then redraped and the infected groin is exposed and again prepared with povidone-iodine solution. The fistulous tract is excised and the graft is exposed. The graft is then disconnected from its anastomosis to the femoral artery and arterial back bleeding is controlled with balloon catheters and three-way stopcocks. Simple running closure of the femoral artery is performed with 3/0 prolene. The graft is then gently dissected proximally and forcefully withdrawn from its retroperitoneal tunnel. The entire area is then irrigated copiously with antibiotic solution (neomycin-bacitracin-polymyxin) and a suction catheter is left in the tract from which the graft was removed. The wound is then loosely reapproximated to cover the femoral vessels and the skin is packed open with iodoform gauze (c).

All patients undergoing such reconstruction for graft infection are administered intravenous antibiotics preoperatively which are continued for 4–5 days postoperatively. The suction catheter is generally removed after 24 h and local wound care is continued until healing is complete.

1a

1b

1c

2a, b & c

Isolated bilateral groin infection

The development of bilateral groin infection should strongly suggest that the entire aortic graft is infected. However, if careful evaluation by sinugram, purified white cell indium scan and computerized tomography are all indicative of infections isolated to the groins alone and not the body of the graft, selective proximal graft preservation may be indicated (a).

In a fashion similar to the management of unilateral groin infection, the draining sinuses in the groin are carefully sealed, usually by placing a povidone-iodine soaked sponge over the draining sinus and suturing it circumferentially to the skin. The abdomen and lower extremities are then prepared and draped and a midline incision is made in the abdomen. The distal area of the graft bifurcation in each limb is isolated proximally. Again, a Gram stain is made of any perigraft fluid and routine cultures are submitted. The graft is doubly clamped, transected, and the distal portion oversewn. Each limb is then pushed distally into its retroperitoneal tunnel and the distal portion of the tunnel is sealed. Externally supported thin-wall 8-mm GoreTex grafts are then sutured end-to-end to the proximal limbs of the bifurcation graft and, as described for unilateral groin infections,

the grafts are passed through the obturator tunnel and sutured distally to the popliteal arteries (b). The abdominal and thigh incisions are then closed and sterile dressings are applied.

Adhesive drapes are then placed on the patient to completely seal away these previous operative sites. The groin areas are left exposed and the occlusive dressings on the groins are removed. The groins are then prepared with povidone-iodine solution and vertical incisions are made in each groin exposing the infected graft segments. The anastomosis is taken down on each side, with control of bleeding from the femoral vessels obtained by balloon catheters with three-way stopcocks. The femoral arteries are closed primarily with running sutures of 3/0 prolene. The proximal extension of the infected graft segments are then gently mobilized and forcefully removed from their tunnel proximal to the inguinal ligament. The areas of dissection are then copiously irrigated with antibiotic solution and suction catheters are left in each tract and brought out through separate staff incisions in each groin. Deep tissue is closed over the femoral vessels themselves and superficial layers are generally packed open with iodoform gauze. The suction catheters are removed after 24–48 h and the wounds are allowed to heal by secondary intention.

2a

2b

2c

3a, b & c

Proximal graft infection

Aortic graft infection may occur but may be confined to the abdomen if a straight aortic graft has been placed, or if a bifurcation graft has been anastomosed distally to the common iliac or external iliac arteries. In these situations, the groins and the vessels distal to the inguinal ligament are considered to be uninfected (a). Occasionally, patients with aortobifemoral grafts develop isolated proximal graft infections, but with the distal limbs, i.e. the femoral anastomoses, free of infection. This is perhaps most commonly seen in patients who develop aortoenteric fistula from simple graft erosion. Although one might selectively treat some of these patients by removal of the infected graft and direct reimplantation of another Dacron graft, we would generally perform extra-anatomic bypass and complete removal of the infected intra-abdominal graft.

In patients with aortic graft infection isolated to the abdomen, we prefer to do preliminary axillofemoral–cross-femoral bypass as the initial procedure, followed by graft excision either at the same operation or with an interval of 1–2 days, depending upon the stability of the patient. For axillofemoral–cross-femoral bypass, the patient is generally placed under general endotracheal anaesthesia. However, in very high-risk patients, we have performed this procedure under local infiltration anaesthesia for the axillary dissection and epidural anaesthesia for the groin dissection.

The patient is placed on the table in a supine position and prepped from the chin to the knees with povidone-iodine solution. Determination of which axillary artery to use as the donor or inflow vessel is made preoperatively by measuring blood pressure in each arm and selecting the axillary artery with the higher blood pressure. In most cases, the right axillary artery is used. A small roll is placed vertically under the right posterior hemithorax to elevate that side of the chest slightly off of the table and to allow more thorough prepping. The arm is placed outward on an armboard. In these patients, we frequently use a multi-team approach with one surgeon exposing the axillary artery and other surgeons exposing each femoral artery.

The axillary incision is made transversely in the intraclavicular area and the underlying pectoralis major muscle is split in the direction of its fibres. The pectoralis minor muscle is identified and, after dividing the clavipectoral fascia, the insertion of the pectoralis minor on the coracoid process is divided with the electrocautery unit. The underlying axillary artery is thus exposed. The axillary artery at this level must be carefully dissected away from the adjacent nerve trunks. Small bridging veins will sometimes run across the axillary

artery in this area and these should be doubly ligated or divided. It is sometimes helpful to divide the artery to the pectoralis major muscle as it arises from the axillary artery. This allows better mobilization of the axillary artery and a more proximal placement of the graft anastomosis can be accomplished. An 8-mm or 10-mm thin-walled externally supported GoreTex graft is then sutured end-to-side to the axillary artery. A long metal tunneller is passed cephalad from the right groin without any counter-incision being made laterally. Every attempt is made to place this tunnel in the mid-axillary line rather than directly anterior over the chest and abdomen. Several rings of the externally supported graft are removed in the proximal-most portion of the femoral incision and a tangential segment of the graft is excised medially. Another segment of externally supported 8-mm GoreTex graft is then sutured end-to-side to the axillofemoral graft at this level and this side limb is then tunnelled subcutaneously just above the level of the pubis and brought into the opposite groin. Each limb is then sutured end-to-side to the femoral artery and flow can be restored to both lower extremities in this fashion. If the patient has had a previous aortobifemoral graft placed but the femoral portions are free of infection, the previous Dacron graft on each side is simply transected and the proximal portions are oversewn. The proximal graft limbs are then pushed cephalad into their tunnel and are made to lie proximal to the inguinal ligament. The inguinal ligament is then sutured posteriorly to the underlying tissue to separate these tunnels completely from the groin. The axillofemoral–cross femoral limbs can then be sewn directly, end-to-end, to the previous graft just proximal to their femoral anastomoses (b). These wounds are then closed in layers and sterile dressings are applied.

Removal of the infected abdominal graft may be performed either at this time or deferred to a separate operation 24–48 h later. At that time, the abdomen is prepared and draped in the usual fashion and a midline incision is performed. The infected graft is exposed and removed completely (c). Proximally, the aorta is debrided back from the original suture line and closed with interrupted mattress sutures of 3/0 or 0 prolene. A pedicle of omentum is then mobilized and passed through the transverse mesocolon so that it can be carefully wrapped around the aortic stump. If there has been extensive purulence in the peritoneal perigraft space, irrigating and suction catheters may be placed and brought out through separate stab incisions in the flank opposite the axillofemoral–cross-femoral graft (c).

3a

3b

3c

4a, b & c

Aortoenteric fistula

Aortoenteric fistula may present as a sudden, severe, near-exsanguinating haemorrhage or may present as several episodes of lesser gastrointestinal bleeding. If the patient has an unequivocal diagnosis and remains relatively stable, we would prefer to do an axillofemoral–cross-femoral bypass as the preliminary step followed by immediate graft removal and repair of the fistula. However, if exsanguinating haemorrhage is the overriding clinical feature, or if the diagnosis is in question, primary laparotomy would be preferred, with revascularization by axillofemoral–cross-femoral graft deferred until after removal of the infected abdominal graft.

For repair of aortoenteric fistula, a transperitoneal approach is made. After entering the abdomen, the peritoneal reflection on the right lateral aspect of the ascending colon is incised and continued medially around the cecum and extended cephalad to mobilize the hepatic flexure of the colon. A Kocher manoeuvre is then performed mobilizing the second portion of the duodenum and the head of the pancreas. This approach allows rapid dissection in previously undissected planes and minimizes the amount of time required to expose the aorta for control. By mobilizing the abdominal viscera to the left, one exposes the inferior vena cava and easily approaches the aorta above the level of the left renal vein where, in most cases, it has been spared the extensive scarring

that would be evident in the infrarenal portion. This allows rapid placement of a clamp, suprarenally if necessary (a). After proximal control is obtained, the duodenum can be further mobilized and the site of erosion of the duodenum by the graft can be approached in this fashion. Once the aortoenteric fistula is adequately exposed the clamps may be moved to the infrarenal position if adequate infrarenal aorta remains. If not, the aorta may be locally debrided and closed at this point so that the aortic clamp may be removed and flow restored to the renal arteries.

The opening in the duodenum is then gently debrided and the duodenum is closed in two layers. The distal graft is then removed entirely. If the distal anastomoses had been made to the common iliac or external iliac arteries, the anastomotic sites are simply oversewn with 3/0 prolene sutures (b).

After closure of the aortic stump and removal of the graft, the right colon is returned to its normal anatomic position. A pedicle of omentum is mobilized and passed through the transverse mesocolon. The omental pedicle is then carefully tacked around the aortic stump to help in the prevention of stump blow-out. Irrigating and suction catheters are then left in the retroperitoneum and brought out through a flank incision opposite to the side of the previous or planned axillofemoral–cross-femoral graft (c).

4a

4b

4c

5a & b

Aortofemoral graft infection

When an aortobifemoral graft infection is identified with infection evident both in the groin and intra-abdominally, we generally manage this by bilateral axilloprofunda or axillopopliteal bypasses with subsequent removal of the entire aortobifemoral graft. Any draining sinuses are carefully sealed as previously described and the patient is placed in a supine position with both arms extended laterally on armboards (*a*). The patient is prepped with povidone-iodine solution from the chin to toes so that complete exposure can be facilitated. Since both groins are infected, we avoid any incision in those areas and plan to bring the graft more laterally down to the popliteal artery.

Occasionally, however, if the superficial femoral arteries are patent and the infected graft is placed high on the common femoral artery, one might perform a distal anastomosis to the profunda vessels with expectation of a retrograde filling of the profunda and the superficial femoral artery after ligation of the common femoral artery. If the infected graft is anastomosed to the femoral bifurcation or if the superficial femoral arteries are occluded, the lower extremities are revascularized by bilateral axillopopliteal grafts.

Bilateral infraclavicular incisions are made and the axillary arteries are exposed as previously described. Bilateral inci-

sions are then made laterally just above each knee and the popliteal arteries are exposed and isolated. Because of the distance between the axillary and popliteal incisions, a small counter-incision is usually required to facilitate passage of the graft. This counter-incision is made lateral to the posterior superior iliac spine and a tunnel is made subcutaneously cephalad and caudad from this area. Externally supported 8-mm thin-wall GoreTex grafts are then obtained and a graft is sutured to each axillary artery as previously described. Each graft is then passed through the subcutaneous tunnel with the grafts placed along the mid-axillary line and lateral aspect of the thigh. The grafts are then sutured to the popliteal artery above the knee in each thigh and flow is restored to the lower extremities. These incisions are closed and sterile dressings are applied (*b*).

The groins are then opened and the infected grafts are removed from their anastomosis to the femoral vessels. The femoral arteries are closed with prolene and every attempt is made to maintain a patent femoral bifurcation if possible. The abdomen is then opened and the graft is removed as previously described. As always, an attempt is made to provide coverage of the aortic stump by a pedicle of omentum.

5a

5b

Additional approaches

Obviously, many techniques have been devised for the management of aortic graft infection. These include direct replacement of the infected graft with a new prosthesis, rotation of muscle flaps to cover the infected graft, replacement of infected grafts with autogenous tissue, and graft removal without any revascularization whatsoever. While each of these techniques is occasionally applicable to a specific patient, they are not always feasible. Thus, this discussion has centred primarily on extra-anatomic revascularization and graft removal.

We have inadequate experience with direct replacement of an infected graft by a new prosthesis and are unable to comment about its safety. We have used rotation of muscle flaps to cover grafts in approximately 30 patients, but have been disappointed with the results. Although one can occasionally get healing of a graft that has been exposed by breakdown of overlying tissues, we have found it less helpful in eradicating established graft infection. Similarly, we have used autogenous reconstruction on several patients and found that it is satisfactory for revascularization in contaminated fields but, unfortunately, blow-out of autogenous tissue occurs when it has been placed in areas of established infection. Because of the high incidence of lower extremity ischaemia following simple removal of an infected aortic graft without revascularization, we have abandoned that technique entirely.

Although specific situations may allow the vascular surgeon to utilize a lesser procedure for the management of graft infection, we believe that most patients with established aortic graft infection are best managed by preliminary revascularization by an extra-anatomic route, followed by removal of all infected graft material.

References

Brown, O. W., Stanson, A. W., Pairolero, P. C. and Hollier, L. H. (1982). Computerized tomography following abdominal aortic surgery. *Surgery* 91(6), 716.

Cherry, K. J. and Hollier L. H. (1982). Prophylactic antibiotics in vascular surgery. In *Extra-anatomic and Secondary Arterial Reconstruction*. Greenhalgh, R. M., ed. London: Pitman.

Goldstone, J. and Moore, W. S. (1974). Infection in vascular prostheses. *American Journal of Surgery* 128, 225.

Paaske, W. P. and Buchart Hansen, J. H. (1985). Graft enteric fistulas and erosions. *Surgery, Gynecology and Obstetrics* 161, 161.

Perdue, G. D., Smith, R. B., Ansley, J. D. and Constantine, M. J. (1983). Impending aorto-enteric hemorrhage: The effect of early recognition on improved outcome. *Annals of Surgery* 192, 237.

Shue, W. B., Worosilo, S. C., Donetz, A. P., Trooskin, S. Z., Harvey, R. A. and Greco, R. S. (1988). Prevention of vascular prosthetic infection with an antibiotic-bonded Dacron graft. *Journal of Vascular Surgery* 8(5), 600.

Szilagyi, D. E., Smith, R. F., Elliot, J. P. and Vrandecic, M. P. (1972). Infection in arterial reconstruction with synthetic grafts. *Annals of Surgery* 176, 321.

Reilly, L. M., Altman, H., Lusby, R. J., Kersh, R. A., Ehrenfeld, W. K. and Stoney, R. J. (1984). *Journal of Vascular Surgery* 1, 36.

Reilly, L. M., Stoney, R. J., Goldstone, J. and Ehrenfeld, W. K. (1987). Improved management of aortic graft infection: The influence of operative sequence and staging. *Journal of Vascular Surgery* 5, 421.

Wilson, S. E., Wang, S. and Gordon, H. E. (1977). Perioperative antibiotic prophylaxis against vascular graft infection. *Southern Medical Journal* 70, 68.

Basic principles in the surgical management of vascular trauma

John V. Robbs   ChM (CT), FRCSEd

Chief, Vascular Service and Head, Division of Surgery, University of Natal Medical School, Durban, South Africa

Introduction

Trauma to the major arteries and veins may present the most taxing technical problems encountered by the operating surgeon. This entails not only access to the major vessels in certain areas, but also control of haemorrhage and the sometimes exacting exercise of accurately restoring continuity of the involved vessels. There are few areas in surgery less forgiving of imperfect technique. The major thrust of this chapter will be towards management of arterial injury.

Mechanisms and pathology of arterial injury

1a, b & c

An understanding of the mechanisms of injury and pathology encountered is essential in order to treat these injuries rationally. In Table 1, mechanisms of injury, each of which results in a specific type of pathology, are summarized. The pathology encountered is illustrated in *Illustration 1a–f*. Following penetration by a sharp instrument or a low-velocity missile (for example, from a small-calibre hand gun) the tissue damage is essentially confined to the track of the penetrating agent. Low-velocity missiles may, however, compound the injury by fragmentation of soft-nosed bullets or fragments of bone; ricochet may also be responsible for more extensive damage.

High-velocity missiles are defined as those in which the muzzle velocity exceeds 2000 feet/s (approximately 600 m/s). Under these circumstances, there is a highly significant energy release during passage through the tissues which causes a cavitation effect resulting in a great deal of soft tissue damage around the track. In addition, extraneous material such as clothing is drawn into the wound.

Penetrating trauma may result in a lateral perforation of the artery with formation of a false aneurysm. Total transection with or without loss of substance of the vessel may also occur and the artery frequently develops spasm at its severed ends (*b*) with resultant thrombosis. Simultaneous lateral perforation of artery and adjacent vein may result in the formation of an acute arteriovenous fistula, with or without an associated false aneurysm (*c*).

Table 1 Mechanisms of vascular injury

Penetrating	Stab
	Missile
	high-velocity (600 m/s or 2000 m/s)
	low-velocity
Blunt	Direct
	Indirect
Blast	Shotgun
	Bomb
Iatrogenic	

1a

1b

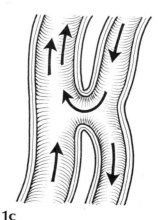

1c

1d & e

Direct blunt trauma is exemplified by a direct localized blow to the vessel against a rigid bony structure. Indirect injuries are caused by distraction which may occur with joint dislocation or acceleration–deceleration trauma with its associated shearing forces at areas of fixity of the artery. An example of the latter is the aortic disruption found at the isthmus or aortic valve ring in road traffic accident victims. The intima and media of the vessel wall are less elastic than the overlying adventitia and when the vessel is subjected to the type of forces described, it tends to disrupt from the less elastic layers on the inside towards the adventitia in proportion to the degree of violence. If the adventitia remains intact with an intimomedial tear in smaller calibre vessels, superimposed thrombosis occurs due to a combination of exposure of blood to the thrombogenic raw surface and the elevation of a distally based flap (d). In larger vessels such as the aorta, thrombosis does not occur to any great extent but an aneurysm tends to form at that site. Obviously with this type of trauma, if the forces are great enough all layers disrupt through part or all of the circumference, with perforation of the artery.

Shotgun blast injuries result in extensive soft tissue destruction which is contaminated by multiple small pellets which remain firmly embedded in the tissues. This is particularly noticeable when birdshot has been used. In addition, there are frequently multiple sites of perforation within the neurovascular bundle.

Bomb explosions may produce similar multiple penetrating wounds and soft tissue trauma but, in victims close to the explosion, high-velocity fragments may result in extensive cavitating injury and the situation may be compounded by surface flash burns.

Iatrogenic vascular injuries warrant separate consideration. The most frequently encountered is catheter trauma associated with diagnostic radiological procedures. Laceration at the arterial puncture site may occur with the formation of false aneurysm or free haemorrhage. However, in smaller vessels (as in children), or the brachial artery in adults, thrombosis may occur at the site of the puncture due to the associated intimal damage. In atherosclerotic vessels, dislodgement of plaque and the formation of a flap with subsequent thrombosis or even distal embolization of atheromatous debris may occur (e). Passage of the catheter between the layers of a diseased vessel with subintimal injection of contrast resulting in superimposed thrombosis is also occasionally seen following diagnostic radiological procedures.

Excessive inflation of the balloon of an embolectomy catheter may result in significant arterial injury. This applies particularly when the balloon is filled with fluid, thus creating a hydraulic system which is capable of transmitting extremely high pressures. The types of lesions caused range from intimomedial tears or stripping with subsequent thrombosis to transmural rupture with perforation. It is strongly recommended that air be used to inflate the catheter balloon during its use.

Intra-arterial injection of lipid-soluble substances may be responsible for injury to the arterioles by fixing in the intimal tissues with superimposed intense spasm and thrombosis. In clinical practice this is occasionally seen following inadvertent injection of sodium pentothal or diazepam which are both widely used for premedication purposes during anaesthesia or invasive diagnostic procedures. A similar spectrum of pathologies is seen in drug abusers following intra-arterial injection of a variety of agents. These lesions are not amenable to direct arterial reconstructive surgery.

1f

Arterial spasm

This is always associated with trauma to an artery whatever mechanism may have been responsible and whatever the underlying pathology may be. In addition, the lack of intraluminal pressure in the arterial tree distal to the site of injury results in marked diminution in calibre of these vessels due to the unopposed sympathetic tone which further aggravates distal ischaemia. Spasm occurring in isolation as a cause of distal ischaemia is exceptionally rare and in our own series, which numbers well in excess of 1000 cases of arterial trauma, it has been found to be the sole cause of the problem in less than 1%. Spasm as a cause of distal ischaemia is therefore a retrospective diagnosis made at the time of surgical exploration.

1d

1e

1f

Preoperative evaluation and diagnosis

Diagnosis rests upon a high index of clinical suspicion, and vascular injury should be entertained in every patient who has a penetrating wound of the neck and extremities and in every long-bone fracture or joint dislocation. In patients with multiple injuries, once ventilatory and haemodynamic deficits have been stabilized, every injury must be considered on its particular merit and remote injuries should not be allowed to distract from the possibility of an arterial injury, particularly in the extremities. An accurate assessment of peripheral perfusion cannot be made in a hypovolaemic peripherally vasoconstricted patient and it is important to reserve final clinical assessment of peripheral perfusion until the patient has been adequately volume resuscitated.

Arterial injuries *per se* present in principle with either occlusion, haemorrhage or arteriovenous fistulation. Occlusion invariably results in a pulse deficit with or without significant signs of ischaemia. It must be re-emphasized that in isolation, arterial spasm will never cause significant peripheral ischaemia. Another important pitfall which must be avoided in patients who have sustained blunt trauma is the entity of delayed thrombosis, as it may take several hours of occlusive thrombus to develop on an area of intimal disruption and patients with high-risk injuries such as knee dislocation or lower third femoral fractures must be continually reassessed during the first 24 h following injury.

Haemorrhage may be overt with obvious arterial or venous bleeding occurring through a wound; contained haemorrhage may manifest as a false aneurysm. Bleeding may also be concealed and occur into the pleural or peritoneal cavity or the retroperitoneum. A fairly frequent occurrence, particularly in patients with penetrating wounds, is the finding of unexplained shock or a low haematocrit with no obvious site of haemorrhage, which is encountered in patients who have sustained transection of a major vessel which has ultimately thrombosed. Arteriovenous fistulae are always associated with a machinery-type murmur. However, this may be subtle, and unless specifically sought will be missed. This is the most common pathology found in patients with arterial trauma who present late.

Place of preoperative angiography

While Doppler ultrasound is an extremely useful screening test when there is doubt, angiography provides the definitive diagnosis. In addition, angiography is essential for the localization of, and hence operative planning in, inaccessible areas such as the superior mediastinum, the base of the skull and the abdominal vasculature. In general, in the presence of focal trauma to the mid-cervical region or the extremities, the performance of angiography is time-wasting, as the injury is easily located on clinical grounds. However, in an ischaemic limb which has multiple fractures, it is essential to image the vascular tree at every fracture site as it is not uncommon to find arterial disruption in more than one area. It is best under these circumstances to perform the investigation on the operating table before embarking upon exploration. It must be emphasized that the patient must be volume resuscitated and haemodynamically stable before angiography is performed. In our own experience, the retrograde femoral route is usually preferable utilizing the digital subtraction technique. In young healthy adults, the complication rate is negligible. In children, as far as possible, digital subtraction angiography via the intravenous injection technique has been found adequate. An overview of the indications for preoperative angiography in our practice is summarized in Table 2.

Table 2 Indications for arteriography in trauma

Suspected cervicomediastinal injury
Pulse deficit
False aneurysm
Haemorrhage
    Overt
    Unexplained shock
    Low haematocrit/haemoglobin value
Bruit
Injury to anatomically related nerves
First rib fracture
Widened mediastinum on chest radiograph

Suspected renal artery injury
Upper quadrant/loin pain
Proteinuria
Non-function on intravenous pyelography

Suspected intraperitoneal haemorrhage

Pelvic fracture
Ongoing haemorrhage
Pulsating or expanding retroperitoneal haematoma

Ischaemic extremity
Severe soft tissue injury
Multiple fractures

Indications for operation and prioritization

The urgency for the operative procedure ranges from the 'crash' exploration in the 'clinically dead' patient, to the stabilized patient in whom a planned urgent procedure can be conducted, to the individual who presents months or years later with the long-term complications of a misdiagnosed or conservatively treated lesion. The question often arises in the stable patient without distal ischaemia or any other significant manifestations of arterial disruption other than an abnormal arteriogram, whether repair should be undertaken. While the precise incidence of complications in injuries that have been misdiagnosed or treated non-operatively is not known, when they do occur they may be life-threatening and indeed cause considerable morbidity. With penetrating wounds, secondary haemorrhage may occur between 5 days and 3 weeks after injury. This is probably due to low-grade sepsis with clot lysis resulting in active haemorrhage, or the acute onset of a false aneurysm which compresses surrounding structures. This most frequently applies to nerves and, in particular, to the brachial plexus. The prognosis for nerve recovery under these circumstances is guarded and when it does occur it may take anything up to 1 year for full function to be restored. Similarly, neglected false aneurysms or haematomas are susceptible to infection. Arteriovenous fistulae with a significant shunt may return with cardiac problems, due to the hyperdynamic circulation and when situated in the extremities with associated distal ischaemia and venous hypertension. Claudication or growth disparity in children are important long-term considerations with occluded arteries in the extremities.

Contraindications to reconstruction

Limb salvagability in the presence of extensive trauma may be an extremely difficult decision to make and should certainly not be left to the junior staff. In general terms, it is probably better to give the patient the benefit of the doubt and to proceed with revascularization under most circumstances. However, in the presence of extensive crush trauma associated with bone comminution and neurological dysfunction, the outlook is generally poor.

Similarly, the decision whether an extremity is irreversibly ischaemic or not may considerably exercise clinical judgement. Fixed skin staining and muscle rigidity in all compartments obviously preclude vascular reconstruction. However, in the presence of localized muscle compartment rigidity, such as the extensor compartment in the lower extremity, for example, a good functional result can still be obtained.

The general approach to the patient with a vascular injury should comprise concerted combined effort on the part of the involved disciplines with rapid resuscitation and definitive therapy as soon as possible. In virtually all instances we believe that the vascular injury should take priority over orthopaedic or plastic surgical intervention. The proviso however is that the vascular surgeons remain in attendance until the procedures are concluded. In our experience, it is exceptionally uncommon for orthopaedic manipulations to disrupt the vascular repair. We believe that this approach is preferable to the use of temporary shunts which serves to prolong the operative procedure considerably.

Operative procedure

Access and positioning

2

Besides meticulous surgical technique the basis for successful surgery is to be on the alert for the unexpected and to provide wide access to the area of injury. It is certainly preferable to overexpose than the converse and there is no place for 'keyhole' or cosmetic surgery. In principle, the aim should be to plan operative exposure to the major vessels in a definitive way in order to obtain control of the vessels proximal and distal to the site of injury. It is ill-advised to attempt to approach the injury by enlarging pre-existing stab wounds, particularly in the root of the neck, because the bony confines of the superior mediastinum make rapid access difficult if torrential haemorrhage from a superior mediastinal vessel is initiated by manipulation through an inadequate incision. The most difficult anatomical areas to deal with from the access point of view are injuries near the base of the skull, the root of the neck and superior mediastinum and the major abdominal vessels, particularly the aorta and its branches above the level of the renal artery. The optimum utility incisions for injuries in these various areas are shown in *Illustration 2*.

In principle, for cervico-mediastinal injuries, the entire neck, sternum and left thoracic cage down to the posterior axillary line should be prepared and draped with the neck in extension and a bolster placed between the scapulae in order to brace the shoulders and thrust the aortic arch and mediastinal vessels forward. An oblique incision placed along the anterior border of the sternomastoid muscle, and extending from the mastoid process to the suprasternal notch is the best utility approach to neck wounds. To expose the distal internal carotid, the sternomastoid muscle can be divided close to its origin from the mastoid process. The incision can be readily extended into a median sternotomy which provides the best access to the superior mediastinum and heart. Left thoracotomy via the fourth or fifth intercostal space provides good exposure of the descending thoracic aorta and structures in the pulmonary hilum. Under certain circumstances the proximal subclavian artery is best approached in this manner.

Similarly, when intra-abdominal vascular injuries are suspected, the entire abdomen and thoracic cage should be prepared and draped and both lower limbs should be free-draped and prepared down to the level of the knee. The initial utility incision is a mid-line from xiphisternum to pubis. There should be no hesitation to extend this incision either by subcostal incisions into the flanks or into the lower

2

thoracic cavity via one of the lower intercostal spaces should this become necessary. The proximal abdominal aorta and its branches are exposed by mobilization of the left colon, spleen and pancreas towards the right side of the patient. The suprarenal inferior vena cava is exposed by mobilization of the right colon to the left, together with Kocher's manoeuvre to the duodenum. For access to the retrohepatic IVC, the right lobe of liver must be mobilized in addition by division of the right triangular ligament.

3a & b

When the injuries are confined to the extremities the entire limb should be prepared and free-draped and there should always be access to the groins in order to obtain a long saphenous vein graft should this be necessary. In every case, arrangements should be made for the ready availability of on-table angiographic facilities. The upper limb should be abducted to 90° and we find it most convenient to place it on a narrow arm board rather than to use a conventional arm table (a). It is also helpful to place a bolster behind the shoulder which serves to thrust the axillary vessels forward. The major access problem is provided by vessels in the vicinity of the shoulder girdle and it is usually necessary to divide the insertions of both pectoralis minor and major muscles in order to obtain adequate exposure and control of the proximal axillary vessels. This applies particularly if the anatomy is distorted by the presence of a large aneurysm which fills the axilla, a frequent accompaniment of penetrating injury. Adequate exposure of the distal subclavian vessels usually requires division of the clavicle mid-shaft. We have never found resection of the clavicle, in part or whole, necessary. The brachial is easily approached directly as illustrated.

The lower limb should be positioned with the knee slightly flexed on a bolster (b). The femoral vessels can be directly exposed via an overlying incision. The optimum approach to the popliteal vasculature is via a medially placed incision. When the injury is situated in the artery behind the knee the hamstrings should be detached as a unit from their insertion on the tibia, together with a cuff of periosteum which can be stapled back into position.

3a

3b

Control of active haemorrhage

Should active bleeding be initiated during dissection it is essential to avoid the blind application of clamps as this will frequently cause unnecessary associated injuries to surrounding nerves or veins. It is usually possible to control bleeding by judicious application of pressure using a finger or sponge stick while resuscitation proceeds, and definitive proximal and distal control can be obtained by dissecting out the relevant vessels and applying atraumatic vascular clamps. Under certain circumstances it may be possible or even desirable to pass intraluminal balloon catheters and to control haemorrhage in this way until more definitive control is obtained.

Principles of repair

Once the pathology has been identified and the vessel controlled the options for repair include lateral suture, patch angioplasty, end-to-end reconstruction and interposition grafting. Under certain circumstances, arterial ligation may be necessary. In order to fully appreciate the significance of the various manoeuvres involved in the techniques or repair, it is important to understand the common reasons for early failure of arterial reconstruction. These may be summarized as follows:

1. Narrowing at the suture lines.
2. Inadequate calibre graft.
3. Anastomotic tension.
4. Failure of intimal apposition with the formation of a distal flap.
5. Adventitial incorporation into the lumen.
6. Inadequate distal run-off due either to undetected thrombosis or additional distal injury.
7. Infection causing thrombosis or disruption of the suture lines.

4

Assessment of inflow and the distal arterial tree

Backbleeding is not a reliable sign of distal patency, as a short collateral network may result in considerable backbleeding even in the presence of propogated thrombus distal to the collateral network. A small (size 3) balloon embolectomy catheter should be routinely passed into the distal vessel, gently inflated with air and withdrawn. This serves to extract any distal thrombus and to break gently co-existing arterial spasm. We do not believe that there is any place for the use of topical vasodilators such as papaverine or local anaesthetic agents. Should the catheter fail to pass the full length of the extremity, an intraoperative angiogram should be obtained. It is also advisable to pass the embolectomy catheter into the proximal artery and ensure that any proximal propagated thrombus is removed and that good pulsatile inflow is obtained. Both proximal and distal segments should be copiously irrigated with dilute heparin solution (10 000 u/litre normal saline); systemic heparin is not recommended in the trauma context.

4

5a

5b

5c

5a, b & c

Preparation of artery for repair

The edges of the artery at the site of injury should be debrided back to healthy intima. The adventitia should be trimmed sufficiently by sharp dissection to prevent incorporation into the suture line; however, care must be taken to avoid excessive adventitial stripping which may result in the sutures cutting out. Thrombosed segments should be excised back to healthy non-oedematous arterial wall; this usually comprises 2–3 cm of vessel wall.

6 & 7

Lateral suture

This can only be performed when closure will not result in narrowing at the site of the suture line. It is important to pick up all layers of the vessel wall and the sutures should be spaced approximately 2 mm apart and about the same distance from the edges. In this way, blocks of tissue are opposed and intimal apposition is secured. The principle applies to any vascular suture line.

Puncture wounds in the aorta compatible with survival are usually relatively small. *Illustration 7* illustrates a useful technique. Bleeding is controlled by digital pressure and the laceration is closed by means of interrupted mattress sutures placed deep to the finger. This technique is, however, not applicable to smaller calibre vessels as it would result in significant narrowing.

6

7

8a, b &c

Patch angioplasty

This should be used whenever simple lateral suture will result in narrowing. Any regional subcutaneous vein may be used and cut to size. Prosthetic material should be avoided in view of the danger of infection. The initial corner suture is of the mattress type in order to evert the suture line and ensure intimal apposition (*a*). The suture line is then completed by an over-and-over technique at approximately 2-mm intervals using the principles described for lateral suture (*b, c*).

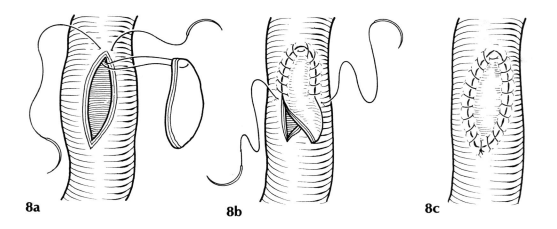

8a   8b   8c

9a–d

End-to-end anastomosis

This can only be performed when apposition between the vessel ends can be maintained without tension. The best parameter to use in this regard is whether the single corner tethering stitch can maintain apposition of the ends with the limb in full extension. If tearing out results under these circumstances it is preferable to insert an interposition graft. After adequate debridement the ends of the vessel are fish-mouthed at opposite ends to prevent narrowing (*a*). It is best to commence the suture line at the posterior corner with a mattress tethering suture (*b*), and it is preferable not to simultaneously tether the opposite corner so that the intimal surface of the suture line can be inspected at all times while the artery is being sutured. In general, interrupted sutures are preferable, placed approximately 2 mm apart as described for lateral suture (*c*). In larger vessels a continuous over-and-over suturing technique may be used. In deeply situated vessels in which ready access to the posterior wall is difficult, e.g. the great vessels in the superior mediastinum, it is possible to suture the posterior third of the anastomosis intraluminally (*d*). The initial suture is placed posterolaterally at approximately the four o'clock point on the circumference and knotted outside the lumen. The lumen is re-entered and a full thickness over-and-over suture placed from within the lumen. Once the posterior part of the suture line is complete (approximately one-third of the circumference) this can be knotted on the adventitial surface at about the seven o'clock point on the circumference and the anastomosis completed in the conventional manner, preferably with interrupted sutures. Whatever technique is used, it is important that the ends be accurately approximated without obliquity of the suture line, the sutures should be evenly spaced, and should always lie at right-angles to the cut ends of the artery.

9a   9b

9c   9d

10

Interposition graft

10

The long saphenous vein taken from the groin area provides the most suitable graft in terms of calibre and ease of handling. We have used the cephalic and internal jugular veins on occasion, but found these to be too thin-walled and, in the case of the cephalic vein, too small under most circumstances. Regarded as being of adequate calibre for reconstruction in the extremities is a vein which measures 4–6 cm in diameter in its native state. It is possible on occasion to fashion a larger calibre vein graft by suturing a panel taken from another vein into the circumference. In most instances, the graft is short and can be seen in its entirety at completion of the procedure, so that in preparation it is not necessary to distend it with saline but preferable to allow arterial blood pressure to distend the graft once the clamps have been released, thus avoiding excessive trauma to the graft. It is also unnecessary to totally denude the graft of adventitia and just sufficient should be dissected free from the anastomotic areas to allow suture without adventitial incorporation into the lumen. The principles of anastomosis are identical to those described for end-to-end reconstruction.

11a & b

As a general rule, prosthetic grafts should be avoided in view of the hazards of infection, particularly following penetrating wounds. An exception to this rule is to be found with injuries to the great vessels close to the aortic arch, paricularly when a through-and-through perforation of both anterior and posterior walls has occurred (*a*). Attempts to restore in-line continuity invariably results in difficulty in closing the posterior wall as the aorta tends to slip out of the clamp as the medial layer retracts. It is therefore preferable to obtain initial control by means of a side-biting clamp and to oversew the origin of the vessel. Continuity is then restored by means of a Dacron graft which takes origin from the intrapericardial ascending aorta (*b*). Should a prosthetic graft be required elsewhere as a last resort, we have found PTFE to be the most satisfactory substitute.

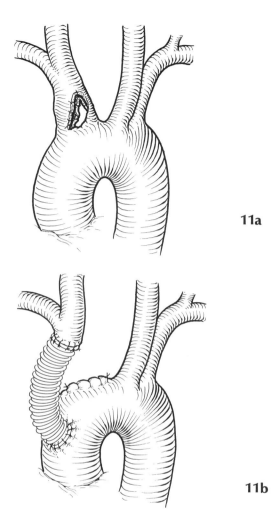

11a

11b

Ligation

Arterial ligation should be limited to 'non-essential' vessels, e.g. branches of the external carotid, or an intercostal vessel. An additional consideration is the situation in which prolonged reconstructive operation is inappropriate to the general clinical condition of the patient ('life or limb').

In a grossly contaminated operative field, attempts at in-line reconstruction are ill-advised. A fairly common example would be the combination of colonic and iliac vessel disruption with gross faecal soiling. When this situation pertains, the injured artery should be ligated and flow to the lower limb restored by means of an extra-anatomical bypass, such as an axillofemoral graft. Once the infection has settled the latter may be taken down and anatomical continuity restored, which may be many months later. The same principles apply in any grossly contaminated operative field and ingenuity may be sorely taxed in finding an extra-anatomical route.

Venous reconstruction

In general, repair in the venous system does not yield equivalent results to arterial construction. This is due mainly to the slower blood flow velocity which makes any technical errors such as stenosis, adventitial invagination or intimal irregularity assume far greater significance in terms of subsequent thrombosis. In addition, the thin-walled delicate structure of the venous system makes it far more susceptible to trauma from clamps or rough handling. There is also a tendency for these vessels to collapse because of their low intraluminal pressure which makes localization and hence control of the bleeding area more difficult. Bleeding from large veins should in most cases be controlled by the use of proximal and distal pressure using sponge sticks or intraluminal balloons in order to avoid tearing collaterals and small branches which aggravate the bleeding and make localization still more hazardous by attempts to encircle and mobilize the vein proximal and distal to the injury. An additional important consideration in dealing with injuries to the neck, mediastinum and abdomen is the danger of significant air embolism. Definitive repair of venous lacerations follows the principles outlined for arterial trauma and entails debridement of the edges and closure by means of lateral suture, patch angioplasty or reanastomosis. Suture technique must be fine and meticulous with close attention to detail. Complex injuries present a great problem and if an interposition graft is required the long saphenous or jugular system make the best grafts. We have found prosthetic grafts in the venous system to be uniformly unsatisfactory and thrombosis is the inevitable result. However, the use of temporary arteriovenous fistulae to improve flow has been shown to be effective in improving patency rates. An example of this technique is the anastomosis of the long saphenous vein to the superficial femoral artery to maintain patency in the iliac system or inferior vena cava. Haemodynamic problems may, however, result if these fistulae exceed 5 mm in diameter and they should be closed within 4–8 weeks. Prolonged reconstructive manoeuvres for complex venous injuries are seldom indicated, as these patients frequently have associated arterial and other injuries that mandate reconstruction and, under most circumstances, ligation of the major veins may be performed without immediate adverse effects. For example, in the superior mediastinum, an extensive analysis of our own experience has shown that any major veins cephalad to the azygous confluence may be ligated with safety, with minimal, if any, postoperative sequelae with regard to oedema. An additional problem in treating inferior vena caval and iliac venous injuries is that a thrombosed repair might theoretically result in pulmonary embolism. The morbidity from chronic venous insufficiency in the lower extremity following failure to repair femoral and distal venous injuries is well established, and every attempt should be made to repair these. On the other hand, more recent reports on long-term follow-up of these patients in civilian practice has indicated a more benign course in those in whom veins have been ligated at this level. Following venous repair to the great veins, in view of the theoretical possibility of pulmonary embolism, it is probably advisable to heparinize these patients until they are fully mobile.

Arteriovenous fistula

In our own experience, these have always occurred as a complication of penetrating trauma and the usual pathology is a lateral perforation of adjacent artery and vein with or without an interposed false aneurysm. Perforations are usually relatively small and the most frequent area involved is the neck and mediastinum. In most instances, the diagnosis is made soon after injury, but in a significant proportion in whom arterial haemorrhage is not a major presenting feature due to immediate decompression into the vein, the fistula only becomes evident some time later with the emergence of haemodynamic complications or the detection of a bruit. Patients frequently notice the latter themselves. The sooner repair is effected after injury, the easier it is technically. Once fibrosis has become established, it adds greatly to the difficulty of control and repair of the component vessels and the concept of waiting for a fistula to mature is historical. Ideally, control of both afferent and efferent arterial and venous components should be obtained and can usually be performed without difficulty in the recently acquired lesion. However, when extensive fibrosis has occured, this may prove hazardous or, indeed, impossible. Under these circumstances, the venous components can usually be readily identified and isolated by palpation of the thrill as they lie on a more superficial plane to the artery. In addition, in the extremities and cervico-mediastinal areas, no vital structures cross the major veins. The thrill pinpoints the situation of the fistula which can then in most cases be occluded by direct transvenous pressure using a finger. Arterial control may then be obtained by sharp dissection proximal and distal to this site. Distal control may on occasion prove difficult, especially when the vessels involved are close to the base of the skull. Under these circumstances, once arterial inflow has been isolated and controlled, and proximal and distal venous control obtained, the fistula should be exposed transvenously and arterial backbleeding controlled digitally. More definitive distal control may then be obtained by means of an intraluminally placed inflated balloon embolectomy catheter. Arterial and venous injuries should be repaired on their respective merits as described in some detail earlier.

While recurrent fistulae undoubtedly occur, in our own experience we have found this to be usually due to a second fistula which remained undetected at the original operation. These have more frequently been a consequence of gunshot or, in particular, shotgun wounds. It is therefore important to study and trace the trajectory of the penetrating agent and ensure that the machinery bruit has disappeared at the conclusion of the operation. While the classically held concept

is that soft tissue should be interposed between the arterial and venous repairs, we have not made this standard practice as this proves difficult on occasion unless considerable tissue mobilization is performed.

Interventional radiology

Occlusion of fistulae by embolization using thrombin pellets, detachable balloons or various coil devices via transarterial catheters are well adapted to the treatment of surgically inaccessible post-traumatic arteriovenous fistulae involving smaller vessels. Particular application is found in the kidney, smaller intra-abdominal vessels such as the pancreatico-duodenal, and the vertebral and carotid near the skull base. In the latter instance, virtually all afferent flow enters the fistula with very little distal flow into the brain, which makes occlusion safe from the point of view of cerebral blood supply.

These embolization techniques have also proved invaluable in arresting haemorrhage arising from branches of the internal iliac artery as a complication of pelvic fracture or penetrating wounds in the buttock or perineal area.

Wound management

Primary closure of a contaminated wound invites septic complications. The most serious of these is disruption of suture lines with massive exsanguinating secondary haemorrhage. In the presence of a compound wound with false aneurysm formation, significant associated blunt tissue injury, multiple foreign bodies (e.g. shotgun wound), and patients with penetrating trauma presenting more than 8–12 h after injury, primarily suture of the wound is inadvisable. Under these circumstances, the deep fascia and skin should be left unsutured and the wound covered with an absorbent, non-adherent dressing. Copious irrigation with antiseptic or antibiotic solution should be performed. Vascular repairs must not be left exposed in the wound but should be covered with muscle or, under certain circumstances, a split skin graft.

The wound should be inspected under sterile conditions 48 h later and further debridement performed if necessary. This should be repeated at regular intervals until the wound is healthy, at which stage formal closure is effected. This regimen significantly reduces the infection rate and hence secondary haemorrhage from the repair site in our own experience.

Postoperative management and complications

Careful monitoring of peripheral pulse status and for evidence of excessive haemorrhage is essential during the postoperative period as a routine. Early complications occur within 5–10 days of operation and may be local or systemic. Local complications are thrombosis, haemorrhage, compartment syndrome, infection and recurrent arteriovenous fistula. Graft thrombosis usually has a mechanical cause and occurs within 24–48 h of operation. Haemorrhage may result from inadequate haemostasis due often to reperfusion of traumatized tissues, but may also occur 5–7 days later due to infection with disruption of the anastomosis. Compartment syndrome may become manifest within the following 6–24 h and must be anticipated, particularly if there has been prolonged preoperative ischaemia or extensive soft tissue injury; its development demands urgent fasciotomy. Compound injuries are contaminated by their very nature and significant infection usually supervenes in the presence of non-viable tissue. Open wound management and frequent inspections with a view to debridement are important. Recurrent arteriovenous fistula as such is rare and persistence of the physical signs usually indicates failure to detect additional fistulae which are not uncommon after missile wounds.

Systemic complications such as adult respiratory distress syndrome and disseminated intravascular coagulation are complications of severe multiple trauma and massive blood transfusion must be anticipated in these patients. The myonephropathic syndrome (crush syndrome) accompanies severe crush trauma or revascularization of necrotic tissue.

The major issue is acute renal failure due to the deposition of myoglobin crystals in the renal tubules. In addition, at the time of allowing reperfusion to occur, the patient undergoes a severe metabolic insult in that a bolus of 'metabolic debris' including potassium and lactic acid which in turn may cause diffuse vasodilatation and myocardial depression with hypotension. It is therefore vital to anticipate this complication in the severely traumatized patient in the appropriate clinical setting. Prior to release of the clamp with reperfusion of the limb, the patient should be well volume resuscitated, should be rendered alkalotic by means of bicarbonate infusion and an osmotic diuresis initiated by means of mannitol infusion. The clamp should then be gradually released and reapplied should the blood pressure fall. At this stage the metabolic acidosis should also be carefully monitored. During the postoperative period, diuresis must be maintained at a level of at least 150–200 ml/h by means of adequate crystalloid volume replacement and, if necessary, mannitol administration. The urine should also be carefully monitored for the presence of myoglobin which has a characteristic brown discolouration. Renal failure can be largely eliminated by this regimen.

References

Costa, M. and Robbs, J.V. (1988). Nonpenetrating subclavian artery trauma. *Journal of Vascular Surgery* **8**(1), 71.

Hirshberg, A., Thomson, S.R. and Robbs, J.V. (1988). Vascular complications of diagnostic angiography via limb arteries. *Journal of Royal College of Surgeons of Edinburgh* **33**, 196.

Meek, A.C. and Robbs, J.V. (1984). Vascular injury with associated bone and joint trauma. *British Journal of Surgery* **71**, 341.

Robbs, J.V. and Baker, L.W. (1979). Late revascularisation of the lower limb following acute arterial occlusion. *British Journal of Surgery* **66**, 129.

Robbs, J.V. and Baker, L.W. (1984). Cardiovascular trauma. *Current Problems in Surgery* **XXI**(4).

Robbs, J.V. and Costa, M. (1984). Injuries to the great veins of the abdomen. *South African Journal of Surgery* **22**(4), 223.

Robbs, J.V. and Naidoo, K.S. (1984). Nerve compression injuries due to traumatic false aneurysm. *Annals of Surgery* **200**(1), 80.

Robbs, J.V. and Reddy, E. (1987). Management options for penetrating injuries to the great veins of the neck and superior mediastinum. *Surgery, Gynecology, and Obstetrics* **165**, 323.

Robbs, J.V. *et al.* (1981). Cervicomediastinal arterial injuries: A surgical challenge. *Archives of Surgery* **116**, 663.

Cervical trauma

Malcolm O. Perry MD
Department of Surgery, Division of Vascular Surgery, Vanderbilt University School of Medicine, Nashville, Tennessee, USA
M. Kathleen Reilly PhD, MD
Department of Surgery, Division of Vascular Surgery, Vanderbilt University School of Medicine, Nashville, Tennessee, USA

Introduction

Most cervical injuries are caused by penetrating trauma, usually from knives or low-velocity bullets and the damage therefore is usually confined to the wound tract. High-velocity weapons are capable of causing considerable damage because of the blast effect. Vascular injuries caused by blunt trauma are more difficult to manage and can be easily overlooked because often there is no superficial evidence of injury to the neck. Moreover, patients sustaining blunt trauma sometimes have associated closed head injuries and other wounds that require an array of diagnostic tests.

Most patients sustaining penetrating cervical trama are males. In the authors' series, 14% of the vascular wounds were in the cervical region, but there is a trend seen in recent publications suggesting that the incidence of penetrating cervical trauma may be as high as 38% (Fry and Fry, 1987; McCormack and Burch, 1979).

1

In evaluating patients with penetrating cervical trauma it is useful to divide the neck into three zones as described by Monson *et al.* (1969). Zone 1 extends from 1 cm above the clavicle down to include the base of the neck and the thoracic outlet. Zone 2 is from 1 cm above the clavicle to the angle of the mandible and Zone 3 extends from the angle of the mandible to the base of the skull.

It is the authors' practice to explore all penetrating wounds of the anterior triangle of the neck that pierce the platysma muscle (Perry, 1981). This is controversial, and if the patient does not have an obvious injury, some surgeons prefer to observe the patient and perform various diagnostic manoeuvres. Patients with injuries of the oesophagus or trachea may have subcutaneous air or drainage; surgical exploration is mandatory. In patients who do not have clear evidence of injury to the aerodigestive tract, endoscopy and contrast studies have been used to exclude injury. These tests have an incidence of false-negative results and cannot be relied upon to exclude damage, particularly to the hypopharynx.

A thorough neurological examination is mandatory in all patients because of the anatomic relationships of the major nerves and vessels. It is important to identify injuries to the cranial nerves or brachial plexus preoperatively, not only to assess the extent of injury, but to document pre-existing damage prior to an operative procedure.

Arteriography may be used to exclude the need for an operation in patients with no obvious injuries. In others, an arteriogram may be helpful in planning the operation, or perhaps will identify a clinically unsuspected injury (Perry *et al.*, 1980). It is the authors' practice to obtain four vessel arteriography in all patients in stable condition who have penetrating trauma to the neck in Zones 1 and 3, as well as in patients with neurological deficits from injuries in Zone 2. Patients with penetrating injuries in Zone 2, but who have no neurological deficit, can safely undergo operative exploration without arteriography.

Because the main concern in these patients is the possibility of a carotid artery injury, it is useful in planning treatment to divide them into three neurological groups (Thal *et al.*, 1974) (Table 1). The majority of patients fall into the first group – those who have no neurological deficit. Their prognosis is good and one can anticipate a successful surgical repair. The second group contains those patients with a moderate neurological deficit, generally manifested by hemiparesis or monoparesis, or transient episodes of cerebral ischaemia. Repair of carotid injuries in these patients is also expected to be successful. Group 3 consists of patients who have severe neurological deficits, and often have carotid artery occlusion. In this group the eventual outcome is directly related to the severity of the neurological deficit before surgical treatment. It is the authors' practice to repair all carotid injuries in patients in Groups 1 and 2. We recommend repair of carotid injuries in Group 3 if prograde arterial flow is preserved and if the patient does not have an acute severe stroke with coma.

Most injuries of the vertebral artery are treated by ligation, but if the injured artery is a large dominant vessel it should be repaired. Those methods described for the carotid artery are used in this situation as well (Fry and Fry, 1987).

Jugular vein wounds are also usually treated by simple ligation. If both veins are damaged, it is prudent to repair the larger of the two. The vessel is often of a size that will permit lateral venography, but vein patch venoplasty may be needed.

1

2

A standard oblique neck incision is made along the anterior of the sternocleidomastoid muscle. The dissection continues through the plastysma muscle, reflecting the sternocleidomastoid muscle posteriorly, thus exposing the carotid sheath. The exposure of the carotid artery is begun at the base of the neck. If haematoma is identified in the sheath or in the periadventitial tissue surrounding the carotid artery at this level, the incision may be extended as a median sternotomy as demonstrated by the dotted lines. This will enable the surgeon to obtain proximal control of the great vessels in the thoracic outlet.

2

3

As the bifurcation of the carotid artery is approached, the jugular vein and sternomastoid muscles are retracted laterally. Beginning the dissection of the common carotid artery first enables the surgeon to establish proximal control. This step also centres the dissection at the proper depth (deep to the visceral fascia) to identify and protect the vagus and hypoglossal nerves, and their branches. The superior laryngeal nerve is hidden by the carotid bifurcation, and if the artery must be freed from its bed, that nerve is protected – it passes forward and medially adjacent and behind the bulb.

3

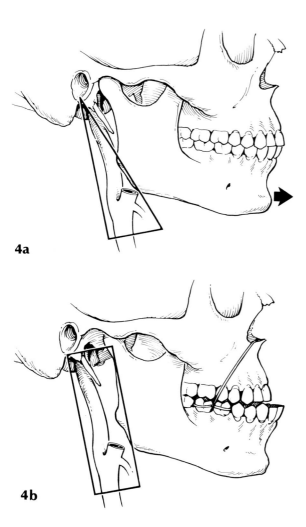

4a

4b

4

This demonstrates the exposure obtained by anterior subluxation of the mandible. This manoeuvre is useful when arteriograms show injuries to the internal carotid above the level of the angle of the mandible. With the mandible in the normal anatomic position (a), the dissection enters a progressively smaller area at the apex of the triangle near the base of the skull. If the mandible is moved anteriorly (b), this narrow apex of the triangle can be expanded by 1.5–2 cm, thus facilitating exposure up to the base of the skull. This eliminates the need for mandibular osteotomies. It is usually helpful to divide the digastric muscle and perhaps excise the styloid process.

There are several methods of obtaining and holding mandibular subluxation. The maxillary wires shown eliminate the need for continuous traction that is required when only mandibular wires are placed at the mentum.

The mandible should be brought directly and evenly forward, and not permitted to assume an angled position because this may compress the opposite carotid artery. Little disability has been seen in these patients after subluxation.

5

Simple oblique lacerations – the kind often seen from a knife injury – are best repaired by simple suture repair after debridement of devitalized wound edges. Intimal coaptation is particularly important in the carotid artery because of the damage to the brain from microemboli.

Most surgeons prefer small monofilament sutures. Often these lacerations are best managed by interrupted suture techniques.

5

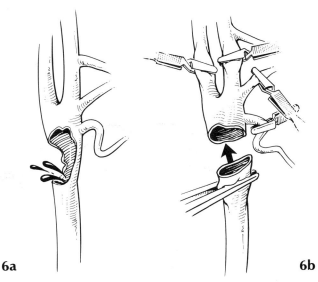

6a   **6b**

6

An extensive injury involving the carotid bifurcation, with loss of most of the circumference of the vessel, generally results from a bullet wound. It is most easily treated by resection of the involved segment as shown in (*b*), and then a simple end-to-end anastomosis is performed (*c*). Injuries to the internal carotid artery involving extensive loss of vessel may be treated by similar technique.

If the artery has a small diameter (4 mm), interrupted sutures are preferred but, alternatively, a spatulated, running suture anastomosis may be chosen.

6c

7

When the internal carotid artery cannot be repaired directly, continuity may be obtained by substituting the external carotid artery. A standard end-to-end anastomosis is constructed between the proximal external carotid and the undamaged distal part of the internal carotid artery. In patients who have multifocal arterial occlusvie disease, the external carotid may be an important collateral pathway, and should be preserved. In this situation, an interposition saphenous vein graft is preferred.

7

8

8

When the internal carotid artery is severely damaged, direct repair or vein patch graft angioplasty may not be possible. An interposition saphenous vein graft is obtained from the groin (these areas should be prepared in all of these cases, since vein grafts may be needed in several situations).

If there is scanty backflow from the internal carotid artery, rather than bright red, brisk, pulsatile flow, a temporary inlying shunt is threaded through the prepared vein graft and put in place to support cerebral blood flow. Alternatively, the surgeon can measure the back pressure in the internal carotid artery. If it is greater than 70 torr, it is thought to be safe to proceed without a shunt. Some surgeons do not employ a shunt in any of these situations.

During these operations a dilute heparin-saline solution (1:10) is used to prevent local thrombosis. Since many of these patients have multiple injuries, full systemic doses of heparin my be contraindicated. If there is only the isolated carotid artery wound, 5000 u of heparin are administered intravenously as soon as control of the bleeding is obtained.

Summary

Although thromboembolic events following the repair of carotid artery injuries are unusual they may cause serious neurological problems on rare occasions if frequent evaluation of the haemodynamic and neurological status of these patients is mandatory. Any alteration in the neurological findings is a clear indication for further studies, usually arteriograms. If a build-up of thrombus in the arteries is suspected, some of the non-invasive tests may be helpful, but often an arteriogram would be required to be certain. If a patient has a frank stroke it is best not to delay for confirmatory studies, but return the patient to the operating room for exploration and restoration of cerebral blood flow as rapidly as possible. The problem is most likely a clot at the site of the repair, and if this is treated before cerebral infarction supervenes, the outcome is usually satisfactory.

Long-term results of repairing carotid artery injuries are quite good (Table 2). In the absence of infection and if the patient does not have a neurological deficit prior to operation, a majority of the patients recover without incident. As seen in Table 2 carotid injuries caused by penetrating trauma have a more favourable outlook than those caused by blunt trauma (Table 3). As indicated in the preliminary remarks of this section, if the patients can be successfully operated upon prior to the develpoment of a neurological deficit, the prognosis is usually favourable. Once the patient has a cerebral infarction then the amount of recovery will depend on the extent of brain damage.

Table 1
Carotid injuries

Group	Degree of neurological deficit	n
1	None	49
2	Mild	8
3	Severe	15

Table 2
Carotid injuries: penetrating trauma

Group	Mortality	
	n	%
1	0	0.0
2	1	1.3
3	5	6.9

Table 3
Carotid injuries: blunt trauma

	Mortality	
	n	%
All cases	4/17	23
Carotid operations	2/14	14
Successful repair	0/7	0

References

Fry, W. J. and Fry, R. E. (1987). Management of carotid artery injury. In *Vascular Surgical Emergencies*. Bergan, J. J. and Yao, J. S. T., eds. New York: Grune and Stratton.

McCormack, T. M. and Burch, B. H. (1979). Routine angiographic evaluation of neck and extremity injuries. *Journal of Trauma* **19**, 384.

Monson, D. O., Saletta, J. D. and Freeark, R. J. (1969). Carotid-vertebral trauma. *Journal of Trauma* **9**, 987.

Perry, M. O. (1981). *The Management of Acute Vascular Injuries*. Baltimore: Williams and Wilkins.

Perry, M. O., Snyder, W. H. and Thal, E. R. (1980). Carotid artery injuries caused by blunt trauma. *Annals of Surgery* **192**, 74.

Thal, E. R., Snyder, W. H., Hays, R. J. and Perry, M. O. (1974). Management of carotid artery injuries. *Surgery* **76**, 955.

Upper and lower limb vascular trauma

Aires A. B. Barros D'Sa   MD, FRCS, FRCSEd
Consultant Vascular Surgeon, Vascular Surgical Unit, Royal Victoria Hospital, Belfast, UK

Introduction

Vascular injuries of the limbs which once occurred almost exclusively in wartime, are now observed not only on the field of battle and following criminal violence so typical of large conurbations, but also as a consequence of road traffic and industrial accidents. Blood vessel injuries of the extremities represent approximately two-thirds of all vascular trauma. Confronted with these undoubtedly challenging injuries, the vascular surgeon must swiftly control life-endangering haemorrhage and initiate resuscitation which proceeds in concert with definitive operative treatment. The objective of surgery is to preserve the viability of a limb by precise repair of damaged arteries and veins using accepted principles in the knowledge that failure may lead to crippling disability, amputation and sometimes to death.

The scenario within which penetrating vascular injury of the extremities takes place, i.e. the nature of the wounding agent, the mode of injury and the lapse of time before admission, will strongly influence operative management. Knives, splinters of glass, shards of metal, bullets, shrapnel and fragments from a variety of explosive devices, account for injuries ranging from mere contusion or puncture to complete transection of a vessel. Stab wounds, usually sustained by the upper limb, may sever major vessels quite cleanly with minimal soft tissue injury. In contrast, a missile has a considerable wounding capacity which is proportional to its mass, muzzle velocity and distance before impact. Whereas a low-velocity missile usually only disrupts a vessel segment lying in its path, the temporary cavitational effect of a high-velocity missile will cause traumatic displacement and destruction of tissues sufficient to stretch and tear neighbouring arteries. If bone is struck, dissipating most of the energy of such a missile, the resulting fragments of bone, now behaving as secondary missiles, will wreak havoc on the soft tissues. A shotgun fired at close range can inflict massive damage to a limb, particularly to soft tissues, including blood vessels. Survivors of bomb explosions sustain a multiplicity of injuries with widespread destruction of all body tissues caused not only by the blast wave, initially faster than the speed of sound, but also by flying fragments, secondary missiles, and falling masonry. A few of the thousands of transfemoral and transaxillary diagnostic procedures undertaken by cardiologists and radiologists in modern hospital practice, represent a further iatrogenic source of penetrating limb vascular trauma.

In road traffic accidents, a sharp bony fragment may directly lacerate a vessel, but more frequently indirect damage may ensue as a result of the intense shearing forces generated by the sudden fracture of long bones. Particularly vulnerable arterial segments are those which lie adjacent to a long bone or at points of relative fixity, especially in close proximity to joints. Sudden violent angulation of the shaft of a long bone or the traction associated with fracture dislocations at the knee, progressively disrupts the layers of the vessel wall beginning with the intima. Crush injuries caused by falling masonry after air raids and bomb explosions are observed in peacetime following industrial, mining and train accidents, and earthquakes. The ischaemia consequent upon injury, whether in the form of extrinsic compression and contusion or division of a vessel, will accelerate the progression of a 'crush syndrome' and renal failure.

Limb vascular trauma may result in blood loss, and hypovolaemic hypotension which compounds the ischaemia of arterial injury. These effects and the impaired drainage due to concomitant vein injury are rapidly overtaken by complex and interdependent pathophysiological events (Barros D'Sa, 1980, 1988). If resuscitatory measures and vascular repair are not forthcoming, the protracted hypoxia will increase capillary permeability, causing a rise in intracompartmental pressure, which may herald a disastrous outcome either in the form of Volkmann's ischaemic contracture or amputation.

Preoperative measures

A firm pad and pressure bandage is preferable to a clamp which, when blindly applied, may add to the injury. The principal resuscitative measure must be the re-expansion of the circulating volume. Prophylactic tetanus toxoid and broad-spectrum antibiotics are prescribed. If the patient is not hypotensive a narcotic analgesic will decrease vasospasm and assist peripheral perfusion.

The surgeon runs through a mental checklist of clinical signs of limb vascular injury: a tense and expanding haematoma in blunt closed injuries, persistent arterial or venous bleeding in penetrating injuries, the presence of a thrill or bruit suggestive of incomplete occlusion or an acute arteriovenous fistula. It should be remembered that pulses may still be palpable beyond an injured artery which on exploration almost invariably reveals intimal damage and mural thrombosis. Doppler ultrasound assessment of pulse waveform and ankle systolic pressure is helpful. Evidence of concomitant bone and nerve injury should be documented.

In the shocked patient, delay in the radiology department may endanger life but in most instances plane films which define the bony injury and identify foreign bodies are of value in planning the best incisional approach. Preoperative angiography wastes valuable time in situations of impending loss of life or limb, whereas a policy of selective angiography based on clinical judgement will rule out arterial injury and prevent unnecessary surgery. In these times the medico-legal implications of not having obtained an arteriogram when the ultimate outcome turns out to be less than ideal, should be emphasized. In institutions unaccustomed to a round-the-clock emergency angiography service, the simple alternative of one-shot percutaneous angiography represents a fast, efficient and effective way of using resources. In certain circumstances such as delayed admission, persistent ischaemia after fracture reduction or doubt as to the trajectory of the wounding agent, a negative angiogram supports the surgeon's decision not to explore the wound and, by the same token, a positive angiogram makes operation mandatory. Biplane arteriograms of good quality will define the site and type of injury, and a lateral projection is of particular value in demonstrating a potentially sinister popliteal injury such as an intimal tear, often missed in an anteroposterior view.

The operation

The operation must be undertaken with the least possible delay, the objectives being control of bleeding, wound toilet, restoration of circulation and prevention of complications. Delay in diagnosis or improper management may result in amputation or lasting functional disability. All wounds in anatomical proximity to a major vessel should be explored.

Emergency amputation

If tissue death and gangrene have supervened due to delayed admission, amputation at the appropriate level must be carried out expeditiously. Following massive destruction and irreparable mutilation of a limb, for example following a bomb explosion, it may be prudent, after careful deliberation, to proceed to immediate amputation so avoiding gas gangrene, sepsis, haemorrhage and renal failure. In such cases, amputation should include vigorous wound toilet and excision of all devitalized tissue, doubly ligating the vessels within viable boundaries and leaving the stump to drain. After inspection, delayed closure, no earlier than 5 days later, is undertaken, using whatever tissue has been preserved to fashion definitive flaps in order to create a functioning rather than cosmetic stump.

Incisions and exposure

1

In upper limb injuries, peripheral and central venous lines should not be inserted on the injured side. The patient lies supine, the upper limb is abducted and extended palm-upwards at right-angles to the body and the draping should provide an operative field with access to the chest, neck and arm if needed. One lower limb should also be prepared and draped in case donor vein is required. The incisional approaches are illustrated.

1

2

In injuries such as stab wounds of the first part of the axillary artery it is wise to secure proximal supraclavicular control of the subclavian artery. Partial division of the clavicular head of the sternocleidomastoid, and identification and delicate retraction of the phrenic nerve medially before careful division of the scalenus anterior will reveal the subclavian artery which can be encircled.

3

The incision to approach the axillary artery commences below the clavicle and is extended laterally down the deltopectoral groove and continued distally if required along the course of the brachial artery. This means that the axillary artery can be approached either above or below the margins of the pectoralis major or by separating the fibres of this muscle, as shown. The pectoralis minor tendon has been divided. For rapid access in occasional exsanguinating situations the pectoralis major tendon may be divided at its insertion. Dissection in this area should be meticulous in view of the intimate proximity of nerves and collateral vessels.

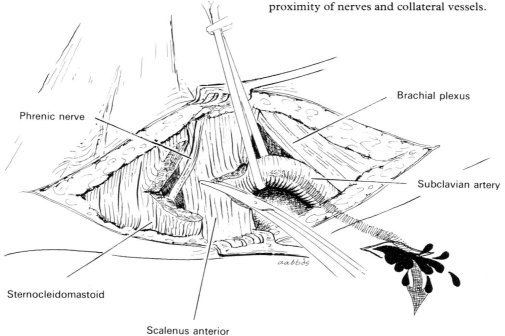

2

Phrenic nerve

Brachial plexus

Subclavian artery

Sternocleidomastoid

Scalenus anterior

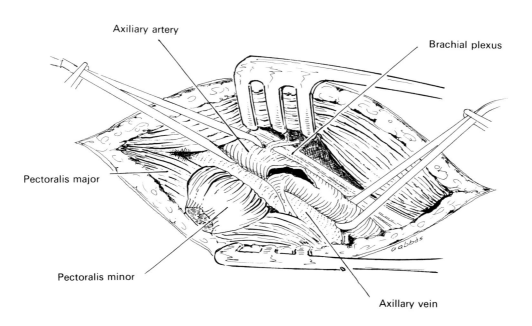

3

Axillary artery

Brachial plexus

Pectoralis major

Pectoralis minor

Axillary vein

4

The brachial artery in the upper arm or at the elbow is exposed via a standard longitudinal incision of sufficient length to expose the injured segment and to establish control. Diagnostic cannulation of this vessel may cause intimal fracture, dissection and thrombosis. Short longitudinal incisions over radial and ulnar arteries are usually quite adequate.

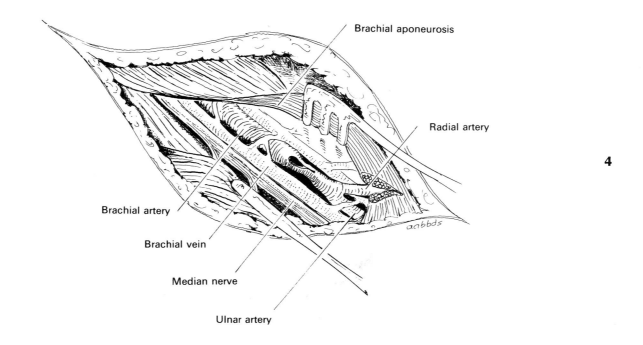

Brachial aponeurosis

Radial artery

Brachial artery

Brachial vein

Median nerve

Ulnar artery

4

5

5

In most instances of lower limb vascular injury the patient lies supine and both lower limbs are prepared and draped to permit proximal and distal extension of longitudinal incisions in the injured leg and to enable the procurement of a donor vein from the contralateral leg.

6

Of particular importance are vascular injuries of the groin associated with torrential bleeding, where control of the external iliac artery may have to be established through an oblique muscle-splitting incision affording retroperitoneal access above the inguinal ligament. While this is in progress, digital pressure over the bleeding artery is maintained and only after the external iliac artery has been clamped can the groin incision be made.

7

Classical longitudinal incisions are employed in the approach to vessels of the lower limb. The common femoral artery and adjacent vein are exposed. Injuries at the common femoral artery bifurcation will also require encirclement and control of the superficial and deep femoral arteries.

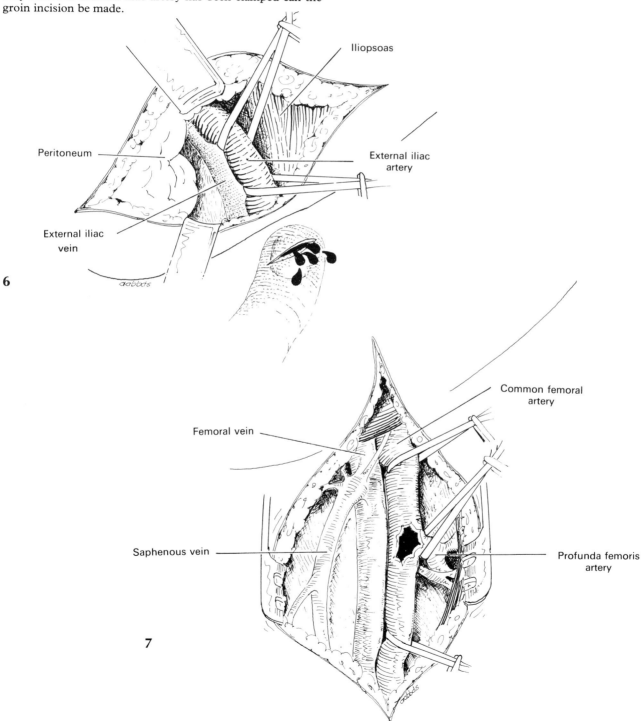

51

8

The medial approach parallel to and preserving the long saphenous vein will expose the entire length of the popliteal vessels. External rotation of the thigh and 50° knee flexion using a pack of two sterile gowns for lateral support at the hip, is the ideal position. This exposure usually necessitates division of the medial head of the gastrocnemius.

9

A posterior approach with the patient lying prone is convenient for localized mid-popliteal artery injuries. A gentle 'S'-shaped incision in an oblique axis, commencing medially above and proceeding laterally downwards provides adequate exposure. In these instances, both legs are routinely prepared enabling a segment of distal long saphenous vein to be removed with moderate ease from the opposite leg when it is flexed at the knee. Alternatively, with the patient supine, the upper long saphenous vein is harvested and the incision closed before turning the patient over for a posterior approach to the popliteal artery. The deep fascia is incised, watching for the short saphenous vein which may be ligated as it enters the popliteal vein. The tibial nerve should be handled gently as it crosses the vessels in the distal fossa. The popliteal vessels lie on the floor of the fossa, the vein superficial to the artery and united to it by dense areolar tissue, which may be carefully snipped to facilitate encirclement.

Control and preparation of vessels

10

The damaged vessels in a wound are quickly exposed and bleeding controlled initially by digital pressure. Using sharp dissecting scissors the segments of an artery above and below are dissected free before encircling them with silastic loops of suitable thickness before clamping. Care is taken to preserve significant branches, which in turn are doubly encircled for control. A sufficient length of artery on either side of the injury is exposed so that it can be trimmed back if necessary to a point where the wall is intact. Minor venous tributaries can be ligated.

10

11

If ischaemia has been prolonged, release of the upper clamp may wash out a plug of clot but a balloon catheter may also be required. Distal balloon exploration, delicately employed, will often recover clot, especially when backbleeding is poor or absent. Lack of backbleeding is ominous, and in these circumstances vigorous upward milking of the limb musculature distal to the injury may express recent propagated clot. In the young patient lacking an established collateral network, backbleeding will be limited making arterial repair even more essential if the limb is to be salvaged. The distal arteries are then perfused with heparinized saline in a ratio of 5000 u of heparin to 250 ml saline. In the absence of other injury, systemic heparinization is both reliable and easily reversible.

11

Shunting

When flow through an artery or vein has been interrupted, a policy of routine intraluminal shunting has contributed to improved operative technique, a reduction in complications and enhanced viability (Barros D'Sa, 1982; 1988). Intraluminal shunts of the Brener, Sundt and Javid type of appropriate size, employed in carotid artery surgery, are reasonably effective and a new purpose-built shunt system for vascular trauma has been designed (Barros D'Sa, in press). When shunts are used, demarcation between viable and dead muscle is more clearly apparent, facilitating accurate debridement and ensuring better haemostasis. In the event of a patient being admitted with multiple injuries, limb-threatening vascular trauma can be safely ignored after shunt insertion, so buying valuable time to complete life-endangering surgery first.

12

A Brener shunt inserted in a torn popliteal artery revitalizes the distal limb and a Javid shunt placed in a severed vein prevents the inevitable rise in intracompartmental pressure, thereby limiting tissue damage and in consequence significantly reducing the need for fasciotomy. The side arm of a Brener shunt forms a convenient port for the delivery of heparinized saline and antibiotics and also for blood sampling, pressure monitoring and on-table angiography if distal injury is suspected.

13

When a long arterial segment in either upper or lower limb is associated with extensive soft tissue trauma, much time may elapse before restoration of flow. In such cases, a long outlying Pudenz shunt, picking up flow proximal to the injured segment and inserted beyond the injury, will revitalize the limb, and if bleeding through damaged veins is excessive the shunt may be clamped intermittently.

12

13

14

When skeletal and vascular injuries co-exist a logical policy formulated around the use of inlying shunts streamlines and co-ordinates operative management. After an agreed incisional approach, if necessary by extending an open wound as when confronted with a case of virtual dismemberment just below mid-thigh level, the vascular surgeon re-establishes flow through artery and vein by means of shunts. He is then relieved by the orthopaedic surgeon who can proceed methodically without undue haste approximating the bone ends and using the most suitable method of fracture stabiliz-ation, which in penetrating trauma is usually by external fixation.

15

The vascular surgeon then returns to execute the vascular repair using long vein grafts to bridge the gaps in the confident knowledge that they will not be disturbed. A great deal of debate still takes place about the order of repair when artery and vein are injured concomitantly, but such controversy is dispelled if both vessels are shunted. In the past an understandable desire to restore limb flow speedily led to exhortations to repair the artery before bony fixation, but this policy was attended by the real fears of suture line disruption of a delicate vessel repair during the robust manipulations necessary to achieve alignment of bone frag-ments. Shunts render this approach almost obsolete.

14

15

Care of the wound

Excision of knife wounds is usually unnecessary and only a small margin of devitalized tissue around the edge of a low-velocity bullet wound is removed. Debridement of high-velocity wounds must be adequate if infection is to be averted, and therefore a liberal longitudinal incision dividing the investing fascia is required. All devitalized muscle, recognized by its deep purplish colour and failure to bleed and contract, is trimmed back to a point where it does. Bone fragments are detached from periosteum and foreign bodies, missiles and contaminants are meticulously removed, aided by copious and if possible pulsatile irrigation. A contused nerve is simply left alone, but if transected in a clean wound accurate primary repair is advisable. If damage is extensive following severe blunt injuries and gunshot wounds, the sheath of each nerve end is simply tagged so that delayed secondary repair can be undertaken as an elective procedure.

Arterial repair

While it may be reasonable to ligate minor arteries and veins, in principle all damaged vessels should be repaired, a precept which is particularly applicable to the small calibre brachial or femoral artery of a child whose limbs require sufficient blood flow for proper growth and development. Tibial arteries should be reconstructed, especially if two of them are known to be damaged. The presumption that axillary or brachial artery ligation will not lead to upper limb amputation due to the protective presence of adequate collateral blood flow should be diminished. Brachial artery injuries should not be regarded as innocuous and left to be repaired by a novice, as opportunities to obtain a good result diminish with each repeated attempt. The Allen test should be used in determining the importance of repairing injured radial and ulnar arteries. The choice of vascular repair indicated will obviously depend on the nature of the injury. The morphological types of injury (Barros D'Sa, 1988) include varying degrees of intimal fracture and dissection with thrombic occlusion, laceration or a lateral defect sometimes complicated by false aneurysm and arteriovenous fistula formation, transection and complete disruption by avulsive forces. In practice, various permutations of these morphologically simple sub-divisions may be present in a single vascular injury. The diagnosis of 'spasm' is both presumptive and dangerous if it leads to inactivity in the presence of limb-threatening arterial injury.

16

Lateral suture

Lateral suture is acceptable in a small puncture wound, especially if it can be performed transversely using interrupted sutures. Transverse and short oblique lacerations with sharp edges may be repaired similarly. When the laceration is longitudinal and particularly if it is contused, adequate excision followed by lateral suture will narrow the lumen and could endanger the extremity, notably in critical vessels such as the brachial and popliteal.

16

17

17

Patch angioplasty

In order to preserve the calibre of the artery an angioplasty using a vein patch is preferable to lateral suture. In a closed or uncontaminated injury to a large vessel such as the iliac or common femoral artery, it would be quite acceptable to employ a suitable prosthetic patch graft in the knowledge that it will heal with an endothelialized flow surface in a matter of a few weeks (Barros D'Sa et al., 1980).

18

Direct anastomosis

Direct end-to-end anastomosis is possible after stab wounds or after excising the edges with limited loss of length. The presence of excessive anastomotic tension may well lead to disruption or thrombotic failure. If a joint has to be flexed and if major collateral channels, particularly in an atherosclerotic artery, have to be sacrificed to permit approximation, then excision and vein grafting is indicated. These limitations are once again particularly applicable to the popliteal artery.

Vein grafts

Autogenous tissue is durable, resistant to infection and can develop nutrient flow from surrounding viable tissue. Long-term promise of patency makes vein the most desirable graft, especially as vascular trauma largely afflicts the young. The indiscriminate use of prosthetic arterial grafts in combat wounds predisposes to infection, secondary haemorrhage and a high amputation rate, and has been avoided with beneficial results (Barros D'Sa, 1980, 1982; Barros D'Sa *et al.*, 1980). An institutional policy of using substitute arterial conduits in the form of polytetrafluorethylene (PTFE) prostheses in gunshot wounds has shown early promise (Feliciano *et al*, 1984), but should not lead to complacency.

18

19

The excision of only a centimetre of apparently normal vessel with a No. 15 scalpel blade on either side of an obvious vascular injury may be inadequate, particularly in high-velocity bullet trauma or the complex traction injury of the popliteal vessels in a motor-cycle accident. The external appearances of an injured artery often belie the extent of damage to the intima, and therefore the arterial wall may have to be trimmed back further with sharp scissors to a point where it is visibly intact. The practice of interposing a reversed vein graft which is easily available encourages adequate excision of a damaged artery. The long saphenous vein of the opposite leg is the usual source for donor graft, the ipsilateral vein representing a precious drainage channel in circumstances where the deep vein may be injured. The vein graft is reversed and is usually used at once but may be stored temporarily in cold Hank's solution or heparinized saline.

19

20

In larger vessels such as the axillary and femoral, a polypropylene everting suture commenced at diametrically opposite points is continued along the suture line, access to which is gained by a measure of rotation on the axis of the vessel. If a shunt is in place, the vein graft can be drawn over it. The shunt then acts conveniently as a stent, permits a more disciplined suture technique and prevents purse-stringing of the anastomosis.

20

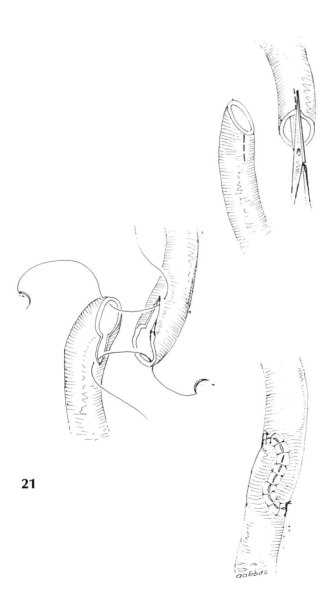

21

If the arterial diameter is less than 4 mm, careful thrombectomy using a size 2 balloon catheter is essential. Meticulous attention is paid to technique in executing the anastomosis using loupes and fine instruments. Small arteries of children are prone to vasospasm which may be abolished by judicious inflation with a fine rounded catheter. The ends of the vein graft and host vessel are cut obliquely and spatulated, a necessary step which will accommodate increasing vessel diameter without stenosis as the child grows. Repair is then undertaken by interrupted 6/0 to 8/0 polypropylene sutures carefully placed without tension so as to prevent constriction at the suture line. Accurate coaptation of intimal surfaces while everting the edges will prevent inward protrusion of adventitial strands.

21

22

If a lengthy segment of atherosclerotic artery is damaged, emergency bypass surgery may be necessary. If soft tissue loss is extensive and if contamination is extreme, then an extra-anatomic vein bypass through clean tissues should be considered. If, for example, a lengthy femoropopliteal segment has been destroyed in a large contaminated wound, the trimmed ends are ligated and an extra-anatomic vein graft, unreversed but with its valves disrupted, is inserted subcutaneously from the common femoral to, for example, the anterior tibial artery.

23

When the calibre of the donor vein is much smaller than that of the host vessel – often a vein – the graft will fail unless a panel compound graft of larger diameter can be constructed to ensure laminar flow. It is fashioned 'on the bench' by taking two segments of vein opened longitudinally to form panels and these are sewn together side by side with 6/0 polypropylene to achieve proportions comparable to the host vessel (Livingston and Wilson, 1975). These grafts have to be made slightly longer than the gap to be bridged.

22

23

24

For larger vessels such as the femoral vein, three rather than two panels may be required. Alternatively, a technique used to replace a segment of the vena cava can be employed and it may have particular value in contaminated wounds. A length of vein is slit open longitudinally and wrapped spirally over a shunt of sufficiently wide bore to act as a stent and then the adjoining margins of vein are sewn together using a continuous 6/0 polypropylene suture.

24

25

False aneurysms

A false aneurysm may develop in a partially penetrating injury which has been missed usually because distal flow did not appear to be compromised. Most frequently, false aneurysms follow diagnostic transfemoral cardiac catheterization. For obvious reasons, these patients may not be fit for general anaesthesia and regional or local anaesthesia may have to be used. After establishing proximal and distal control, the aneurysm is opened and the profunda femoris which could not be exposed initially is now clamped. The thrombus is removed and the aneurysm excised. The vessel lumen is inspected for intimal damage, if necessary by transverse extension of the opening. If a loose atheromatous flap is present on the posterior wall, it is tacked down with a 5/0 or 6/0 polypropylene suture. The laceration is repaired transversely with interrupted 5/0 double-ended sutures, picking upper and lower edges from within outwards. In the case of a chronic larger fusiform aneurysm, patch angioplasty or segmental excision and replacement with an interposed vein graft or prosthetic conduit is preferred.

25

26

Arteriovenous fistulae

Arteriovenous fistulae may be missed both clinically and at operation due to inadequate exploration and will present much later, usually accompanied by one or two false aneurysms. The intraoperative use of a sterile stethoscope may have some value, especially in cases of shotgun wounds, to ensure closure of all fistulae. The artery and vein are exposed, brought under control, the fistulous communication separated by means of a fine scalpel and the false aneurysms excised. The edges of the defects are trimmed back to intact vessel wall. The openings in the artery are best repaired by vein patches and, if required, by excision of a segment and vein graft replacement. The vein is usually repaired successfully either by lateral suture or by insertion of a vein patch. Finally, a flap of fascia may be interposed between adjacent suture lines to prevent recurrence.

26

On-table angiography

Clinical evaluation of the quality of arterial repair in a severely injured and hypotensive patient whose core temperature has fallen may be difficult simply because distal pulses are weak or absent, and even Doppler ultrasound cannot be relied upon. The only way of excluding technical error or distal thrombotic obstruction is by on-table angiography which takes a few minutes and provides visual evidence of the adequacy of surgery.

Venous repair

The mistaken attitude that ligation of a damaged vein, while not helpful, would do no harm, or that venous repair is possibly less important than arterial repair, should not be perpetuated. When both vessels are injured, vein ligation may result in amputation even after successful arterial reconstruction. Conversely, venous repair will enhance arterial patency. Ligation of a main vein causes venous hypertension and can result in acute massive oedema, in some cases leading to gangrene and amputation and in others to deep vein thrombosis and pulmonary embolism or to disabling chronic odema and postphlebitic changes. Every effort must be made to secure at least one good venous channel at axillary, femoral or popliteal level. A vein tolerates lateral suturing much better than an artery, but loss of diameter must still be guarded against. Repair of a major vein is quite valuable when tissue loss is massive and lymph damage is compromised.

27

If both artery and vein are injured and each is shunted, the order of repair of these two vessels is immaterial, but if neither vessel has been shunted then preliminary vein repair will prevent a serious rise in venous pressure when arterial flow is eventually re-established. With shunts in place in this wound, a simple vein graft has been reversed and interposed perfectly adequately to replace a damaged arterial segment of similar calibre, but it would have been too narrow for the adjacent vein of much larger diameter. As time is not of crucial importance, a panel compound vein graft is constructred to match the host vein, drawn over the shunt and sutured in position.

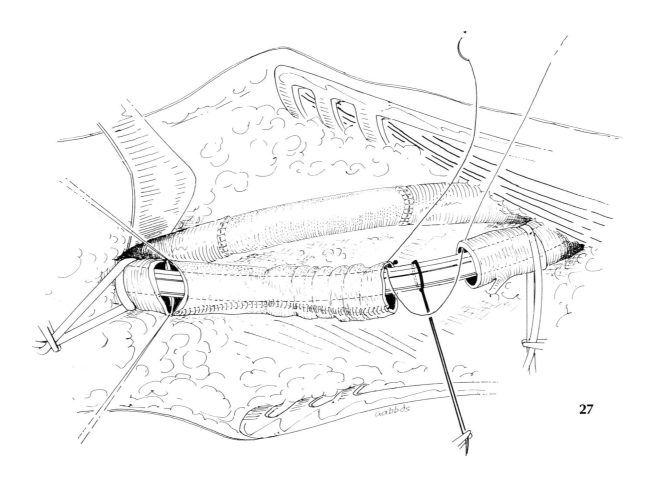

27

Fasciotomy

Restoration of arterial flow, especially if delayed, increases intracompartmental pressure, which in turn aggravates peripheral ischaemia. These considerations are of particular importance in brachial and popliteal artery injury, and in the latter case the anterior compartment which lies within rigid confines is most vulnerable. Adequate pedal pulses, good skin flow and satisfactory Doppler signals may be observed, although the muscle within the compartments is dying. Fasciotomy, if carried out early and effectively, is an invaluable adjunctive measure aimed at forestalling the serious complications of muscle ischaemia. The early use of intra-luminal shunts in both artery and vein diminishes the need for fasciotomy. If shunts have not been employed, fasciotomy should be considered if any one of the following several factors is present: sustained hypotension, an interval of more than 4 h between injury and surgical intervention, evident oedema or patchy muscle necrosis, concurrent injury to a main vein, marked injury of distal soft tissue, subfascial haematoma and bleeding, muscle paralysis and fixed flexion deformity after initial vascular repair or a compartment pressure in excess of 40 mmHg.

28

The classical percutaneous or closed fasciotomy is employed as a rule by using 5-cm vertical incisions into the deep fascia through which muscle tends to bulge. These incisions are made in the centre of the upper anterior compartment, further laterally in the middle of the upper lateral compartment and, finally, medial to the short saphenous vein over the upper posterior compartment. A pair of long curved blunt-tipped scissors is held slightly open to grasp the lower corner of the divided fascia and advanced, slitting it down the length of each compartment. Care is taken to avoid damaging the common peroneal nerve at the neck of the fibula as well as the distal superficial peroneal and sural nerves.

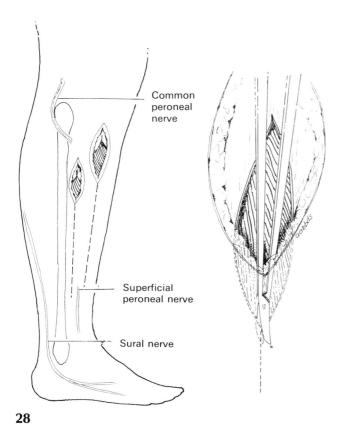

Common peroneal nerve

Superficial peroneal nerve

Sural nerve

28

29

If the muscle is pale, grey and firm, or if obvious compartmental tension is still present, the skin and subcutaneous tissues are incised converting it to an open fasciotomy. As tension decreases, these transcutaneous fasciotomy incisions will gradually approximate, but during this period utmost care must be taken to prevent infection within relatively ischaemic tissues.

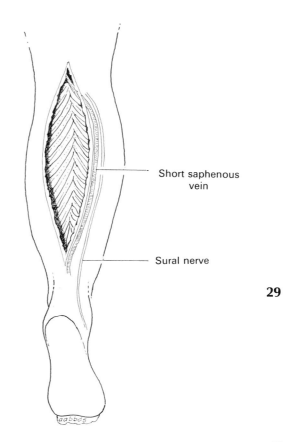

Short saphenous vein

Sural nerve

29

30

Open fasciotomy is the technique of choice in severe compression of the muscles of the forearm. The extensor compartment is released by a longitudinal centrally placed incision, while the flexor compartment is decompressed by a long curvilinear incision commencing in the antecubital fossa and crossing the wrist onto the palm along the thenar crease.

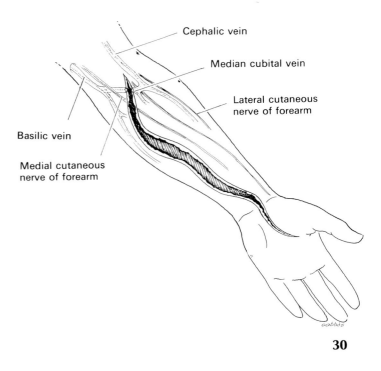

Cephalic vein

Median cubital vein

Lateral cutaneous nerve of forearm

Basilic vein

Medial cutaneous nerve of forearm

30

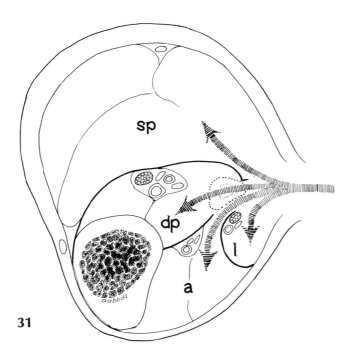

31

31

It should be remembered that a fourth deep posterior compartment is present in the lower leg in addition to the other three, and all four can be decompressed simultaneously after first resecting the mid-third of the shaft of the fibula subperiosteally (Patman and Thompson, 1970). The relationship of the superficial posterior (sp), deep posterior (dp), anterior (a) and lateral (l) compartments to the fibula when imagined in transverse section show how this route of entry can achieve the desired result.

Wound closure and vessel cover

It is important to ensure adequate cover of repaired vessels by adjacent tissues. In closed injuries primary suture of the wound is acceptable, leaving a vacuum suction drain *in situ* for a short period. In contaminated wounds the wisdom of a policy of delayed primary suture 5–7 days later has been borne out by experience (Barros D'Sa, 1980), but that should not be an excuse for slipshod wound excision and toilet.

In situations of extensive loss of skin and soft tissue over a site of arterial repair, the wall of a vein graft or adjacent artery may conceivably undergo ischaemia, desiccation and degeneration followed by catastrophic haemorrhage. While prosthetic grafts are immune to these influences they still represent alien material and if the field is contaminated then infection, thrombosis and suture line dehiscence could follow. This observation has a special bearing on the management of large dirty wounds which have to be left open to drain, making graft cover difficult. Biological dressings, such as porcine heterografts and amniotic membrane, have been tried but the alternative of a vascularized muscle flap requiring the skills of a plastic surgeon is preferable. Many of these difficulties will, of course, have been countered by the employment of the extra-anatomic vein bypass described.

Postoperative management

Ordinarily, following arterial repair, a limb is nursed in a horizontal position, but when the adjacent vein has been repaired, some degree of elevation is justified. As the patient rewarms, a deficiency in fluid replacement, evident from general observation and vital signs, must be corrected to ensure adequate flow through the reconstructed vessels. Anticoagulation with low-dose heparin (5000 u every 6 h subcutaneously) will aid graft patency and prevent deep vein thrombosis.

Failure of repair

Utmost vigilance must be exercised in monitoring flow by checking pulses, skin circulation and Doppler signals. Their absence may be a prelude to amputation unless urgent angiography and further reconstruction are undertaken. In such cases, classical weaknesses of technique are observed, namely, constriction caused by lateral suture, tension at the suture line of a direct anastomosis, insufficient excision of damaged artery, too narrow or too long vein grafts, 'purse-string' effect of a continuous anastomotic suture and poor intimal coaptation. In dealing with graft failure the most reliable sequence of measures is as follows: excise the segment concerned liberally, confirm the quality of the freshly trimmed vessel, perform an adequate balloon thrombectomy, reperfuse the distal artery with heparinized saline and very precisely revise the repair with a fresh vein graft of suitable calibre and length. Systemic heparinization and close observation will avert an unfavourable outcome.

In summary, a number of factors play a role in minimizing the complication rate and incidence of limb loss: routine use of intraluminal shunts in both injured artery and vein, vascular repair after skeletal fixation, early and definitive repair of both artery and vein injury, avoidance of lateral suture and direct anastomosis, use of vein grafts and of panel compound grafts of appropriate diameter when required, immediate fasciotomy when indicated, postoperative vigilance and, in cases of graft failure, expeditious re-exploration and fresh repair.

References

Barros D'Sa, A. A. B. (1980). Missile-induced vascular trauma. *Injury* **12**, 13.

Barros D'Sa, A. A. B. (1982). A decade of missile-induced vascular trauma. *Annals of the Royal College of Surgeons of England* **64**, 37.

Barros D'Sa, A. A. B. (1988). How should we manage acute ischaemia associated with trauma? In *Limb Salvage and Amputation for Vascular Disease*. Greenhalgh, R. M., Jamieson, C. W., Nicolaides, A. N., eds. London and Philadelphia: W. B. Saunders.

Barros D'Sa, A. A. B., (in press). Arterial and venous shunting in the management of limb vessel injury.

Barros D'Sa, A. A. B., Berger, K., DiBenedetto, G., *et al.*, (1980). A healable filamentous Dacron surgical fabric. *Annals of Surgery* **192**, 645.

Feliciano, D. V., Carmel, G., Bitondo, P. A. C., *et al.* (1984). Civilian trauma in the 1980's. A 1-year experience with 456 vascular and cardiac injuries. *Annals of Surgery* **199**, 717.

Patman, R. D. and Thompson, J. E. (1970). Fasciotomy in peripheral arterial injury. *Archives of Surgery* **101**, 633.

Direct reconstruction of intrathoracic great vessels

E. Kieffer
C. Petitjean
Y. Bensaïd
J. Natali
Service de Chirurgie Vasculaire.
Groupe Hospitalier Pitié-Salpétrière, Paris, France

Introduction

Direct surgical management of intrathoracic great vessel disease was used exclusively in the first years following the pioneering work of Bahnson, Spencer and Quattlebaum (1959) and Davis, Grove and Julian (1956). Reconstruction of the innominate artery, left common carotid artery or multiple lesions was performed through a median sternotomy, and a posterolateral thoracotomy was used for left subclavian artery procedures. However, owing to the magnitude of these operations in poor-risk patients, operative mortality remained high (Crawford *et al.*, 1969), leading to a progressive decrease in indications for intrathoracic procedures and the introduction of extrathoracic reconstructions. By far the most popular of these has been the carotid-subclavian bypass (Dietrich *et al.*, 1967), but other operations have been developed including direct reimplantation of subclavian artery into the common carotid artery (Edwards and Wright, 1972) and various types of cross-over cervical bypasses (Finkelstein, Byer and Rush, 1972; Sethi, Scott and Takaro, 1975; Manart and Kempczinski, 1980).

The cervical procedures facilitate surgical management of most isolated lesions of the intrathoracic great vessels. Their low operative risk and clinical effectiveness certainly make their use valid and logical in the management of isolated subclavian or common carotid lesions, particularly left subclavian artery lesions, which are the most commonly found and whose direct surgical management is possible only through left thoracotomy. However, it is our opinion that most cases of innominate artery and multiple lesions are best treated using direct reconstruction through a median sternotomy.

The purpose of this chapter is to describe the most commonly performed procedures in our 10-year experience including 142 patients treated by direct intrathoracic procedures.

Patterns of intrathoracic arterial lesions

A knowledge of arterial pathology is important as it governs the type of reconstructive procedure to be used.

Most occlusive lesions are atherosclerotic in origin. They are usually very localized, although sometimes multiple.

Atherosclerotic involvement of the aortic arch, leading to ostial stenosis, is the most frequently encountered lesion. Each of the three intrathoracic great vessels – the innominate artery, the left common carotid artery (LCCA) and the left subclavian artery (LSCA) – may be involved. Different combinations of these lesions are possible, but when all three are involved it is called the 'aortic arch syndrome'. Lesions of the middle part of the innominate artery or the LSCA, not involving the aortic origin of these vessels, are much rarer, as are localized lesions of the bifurcation of the innominate artery, extending in various degrees to the right subclavian artery (RSCA) and/or to the right common carotid artery (RCCA).

Ulcerated atherosclerotic lesions, especially in the innominate artery, may lead to embolization in the brain, eye or upper extremity. Haemodynamic consequences are to be expected only in the presence of tightly stenosing and/or completely occluding lesions, especially when multiple. Innominate artery and LSCA occlusions are usually segmental, sparing the bifurcation of the artery or remaining proximal to the origin of the left vertebral artery (VA). In such cases some form of reversed flow in the VA and RCCA is present. Occlusion of the LCCA always extends at least up to the carotid bifurcation. The presence of a significant stenotic lesion at this level usually leads to an extensive occlusion including the whole length of the internal carotid artery (ICA), sparing the external carotid artery (ECA), whose distal part is revascularized by numerous collateral branches coming from the ipsilateral SCA and contralateral ECA. In the presence of a normal carotid bifurcation, LCCA occlusion is usually only segmental, with the ICA remaining patent, often with a reversed flow to the ECA.

Takayasu's arteritis is usually localized to the middle or distal part of the common carotid and/or subclavian arteries (Kieffer and Natali, 1983). Involvement of the intrathoracic great vessels is less frequent but, when present, it is commonly associated with severe involvement of the aortic arch, leading to a complete form of 'aortoarteritis'.

Traumatic lesions are uncommon. They may be observed following penetrating or blunt deceleration injuries. The latter usually results in avulsion of the artery at its origin on the aortic arch (Kieffer *et al.*, 1977) but rupture of the middle part of the intrathoracic segment is possible. Acute lesions leading to emergency operations are beyond the scope of this chapter. Chronic sequelae include occlusions, false aneurysms and arteriovenous (AV) fistulae.

Congential lesions of the intrathoracic great vessels may be associated with the left or right aortic arch. A retro-oesophageal subclavian artery is present in 0.5% of the normal population but surgery is only indicated in the occasional symptomatic case. Isolation of the innominate or left subclavian artery is much less common. These abnormalities are usually found in association with intracardiac and/or aortic congenital lesions but may be completely isolated.

Although anatomically frequent, especially in the innominate artery, kinking is usually not haemodynamically significant and should lead to surgery only on very rare occasions. Spontaneous aneurysms are atherosclerotic or luetic in origin but remain much rarer than occlusive lesions.

Special preoperative preparation

The intrathoracic nature of the procedure obviously necessitates a precise assessment of the patient's cardiopulmonary status and medical treatment of all treatable abnormalities whenever possible. Pulmonary function should be assessed precisely. Preoperative pulmonary physiotherapy is often indicated in this middle-aged smoking population. Cardiac abnormalities should be looked for carefully through history and a standard ECG. Coronary angiography and cardiac catheterization should have broad indications even in the presence of stable angina, since coronary artery bypass, if indicated, should be performed in the same operative session. Arterial hypertension should be treated preoperatively in order to allow for safe lateral clamping of the aorta and prevent cardiac and cerebral complications. A CT scan should be obtained in the presence of any permanent neurological symptoms.

Although non-invasive ultrasonic techniques are of great value and should be obtained routinely, angiography is necessary for a precise assessment of the cerebral circulation.

Arch aortography should visualize not only the intrathoracic vessels but also the carotid bifurcations and vertebral arteries. Distal arteries may be difficult to visualize in the presence of multiple extensive occlusions. In rare cases we used to begin the operation with surgical exploration of one or both of the carotid bifurcations. More recently, most of these problems have been overcome using non-invasive techniques and intra-arterial digitalized subtraction angiography.

Special intraoperative monitoring for these procedures

Much of this is as described in the chapter on 'Operative planning'. Blood pressure is recorded through an intra-arterial line placed either in the radial artery opposite the artery to be revascularized or in either of the femoral arteries in the presence of multiple lesions. Cardiac function assessment by a Swan-Ganz catheter should be routinely used since intraoperative lowering of the blood pressure using halothane or preferably sodium nitroprusside or trinitrin is often necessary to allow for precise and safe lateral clamping of the aorta. Multiple venous lines are also used, avoiding the cervical and left brachial regions because the left innominate vein may have to be transected in order to obtain adequate access to the lesions.

We use no special intraoperative cerebral monitoring such as EEG or pressure measurements. The only routine cerebral protective measures taken are: (1) systemic heparinization during arterial clamping (0.5 mg/kg, with neutralization by protamine sulphate at the end of the procedure); (2) avoidance of hypotension during arterial clamping and of hypertension in the postoperative period; and (3) sequential declamping of the arteries, beginning with the non-cerebral arteries (ECA or distal SCA). In the presence of multiple proximal lesions, revascularization should begin with the most stenotic lesion(s). Similarly, tandem intrathoracic and cervical lesions should be treated sequentially, beginning with the more proximal one.

The use of cardiopulmonary bypass (CPB) may be necessary in a few selected situations, the most frequent of these being simultaneous coronary revascularization. Circulatory arrest using deep hypothermia has been used in a few cases to perform transaortic endarterectomy of multiple proximal lesions of the great vessels (Thevenet, Chaptal and Negre, 1968). However, although this technique seems logical and appealing, reasonable clinical and angiographic indications remain rare and the whole procedure may seem unnecessarily complicated.

Shunting devices such as Gott (Murray, Brawley and Gott, 1971) or Javid shunts inserted into the ascending aorta have no routine indication but may be used in very selected cases in order to avoid a prosthetic bypass if endarterectomy or reimplantation necessitates simultaneous clamping of both the innominate artery and LCCA.

The operations

Incisions and approaches to the great vessels

Anterolateral thoracotomy through the second or third intercostal space has been advised by some surgeons (Crawford *et al.*, 1969). However, this approach only allows for the proximal implantation of a bypass. In addition, tunnelling through the thoracic inlet seems to be a rather blind procedure, carrying the risk of venous trauma. We have used this approach only for very selected indications for subclavian artery reconstruction such as failure or infection of a cervical

procedure or associated extensive lesions of the contralateral subclavian artery and common carotid arteries, precluding their use as an inflow source (Kieffer and Natali, 1983).

Left posterolateral thoracotomy through the fourth intercostal space is unique in providing direct access to the whole length of the intrathoracic portion of the LSCA. However, it has several drawbacks that explain its declining use in recent years: distal exposure is limited to the origin of the VA; associated surgery is not possible: and above all respiratory complications are more frequent than with a median sternotomy. Except for aneurysmal lesions, this route involves an unduly extensive technique for isolated lesions of the LSCA, since they may be managed easily through a much simpler cervical approach.

1a

1b

1c

1a, b & c

The standard approach is through a median sternotomy. Aside from its simplicity, well-known advantages of this route include (1) low rate of respiratory complications (as evidenced by cardiac surgery in the aged patient); (2) possibility of extension to all supra-aortic vessels, either intrathoracic (except perhaps the origin of the LSCA) or cervical, as well as to the abdomen (sternolaparotomy); and (3) possibility of associated cardiac surgery.

One or more complementary cervical incisions are usually necessary, according to the vessel(s) to be revascularized. The innominate and left common carotid arteries are approached by a short presternomastoid incision at the base of the neck, permitting a very easy direct approach (*a*). The proximal subclavian arteries are approached through the same incision, which is sufficient to give access to the subclavian artery medial to the internal jugular vein and to permit its dissection up to the scalenus muscles, beyond the origin of the VA. On the left side, the proximal subclavian artery is reputedly difficult if not impossible to approach through sternotomy. In fact this is possible after section of the vertebral vein and thoracic duct, although this does not allow for safe clamping of the aortic arch at the origin of the artery. The approach to the distal subclavian artery necessitates a complementary supraclavicular incision on either side (*b*), with section of the sternomastoid and scalenus muscles and reclination of the phrenic nerve. The entire aortic arch and its proximal branches may be approached through a low horizontal cervicotomy without sectioning of the sternomastoid muscles, provided the approach to the subclavian arteries does not have to go beyond the scalenus muscles (*b*). The carotid bifurcation is approached by presternomastoid incision either by extending the sternotomy, especially if the neck is short, or by a separate approach (*c*). The axillary arteries are easily reached by deltopectoral incisions (*b*). The transection or removal of the clavicle does not offer any additional advantage. Multiple great vessel lesions can be approached by combining these cervical incisions, particularly if the low horizontal cervicotomy is completed by one or more separate distal approaches to the carotid and/or axillary arteries. For all distal revascularizations (axillary artery or carotid bifurcation), complementary cervicotomies are done at the beginning of the operation in order to confirm the possibility of revascularization suggested by angiography.

2

To approach the arterial axis on either side, it is necessary to transect the subhyoid muscles and the thymic remnants. The left innominate vein hides the aortic arch and the proximal part of the great vessels. It does not have to be isolated for distal revascularization (axillary artery and carotid bifurcation). When revascularizing a proximal artery it is usually sufficient to mobilize the vein by complete dissection and division of its lower (thymic) and upper (thyroid) branches. Detachment of the jugular-subclavian venous confluence from the posterior part of the sternal manubrium is useful to allow for a broad sternal opening without undue tension on the vein. However, it may be divided without hesitation, especially if a wide approach to the aortic arch is required and

surgery on the proximal LSCA in anticipated. Transection of the left innominate vein usually has no long lasting effect except for a transient oedema of the left upper extremity, possibly followed by the development of prethoracic collateral circulation. The latter may be an uncosmetic sequela in young female patients. We do not usually reconstruct the vein at the end of the operation, although this presents no particular difficulty. At the end of the procedure, the thymic remnants and subhyoid muscles are sutured in front of the intrathoracic portion of the reconstruction. If entered, the pericardium is left partially opened. Closure is made according to routine techniques, following pericardial, mediastinal and cervical drainage.

2

Innominate artery reconstruction

Among isolated lesions of the intrathoracic great vessels, those involving the innominate artery present the most logical indications for direct intrathoracic surgery (Kieffer, 1975). In our opinion, cervical bypasses are justified only in very occasional poor-risk patients. Cross-over subclavian-subclavian or axilloaxillary bypasses using the LSCA as an inflow source should be avoided since the artery is the most likely to be or become diseased.

Two reconstructive techniques will be described in detail: endarterectomy and bypass.

3

4

Innominate endarterectomy

This technique is applicable only in selected cases of atherosclerotic occlusive disease. Exposure of the entire length of the innominate artery, proximal parts of the LCCA, RCCA and RSCA, as well as the upper aspect of the aortic arch is necessary (*see Illustrations 1a* and *2*). The left innominate vein is retracted towards the lower part of the incision. The pericardium is usually not opened.

3

The first step is to make sure that wide lateral clamping of the aortic arch is possible safely. The following two conditions must be fulfilled (Kieffer, 1975).

First, sufficient space must be present in the upper aspect of the aortic arch between the origins of the innominate artery and the LCCA. Inadvertent partial clamping of the LCCA may be complicated by left cerebral embolism due to trauma of an associated non-significant lesion frequently involving the proximal part of the artery. Simultaneous complete clamping of both vessels, such as may be necessary in the presence of a common trunk between the innominate artery and the LCCA, will usually be followed by cerebral ischaemia of variable magnitude. In most of these cases aortoinnominate bypass seems preferable. However, endarterectomy remains possible if a shunting device is inserted between the ascending aorta and one of the common carotid arteries.

Secondly, involvement of the upper aspect of the aortic arch by the pathological process must be minimal if endarterectomy is to be performed with complete security. In our opinion, extensive indications for conventional endarterectomy (Carlson *et al.*, 1977) carry the risk of intra- or postoperative haemorrhage or dissection and for this reason should be discouraged. If endarterectomy must be performed despite the risks, CPB with deep hypothermia and circulatory arrest should be used in order to perform a transaortic operation (Thevenet, Chaptal and Negre, 1968), but this somewhat complex technique seems unwarranted for an isolated innominate artery lesion.

4

When the two above-mentioned conditions are fulfilled, one may proceed to innominate endarterectomy. Under controlled hypotension and with the patient systemically heparinized the aortic arch is widely clamped around the origin of the innominate artery using a specially designed J clamp.

5

The RCCA and RSCA are then clamped separately using right-angle clamps, whatever the distal extension of the innominate artery lesion may be. A longitudinal arteriotomy of the innominate artery is made, extending proximally to the aorta in order to obtain adequate visualization of the origin of the innominate artery and aortic lumen.

5

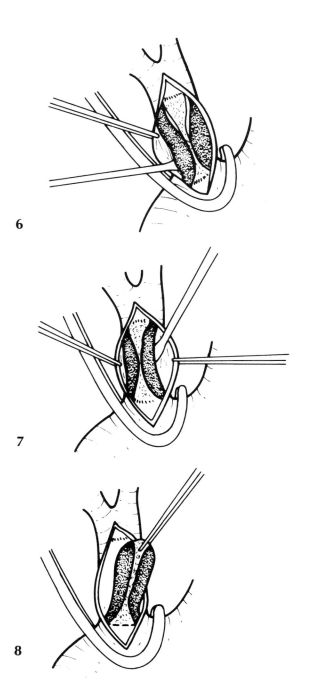

6

7

8

6, 7 & 8

Using an adequate spatula, endarterectomy is begun at the middle part of the innominate artery. The plane of cleavage should not be too external, especially in the proximal part of the artery, if the hazards of aortic dissection, rupture or secondary dilatation of the artery are to be avoided.

The distal limit of the endarterectomy is usually very clear and no intimal fixation is necessary in these circumstances.

9

However, when the distal intima remains thick and easy to mobilize, one should not hesitate to tack it with a few 6/0 monofilament sutures. The proximal intima must usually be transected with scissors at the origin of the vessel, and its posterior aspect tacked using one or two 5/0 monofilament sutures.

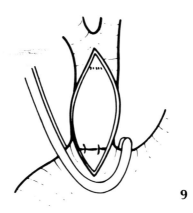

9

10a & b

Closure of the arteriotomy is usually performed using a 5/0 monofilament continuous suture (*a*). Patch angioplasty (*b*) is used in rare cases such as in a small innominate artery or when post-stenotic dilatation would result in relative stenosis of the proximal part of the artery. We prefer to use a knitted Dacron velour patch since a vein patch may lead to late dilatation.

10a

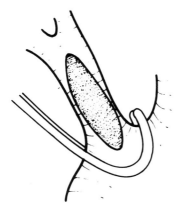

10b

11 & 12

Whichever form of closure is used, declamping is done sequentially, first towards the RSCA and then towards the RCCA.

11

12

13

Distal extension of the lesion may necessitate associated endarterectomy of the RSCA and/or RCCA. However, this extended procedure should not be performed in the presence of SCA lesions extending distal to the **origin** of the VA. Separate clamping of RCCA, distal RSCA and VA is applied distally and the innominate arteriotomy is extended up to the level of the right VA. In most cases lesions stop proximal to the VA and endarterectomy of the proximal SCA is performed easily under direct vision.

13

14   15

14 & 15

Associated stenosis of the VA may be treated by trans-subclavian endarterectomy. On rare occasions tacking the distal intima of the SCA may be indicated. The RCCA is completely transected 1 or 2cm above its origin and endarterectomy of the proximal part of the artery is done using an eversion technique. In the presence of extensive lesions of the RCCA and carotid bifurcation, a conventional endarterectomy of the birfurcation is performed. The middle and distal parts of the RCCA are then endarterectomized using an eversion technique through the distal arteriotomy.

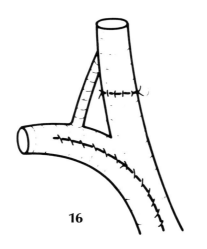

16

16

The two segments of the RCCA are then anastomosed using a 5/0 monofilament continuous suture and the longitudinal innominate-subclavian arteriotomy is closed using either a continuous suture (as shown) or a Dacron patch angioplasty.

Aortoinnominate artery bypass

17

The incision used is shown in *Illustration 1b*. This technique has much broader indications than endarterectomy, since it is nearly always possible. Once the innominate artery and its bifurcation have been freed, the upper part of the pericardium is opened longitudinally and its edges suspended from those of the sternal incision in order to expose the ascending aorta. Palpation of the latter will rarely lead to the unexpected discovery of extensive and/or heavily calcified lesions which preclude use of the procedure. In such exceptional cases, an alternative technique would be to extend the incision to the upper part of the abdomen and to use the supraceliac aorta as an inflow source (Kieffer and Natali, 1983). Although complete transection may be necessary, extensive dissection usually facilitates the appropriate mobilization of the left innominate vein.

17

18

18

A knitted Dacron prosthetic graft of suitable size (8, 10, or sometimes 12 mm) is preclotted. When the chosen calibre is 10 mm or more, a tube graft is used. If the calibre is less than 10 mm, we prefer to use a bifurcated graft, only one of its branches and the adjacent part of its body being used. This permits the performance of a wide proximal anastomosis using large bites without any risk of inadvertent anastomotic stenosis.

19

Palpation of the ascending aorta is performed very carefully in order to avoid either incomplete clamping with its associated risk of uncontrolled haemorrhage or a complete but traumatic clamping with the risk of fracture and/or dissection of the aorta. Heparin is not yet administered. The middle part of the right anterolateral aspect of the ascending aorta is widely clamped using a J clamp. Lowering the blood pressure to around 100 mmHg has the distinct advantages of avoiding aortic clamp trauma and allowing precise placement of the clamp. Indeed, the anterior aspect of the aorta should be avoided since placement of a graft in this position carries the risk of postoperative compression by the sternum. A 2–3 cm longitudinal aortotomy is performed. If the ascending aorta is too thick and rigid a quadrangular or oval-shaped segment has to be excised in order to avoid proximal anastomotic stenosis.

19

20

The graft is bevelled and anastomosed to the aorta using a 3/0 or 4/0 monofilament continuous suture taking large bites through the aortic wall. After slow removal of the clamp, the anastomosis is gently compressed in order to avoid any aortic wall haematoma. The anastomosis is then checked and should any complementary suture be necessary, this is made after reclamping the aorta. Preclotting of the graft is completed as necessary. The precise length necessary to reach the distal innominate artery is calculated with pressure in the graft. The graft is then reclamped close to its origin and any intraluminal clots are carefully removed by aspiration and lavage with non-heparinized saline solution. Any thrombus left on the wall of the graft might cause cerebral embolism when the bypass is made functional.

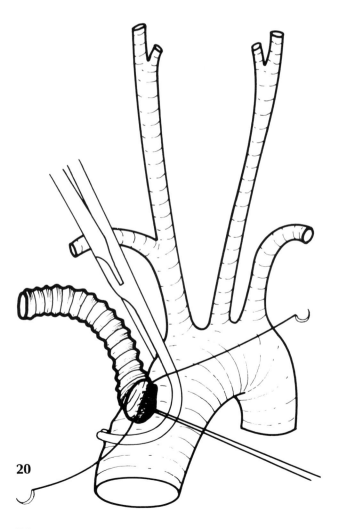

20

21 & 22

Heparin is then administered systemically and the blood pressure is allowed to return to normal levels. The origin of the innominate artery and both its branches are clamped using a straight aortic clamp and two right-angle clamps respectively. If its bifurcation appears normal, the distal part of the innominate artery is completely transected and anastomosed to the graft in an end-to-end fashion using 4/0 or 5/0 monofilament continuous suture.

21

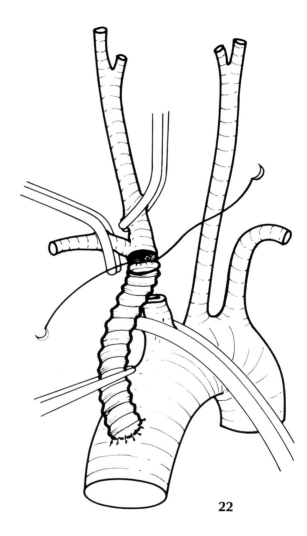

22

In the presence of associated lesions of one or both of the distal branches of the innominate artery, blind distal endarterectomy should be avoided and modifications of the distal anastomosis become necessary.

23 & 24

When one of the branches is stenosed by a smooth localized plaque, a longitudinal incision is made and the graft may be anastomosed in a spatulated end-to-end fashion.

23   **24**

25 & 26

Otherwise, we prefer to transect the two branches distal to the stenotic lesion (Edwards and Wright, 1972) and perform a short sequential bypass.

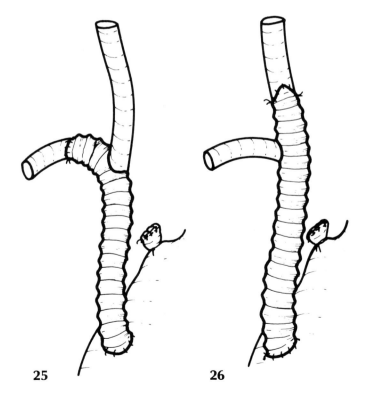

25   **26**

27 & 28

With both methods declamping is done in the usual manner.

27

28

29 & 30

The proximal stump of the innominate artery is then closed using a continuous over-and-over 2/0 braided Dacron or 3/0 monofilament suture, the choice depending on the presence of heavily calcified lesions in the proximal part of the artery.

29

30

Alternative techniques

These are used on rare occasions. Resection and grafting may be done in the presence of aneurysmal or traumatic lesions without involvement of the origin of the artery or in the rare case of intraoperative failure of endarterectomy.

Resection followed by end-to-end anastomosis is the logical technique for managing the very rare cases of kinking in which surgical correction is necessary.

Isolated patch angioplasty may be applicable in a few selected cases of proximal non-ulcerated atherosclerotic lesion, when endarterectomy seems impractical.

Left common carotid artery reconstruction

In many cases an isolated lesion of the LCCA is a good indication for extrathoracic reconstruction using a subclavian-carotid bypass (Dietrich *et al.*, 1967). This is particularly true in poor-risk patients, where the cervical procedure is simpler and much safer. However, the LSCA may already be diseased at the time of initial evaluation or may become diseased afterwards. Conversely, its use as an inflow source seems to be unwarranted in younger patients, leading to consideration of intrathoracic reconstruction.

Endarterectomy is usually impractical because of the difficulty or impossibility of clamping the aortic arch between the innominate artery and the LSCA. Reimplantation into a neighbouring artery is sometimes performed in order to avoid the placement of a prosthetic graft. However, reimplantation into the intrathoracic part of the LSCA is illogical for reasons already mentioned and in any case can be performed through a simpler cervical approach. Reimplantation into the innominate artery is more attractive but necessitates simultaneous clamping of both arteries.

31

Aortocarotid bypass thus appears to be the logical procedure in these cases. A 6-, 7- or 8-mm knitted Dacron graft is selected, using part of a bifurcated graft. Alternatively, a saphenous vein graft may be used in young patients with small arteries, as may be encountered in Takayasu's arteritis (Kieffer and Natali, 1983). The technical steps of the procedure are the same as in the previously described aortoinnominate bypass. The length of the graft must be evaluated after temporary closure of the sternal retractor, in order to avoid overestimation with its attendant hazard of kinking. Although the distal anastomosis may be intrathoracic, in most cases it has to be performed to the carotid bifurcation.

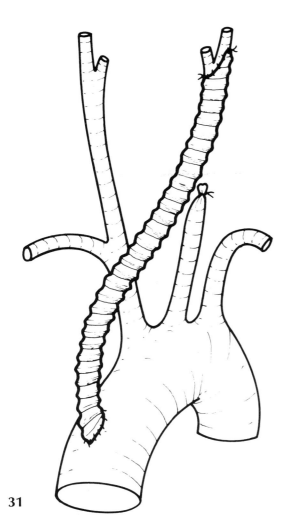

31

Left subclavian artery reconstruction

Isolated lesions of the LSCA are almost always an indication for a cervical approach using either carotid-subclavian bypass (Dietrich *et al.*, 1967) or, preferably, direct reimplantation of the LSCA into the LCCA (Edwards and Wright, 1972). A direct approach using a posterolateral thoracotomy is rarely indicated except for aneurysm or trauma. However, to avoid a cross-over cervical bypass in good-risk patients, atherosclerotic occlusive disease may be best treated through a thoracic incision when the LCCA appears impractical as a source of inflow. Endarterectomy of aortosubclavian bypass may be used. Anatomical indications and technical steps are similar to those described for management of innominate artery lesions.

Management of multiple occlusive lesions

General principles

Whatever their aetiology, multiple lesions constitute a logical indication for intrathoracic procedures (Kieffer, 1975; Thevenet, 1979; Crawford, Stowe and Powers, 1983). A one-stage complete revascularization, including the LSCA, if diseased, is always preferable, since secondary reconstruction of the initially untreated lesion would prove difficult or even necessitate a left thoracotomy.

Multiple revascularizations are usually performed using the bypass principle, according to the following guidelines:

1. Multiple grafts are possible only if the ascending aorta is not too short, too small and/or too thick. This technique is particularly suitable if vein grafts are being used. Multiple prosthetic grafts are more likely to cause compression of the veins and airway in the thoracic inlet, especially in young female patients, and should be avoided.
2. Bifurcated grafts are simpler, but even when small sizes are used (16/8 or preferably 14/7) and the length of the body graft is tailored to be as short as possible, they may be a major cause of compression in the thoracic inlet, leading to serious complications such as venous and tracheoesophageal compression and, at a later stage, stenosis or even occlusion of one or more of the grafts.
3. Sequential grafts are to be preferred in most cases. One large prosthetic tube graft (10–12 mm) is selected to revascularize the largest vessel, usually the innominate artery. The proximal anastomosis is performed first and the graft is sequentially anastomosed to the arteries to be reconstructed, either directly or using an intermediate smaller tube graft (6–8 mm).

Application of these principles to the many possible anatomical combinations is determined mainly by the surgeon's imagination and ingenuity.

References

Bahnson, H. T., Spencer, F. C. and Quattlebaum, K. (1959). Surgical treatment of occlusive disease of the carotid artery. *Annals of Surgery* **149**, 711.

Carlson, R. E., Ehrenfeld, W. K., Stoney, R. J. and Wylie, E. J. (1977). Innominate artery endarterectomy. *Archives of Surgery* **112**, 1389.

Crawford, E. S., DeBakey, M. E., Morris, G. C., Jr and Howell, J. F. (1969). Surgical treatment of occlusion of the innominate, common carotid, and subclavian arteries. *Surgery* **65**, 17.

Crawford, E. S., Stowe, C. L., and Powers, R. W., Jr (1983). Occlusion of the innominate, common carotid, and subclavian arteries: Long-term results of surgical treatment. *Surgery* **94**, 781.

Davis, J. B., Grove, W. J. and Julian, O. C. (1956). Thrombotic occlusion of the branches of the aortic arch. *Annals of Surgery* **144**, 124.

Dietrich, E. B., Garrett, H. E., Ameriso, J., Crawford, E. S., El Bayar, M. and DeBakey, M. E. (1967). Occlusive disease of the common carotid and subclavian arteries treated by carotid subclavian bypass. *American Journal of Surgery* **111**, 800.

Edwards, W. H. and Wright, R. S. (1972). Current concepts in the management of arteriosclerotic lesions of the subclavian and vertebral arteries. *Annals of Surgery* **175**, 975.

Ehrenfeld, W. K., Wilbur, B. G., Olcott, C. N. and Stoney, R. J. (1979). Autogenous tissue reconstruction in the management of infected prosthetic grafts. *Surgery* **85**, 81.

Finkelstein, N. M., Byer, A. and Rush, B. F. (1972). Subclavian-subclavian bypass for the subclavian steal syndrome. *Surgery* **71**, 142.

Kieffer, E. (1975). Stenoses et occlusions atheromateuses du tronc arteriel brachio céphalique. *Journal de Chirurgie* **110**, 493.

Kieffer, E. and Natali, J. (1982). Ascending aorto-abdominal aorta by-pass. Technical considerations, indications and report of 15 cases. In *Extra-anatomic and Secondary Arterial Reconstruction*. Greenhalgh, R. M., ed. London: Pitman, pp. 313–333.

Kieffer, E. and Natali, J. (1983). Supra-aortic trunk lesions in Takayasu's arteritis. In *Cerebrovascular Insufficiency*. Bergan, J. J., Yao, J. S. T., eds. New York: Grune and Stratton, pp. 395–415.

Kieffer, E., Tricot, J. F., Cousin, M. T., Dauptain, J. and Natali, J. (1977). Desinsertions traumatiques du tronc arteriel brachio-céphalique. *Annales de Chirurgie Thoracique et Cardiovasculaire* **16**, 323.

Manart, F. D. and Kempczinski, R. F. (1980). The carotid-carotid bypass graft. *Archives in Surgery* **115**, 669.

Murray, G. F., Brawley, R. K. and Gott, V. L. (1971). Reconstruction of the innominate artery by means of a temporary heparin-coated shunt bypass. *Journal of Thoracic and Cardiovascular Surgery* **62**, 34.

Ochsner, J. L. and Mills, N. L. (1979). Profound hypothermia and circulatory arrest in control and repair of infected aortic prosthesis. *Journal of Cardiovascular Surgery* **20**, 1.

Selle, J. G., Cook, J. W., Elliott, C. M. Robicsek, F., Daugherty, H. K. and Hess, P. J. (1982). Simultaneous revascularization for complex brachiocephalic and coronary artery diseases. *Surgery* **90**, 97.

Sethi, G. K., Scott, S. M. and Takaro, T. (1975). Extrathoracic bypass for stenosis of innominate artery. *Journal of Thoracic and Cardiovascular Surgery* **69**, 213.

Stolf, N. A. G., Bittencourt, D., Verginelli, G. and Zerbini, E. J. (1983). Surgical treatment of ruptured aneurysms of the innominate artery. *American Journal of Thoracic Surgery* **35**, 394.

Thevenet, A., Chaptal, P. A. and Negre, E. (1968). L'arrêt circulatoire en hyppothermie profonde dans la chirurgie des branches de la crosse de l'aorte. *Annals de Chirurgie Thoracique et Cardiovasculaire* **7**, 69.

Thevenet, A. (1979). Surgical management of atheroma of the aortic dome and origin of supra aortic trunks. *World journal of Surgery* **3**, 187.

Carotid endarterectomy

Jesse E. Thompson MD, FACS

Attending Surgeon, Baylor University Medical Center, Dallas, Texas, USA; Clinical Professor of Surgery, University of Texas Southwestern Medical School, Dallas, Texas, USA

Introduction

Carotid endarterectomy is the procedure most frequently employed in the operative treatment of cerebral ischaemic syndromes due to atherosclerotic disease. Clinical considerations determine the indications and contraindications for operation. These are listed in detail in Table 1. The principal indication is transient cerebral ischaemia since strokes can be prevented and troublesome episodes of ischaemia are largely abolished. Indication for operation is also based on a critical evaluation of operative risk, since a high proportion of these patients have hypertension and generalized atherosclerosis, especially coronary disease.

deficits and with crescendo transient ischaemic attacks. Management of these patients is fraught with difficulty. Although CT and MRI scans are helpful, in the absence of totally reliable methods for distinguishing between cerebral infarction and reversible ischaemia without infarction, the results of therapy, whether surgical or medical, are unpredictable. In general, if the deficit is mild and the lesion severe, emergency operation may be justified. Patients with significant bilateral lesions should have bilateral endarterectomies, but in separate stages at least 1–2 weeks apart or even longer.

Table 1
Indications for carotid endarterectomy in cerebrovascular insufficiency

Indications
1. Transient cerebral ischaemia
2. Stable strokes (selected)
3. Asymptomatic bruits (selected)
4. Chronic cerebral ischaemia (selected)

Contraindications
1. Acute profound strokes
2. Progressing strokes
3. Severe intracranial disease
4. Other severe generalized disorders
   (e.g. cancer)

Table 2
Timing of carotid endarterectomy for cerebrovascular insufficiency

*Elective operation**
1. Stable stroke, recent or old
2. Transient cerebral ischaemia
3. Asymptomatic bruit
4. Chronic cerebral ischaemia (rare)

Delayed operation (days to weeks)
1. Mild stroke
2. Fluctuating stroke

Emergency operation (rarely necessary)
1. Frank stroke

   −disappearance of bruit
   −slowly worsening
   −fluctuating

2. Transient cerebral ischaemia

   −severe stenosis, especially if bilateral
   −disappearance of bruit
   −crescendo tia's

3 Carotid thrombosis immediately following arteriography or endarterectomy

Table 2 summarizes the appropriate timing of operation for the various clinical categories. There is considerable difference of opinion regarding operation for acute carotid thrombosis following arteriography or endarterectomy. If operation can be performed immediately (1–2 h), it is probably a justifiable and worthwhile procedure. Controversy has also developed over the advisability of performing emergency endarterectomy on patients with unstable or fluctuating

Technique of carotid endarterectomy

Technical considerations are of the utmost importance in carotid endarterectomy, since the limits of tolerance to temporary occlusion of the blood supply to the brain may be quite narrow. Safety factors must be employed which will eliminate in most instances the occurrence or aggravation of neurological deficits. Any method of carotid endarterectomy should carry low mortality, few complications, satisfactory immediate and long-term anatomical results, and good functional results relative to cerebrovascular insufficiency. The technique to be described has evolved over a period of 30 years and has proved safe and reliable. It involves the routine use of a temporary inlying bypass shunt.

1

Operation is performed under light general anaesthesia. The head is turned away from the side to be operated upon and placed on a rubber ring. The shoulders are elevated slightly using a folded sheet but there should be no undue extension of the neck. An oblique incision is made along the anterior border of the sternocleidomastoid muscle, curving medialward at its lower end, centred over the bifurcation of the common carotid artery, and curved slightly inferior to the lobe of the ear at the upper end.

1

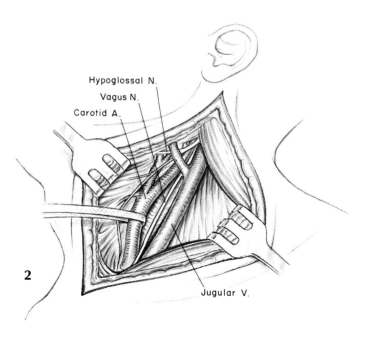

Hypoglossal N.

Vagus N.

Carotid A.

Jugular V.

2

2

Adequate exposure of the common carotid and of the internal and external carotid divisions is essential. The carotid sinus area is infiltrated with 1% lidocaine to prevent hypotension and bradycardia. The artery is freed completely including division of the carotid sinus plexus if necessary.

One must avoid injury to the mandibular branch of the facial nerve and the vagus, hypoglossal and superior laryngeal nerves. A small branch of the external carotid artery, supplying the sternocleidomastoid muscle, usually passes over the hypoglossal nerve holding it down as a sling. This small artery should be ligated and divided to free the hypoglossal nerve off the external and internal carotid divisions. Though rarely necessary, the superior thyroid artery may be ligated and divided to facilitate dissection and exposure. An umbilical tape is first placed around the external carotid artery. Umbilical tapes are then placed around the common and internal carotid arteries and segments of #16 French rubber catheters are threaded over the tapes to act as tourniquets.

3

The occluding plaque is usually located at the bifurcation of the common carotid and extends only a short distance into the internal carotid. The distal internal carotid is ordinarily soft and thin-walled and is freed up for at least 1 cm beyond the palpable distal end of the plaque. Utmost gentleness is used throughout manipulation and the artery is simply palpated, never squeezed, since platelets, thrombi or athero-sclerotic debris may break off and embolize intracranially.

When satisfactory exposure is obtained, systemic herariniz-ation is affected with 3500–5000 u of heparin. The external carotid is occluded with a bulldog clamp and heparinized locally with 10 ml of a solution containing 100 u of heparin per ml. The common carotid is then clamped proximally with an angled vascular clamp. The distal internal carotid is occluded with a soft bulldog clamp and a linear arteriotomy is made from the common carotid into the internal carotid beyond the distal extent of the plaque. It is important that the internal carotid be opened beyond the plaque and that the entire extent of plaque be visualized in order to facilitate the succeeding steps of the operation.

3

4

A plastic catheter shunt is then inserted into the distal internal carotid and the artery allowed to backflow.

4

5

The proximal end of the plastic shunt is then placed into the common carotid lumen and the umbilical tapes with rubber tourniquets are made snug.

5

6

Cerebral blood flow is thus restored through the shunt. This step of the operation requires 45–90 s.

The average size shunt which fits the distal internal carotid is a #10 French plastic catheter about 9 cm in length. A #8 or #12 catheter may be used as a shunt if the artery is smaller or larger than usual. The internal diameter of the #10 catheter used is 2.5 mm. With normal levels of blood pressure this shunt carries approximately 125 ml of blood per min. Experience has shown that this is an adequate flow during the period required for endarterectomy.

6

7

8

The distal end of the plaque in the internal carotid usually feathers off quite smoothly leaving only thin intima above, which should not be disturbed. Small bits of debris may be lifted out with forceps or flushed out with saline. It is of the utmost importance that the distant extent of the endarterectomy be visualized so that no large pieces of intima be left to dissect distalward and produce a postoperative occlusion.

7

With the intraluminal shunt in place one may endarterectomize the vessel without undue haste. The appropriate plane is entered with a fine pointed clamp or other dissector and the plaque dissected from the common carotid, the bifurcation, first portion of the external carotid and that portion of the internal carotid containing the plaque.

8

9

Occasionally, it is advisable to secure the distal intima with a few interrupted stitches to prevent dissection. Some 6/0 polyester sutures serve well to take down the intima as well as to close the arteriotomy. It is also important to endarterectomize carefully the origin of the external carotid, since this artery is an important source of blood supply to the brain.

9

10

The arteriotomy is then closed with running sutures of 6/0 polyester beginning at each end. Immediately prior to placing the final three or four sutures the common carotid and internal carotid are clamped and the shunt removed. The vessels are then flushed. The final sutures are quickly placed and tied. At this point the internal carotid is allowed to backflow and is then reclamped.

Clamps are removed from the external carotid and common carotid arteries and flow restored into the external carotid allowing any debris or air to be flushed into it rather than into the internal carotid. The clamp is then removed from the internal carotid and flow restored to the brain. The occlusion time during this final step is 1–2 min. The heparin is then reversed with protamine, if necessary.

10

11

12

11 & 12

One may vary the technique of arteriotomy closure by using a thin-blade, partially occluding clamp to include the unfinished portion of the suture line after the shunt is removed. In this way cerebral blood flow is quickly re-established and the suture line is then completed.

If one is concerned about completeness of endarterectomy or the quality of pulsation in the internal carotid following restoration of flow, arteriograms may be performed on the operating table. Some surgeons perform this step routinely, but the author has not found its routine use necessary.

It is rarely necessary to use a patch graft for closure of the arteriotomy, but if the artery is quite small, a patch graft of autologous vein or prosthetic material may be used. The wound in the neck is then closed anatomically in two layers with interrupted sutures of fine cotton. A small rubber drain is brought out of the lower end of the wound and is removed 24 h post operatively. Bilateral operations when necessary are done in separate stages about 1 week apart to avoid complications of laryngeal oedema, transient hypoglossal paresis, and cerebral oedema.

It is important that adequate levels of blood pressure be maintained during the operation and in the immediate post-operative period. The most satisfactory way to achieve this is to administer 500–1000 ml of lactated Ringer's solution during the operation and postoperatively. Vasopressors are occasionally necessary even when adequate fluids have been given. Routine postoperative heparinization is not used.

The technique may vary depending upon variation in pathology. If the plaque is a long one and extends quite far distally, a longer arteriotomy is necessary as is a longer shunt. At times it is prudent to close the distal portion of the arteriotomy and move the shunt proximalward before completing the endarterectomy at the common carotid bifurcation. Occasionally, one finds a plaque in the common carotid 1 cm or so proximal to the bifurcation. In this case, the arteriotomy may be extended proximally, as it is important to remove this plaque as well.

Rarely does one encounter patients with bilaterally occluded internal carotid arteries which cannot be opened by operation. Under these circumstances it is important that patency of the external carotid arteries be maintained, and endarterectomy of the orifices of these arteries may be necessary to improve collateral cerebral blood flow. The shunt technique is easily adapted to endarterectomy of the external carotid arteries.

The technique as described depicts carotid endarterectomy with the aid of a temporary inlying shunt, which is the most reliable method for cerebral support. Some surgeons use the shunt routinely in all partially occlusive lesions, some use it selectively based on an assessment of cerebral collateral circulation, while a few rarely if ever use it. Those who advocate selective shunting rely on one of several criteria of inadequacy of cerebral collateral circulation. Some test the patient under local anaesthesia and use a shunt if temporary clamping cannot be tolerated. Others, using general anaesthesia, insert a shunt if internal carotid artery stump pressure is below 50–55 mmHg or if EEG changes occur upon carotid clamping. In the hands of experienced operators, comparable results may be obtained using selective shunting.

Acknowledgements

I would like to thank Little, Brown for Permission to reproduce *Illustrations 1, 2, 4, 5, 6, 7,* and *9* from Thompson (1984), and J. B. Lippincott for permission to reproduce *Illustrations, 3, 8, 10, 11* and *12* from Thompson (1988).

References

Thompson, J. E. (1984). Carotid endarterectomy with shunt. In *Mastery of Surgery*. Nyhus, L. M. and Baker, R. J. eds. Boston: Little, Brown.

Thompson, J. E. (1988). Thrombo-obliterative disease of the vessels of the aortic arch. In *Hardy's Textbook of Surgery*, 2nd ed. Hardy, J. D., ed. Philadelphia: J. B. Lippincott.

Selective shunting during carotid endarterectomy

Roger M. Greenhalgh   MA, MD, MChir, FRCS

Professor of Surgery, Charing Cross and Westminster Medical School, London, UK

Introduction

The previous chapter by Dr Thompson fully discusses indications and his personal incision and mandatory shunting technique for carotid endarterectomy. Here, a curved incision is described which is preferred by some surgeons for cosmetic reasons; arguably this approach allows equivalent access to the carotid artery. The use of an intraluminal shunt for every procedure is not my practice because its very use carries a morbidity from dislodging artereal debris which can embolise to the brain.

The operation

Position of patient and anaesthesia

1

The skin is prepared and the towels are placed so that the whole neck area and the earlobe can be seen. The intended skin incision is marked in ink with cross-stripping marks to show the correct apposition points for the eventual skin closure. It is convenient to secure the towels and maintain sterility by using a plastic drape after the skin has been marked. The skin incision is placed as shown in relation to the anterior border of the sternomastoid muscle. Many surgeons prefer a longitudinal incision down the anterior border of the sternomastoid but this is less cosmetic and does not provide better exposure. The skin crease incision is preferable and care should be taken to ensure that it is at least two fingers' breadth away from the angle of the jaw for fear of damage to the cervical branch of the facial nerve. The great auricular and other cutaneous nerves are shown and these must be avoided as the incision is deepened through the platysma muscle to locate the anterior border of the sternomastoid. This is the vital landmark to find, because the rest of the dissection is continued along the plane of the anterior border of this important muscle.

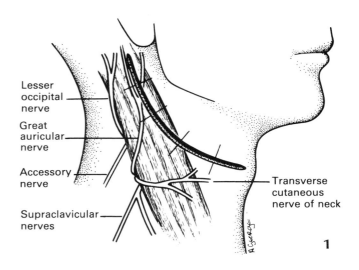

2

The carotid sheath is approached by dividing and transfixing the common facial vein. A simple ligature for this vein is frequently inadequate as tremendous pressures are achieved during extubation and when coughing occurs. The dissection then continues as described in the previous chapter.

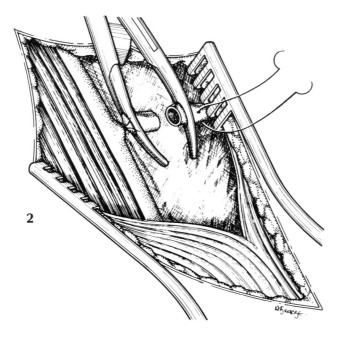

Selective intraluminal shunting

3 & 4

The subsequent figures concentrate on the carotid vessel itself. The patient is given heparin 5000 u intravenously and after 3 min a clamp is placed across the external carotid artery. A needle attached to a monitoring line is placed in the external carotid artery as this avoids risk of embolization to the brain. Pressure in this artery is measured using the monitoring equipment. When the pressure is displayed on the monitoring system the common carotid is cross-clamped using a very soft clamp such as the Fogarty clamp with Silastic implants. This provides a 'back pressure' or 'stump pressure' reading.

At this stage the internal carotid artery is behaving as a side arm to the circle of Willis and this pressure is an estimate of the pressure in that circle. Those surgeons who, like the author, take notice of this reading will, in practice, find that one of two things happens the moment the common carotid artery is clamped: either the pressure falls slightly but stays at around 90 mmHg mean pressure with a pulsatile waveform, or the pressure suddenly falls and the waveform goes flat. As soon as the pressure falls to below 50 mmHg the author waits no longer but inserts an intraluminal shunt. If the pressure is above 50 mmHg and the waveform is pulsatile, no shunting is performed. Others use different methods for deciding whether to use a shunt, such as monitoring with the electro-encephalogram.

3

4

Shunting technique

5

When it is decided that an intraluminal shunt should be used, the author's preference is for the Javid shunt. This is a plastic shunt which fits comfortably into the common carotid below and the internal carotid above. Special ring clamps can be used to hold it in place as shown. As soon as the use of an intraluminal shunt for cerebral protection is indicated, an artery clip is placed across the Javid shunt, the larger end of the shunt is introduced into the common carotid artery below the atheroma and the ring clamp is made secure.

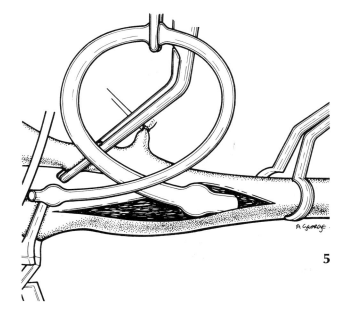

5

6

The artery clip is then momentarily removed to allow forward squirt to occur onto a swab. This clears both the shunt and the common carotid artery of any debris, minimizing the risk of embolization to the brain, and indicates that a good flow can be delivered to the brain.

6

7

7

The artery clip is replaced on the Javid shunt and the bulldog clamp is removed from the internal carotid artery, allowing backbleeding to occur, which removes any debris from this vessel. The shunt is then gently manipulated into the internal carotid artery well above the diseased bifurcation.

8

The smaller ring clamp is now secured and the artery clip is taken off the shunt. This allows blood flow to pass through the shunt from the common carotid to the internal carotid artery so that endarterectomy can be performed without any hurry.

8

9

Suturing is performed as before. The shunt is no hindrance; in fact, it acts as a stent and can be a very useful aid to performing a good suture line. When no more suturing can be performed, the shunt is one again clamped with an artery clip and the ring clamps are removed; the former arterial clamps are then replaced and the shunt is removed. The arteriotomy is closed, the sutures tied and the unclamping procedure is exactly as described previously.

9

Approach to the internal carotid artery at the skull base

Wilhelm Sandmann
Department for Vascular Surgery and Kidney Transplantation, Chirurgische Universitätsklinik Düsseldorf, Düsseldorf, Federal Republic of Germany

Introduction

In contrast to the rather uniform and frequent appearance of atherosclerosis at the carotid bifurcation, the lesions of the internal carotid artery at the skull base show a much more variable morphology and remain a challenge even for the experienced vascular surgeon. In our experience, with 60 reconstructions over 10 years, stenotic lesions have outweighted aneurysms by 2:1. Fibromuscular dysplasia appeared in 31%, chronic trauma in 26%, atherosclerosis in 21%, spontaneous dissection in 10% and other diseases in 12%. Embolism from local thrombus formation was the major cause of preoperative transitory ischaemic attacks or strokes. Therefore, the distal segment of the internal carotid artery is not only difficult to approach for anatomical reasons but delicate to repair. Manipulation at the diseased vessel wall before clamping inevitably causes cerebral embolism. Sometimes the reconstruction has to be performed with a weakened arterial wall. Although indications for reconstruction of the internal carotid artery at the skull base are rather rare and amount to only 0.5% of all carotid operations at our institution, the approach to the skull base and technical details for reconstruction are described in this chapter.

Like other reconstructions in areas difficult to approach, surgery at the skull base requires excellent diagnostic work-up. Large skull-base aneurysms can be palpated through the nasopharynx and may be measured by CT-scanning of the neck. Doppler studies are helpful to detect flow-restricting lesions, but neither extra- or transcranial Doppler examination nor angiography can predict if longer time periods of clamping will be tolerated. The majority of these patients are much younger than the typical atherosclerotic patient. Therefore, collateral flow is not restricted by generalized occlusive disease and the risk of clamping ischaemia is very low. At least in our experience, recurrent or new postoperative deficits could not be attributed to temporary interruption of cerebral blood flow.

Superselective catheterization using conventional techniques or intra-arterial DSA in at least two planes is mandatory to determine the aetiology, anatomical extension and emboligenic potential of the disease and to visualize intracranial circulation.

Applied surgical anatomy

The extracranial portion of the internal carotid artery can be divided into three segments. The first extends from the bifurcation, where the hypoglossal nerve crosses the internal carotid artery at the level of the third vertebra. At the beginning of the second segment the hypoglossal nerve joins the sheath of the vagus nerve. At this level the architecture of the arterial wall changes from the elastic to the muscular type. Spontaneous dissections usually originate from this transition zone. The second segment reaches up to the body of C2, which is about the tip of the styloid process, where the superior laryngeal nerve leaves the vagus nerve in a dorsomedial direction. The internal jugular vein and the vagus nerve accompany the internal carotid artery within the same sheath. At the bifurcation the position of nerve and vein is lateral and not very close to the internal carotid artery, whereas at the skull base both are in a more dorsal position and the vein becomes rather close to the artery. The third segment extends from the tip of the styloid process to the carotid canal, which is entered obliquely. The view into the canal is hampered both caudally and laterally by a squamous portion of the temporal bone, which is located between the styloid process and the petrotympanica fissure below the acoustic canal.

1

The patient is placed in a supine position on the operating table with the head slightly elevated and turned towards the opposite side. The skin is incised vertically along the anterior border of the sternocleidomastoid muscle just behind the ear lobe.

1

2

After transection of the platysma, the posterior facial vein and the posterior belly of the digastric muscle can be seen in front of the carotid artery.

2

3

The internal carotid artery is exposed stepwise. The descendens hypoglossi is seen passing down from the hypoglossal nerve and may be divided if it helps the exposure. Any vessels lying in front of the hypoglossal nerve are divided.

3

4

The digastric muscle is divided using electrocautery. The occipital artery or a major branch, usually located behind the digastric muscle, is ligated to avoid postoperative bleeding. Most of the skull-base arterial lesions begin at about this level.

4

5

Before exposure of the diseased segment, the patient is fully heparinized and the internal carotid artery is clamped near the bifurcation. A long but shallow retractor is placed against the styloid process, which usually breaks at its base. The retractor is pulled towards the skull base and a second retractor is placed more laterally, so that a tunnel is created around the diseased internal carotid artery. The glosso-pharyngeal nerve and the rami pharyngei are identified and mobilized using a silicon vessel loop.

5

6

At this point the internal carotid artery is cross-clamped below the lesion and divided.

6

7

A suitable segment of harvested saphenous vein is pulled over a 3F balloon catheter. The internal carotid artery is opened and backbleeding is controlled by the balloon catheter.

7

8

8

In patients with aneurysms, the aneurysmal sac is partially resected and the graft is anastomosed from the inside (the graft inclusion technique) with absorbable suture material using interrupted sutures to avoid stenosis of the anastomosis.

9

After the distal anastomosis has been performed, the vein graft is pulled through beneath the glossopharyngeal and hypoglossal nerves.

9

10

11

10 & 11

The common and external carotid arteries are cross-clamped and the common carotid artery is incised. The stump of the internal carotid artery is oversewn and the graft is anastomosed further proximally. The graft has to be anastomosed with a certain tension, because the neck is overextended and turned through almost 90°. Before the proximal anastomosis is performed, the optimal length of the graft is determined by turning the head into the normal position.

After the anastomosis, arteriography is performed on the operating table because on occasion a very distal anastomosis cannot otherwise be checked. During cross-clamping, the patient is ventilated with 100% oxygen and anaesthesia is maintained by intravenous methods.

In patients with lesions extending just to the entrance of the carotid canal the lateral wall can be removed using a chisel. It is possible to perform the distal anastomosis 1 cm within the carotid canal. However, at this point, the operation becomes complicated and the surgeon needs to have had great experience of such reconstructions. Early proximal clamping during the dissection avoids embolization. The interrupted suture technique using monofilamentous absorbable suture material avoids stenosis of the anastomosis at the skull base. A shunt cannot be used in extremely high lesions, though through-graft balloon catheter blockage is very helpful. Although I prefer operative angiography, electromagnetic flow measurement is an alternative to detect critical stenoses or distal occlusions during the procedure. Heparinization is necessary throughout clamping to avoid distal thrombosis. Graft length must be checked in the normal head position at the end of the procedure to ensure that kinking and twisting will not occur.

Excision of carotid body chemodectoma

Averil O. Mansfield   ChM, FRCS
Consultant Surgeon, St Mary's Hospital, London;
Honorary Senior Lecturer in Vascular Surgery, Royal Postgraduate Medical School, London, UK

Introduction

1

Paraganglia are widely disseminated organs with sensory and perhaps local neurosecretory function. Those APUD cells with an affinity for chrome salts are known as chromaffin paraganglia and their tumours are phaeochromocytomas. Those without chrome salt affinity are the non-chromaffin paraganglia; their most common tumour affects the carotid body. The most common sites of non-chromaffin paraganglion tumours are illustrated. In the author's experience the second most common paraganglioma in the neck is of vagal origin. On angiography this is seen as a vascular tumour which does not splay the internal and external carotids apart. When vocal cord paralysis also exists the preoperative diagnosis is complete.

Histological distinction between benign and malignant tumours is not possible and only the development of metastases can determine malignancy. This is fortunately uncommon.

There has been much discussion about whether it is necessary to remove these usually benign tumours, but in the author's experience the tumour can be removed safely with little or no risk of recurrence and it is usually easier to deal with this tumour while it is small, rather than to wait until it is an advanced tumour involving local cranial nerves.

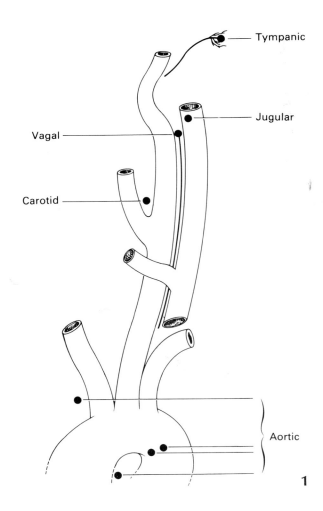

Tympanic

Jugular

Vagal

Carotid

Aortic

1

Investigations

The important and diagnostic investigation is the angiogram. Normally, this consists of a selective carotid injection and views in two planes. Intravenous digital subtraction angiography, where available, avoids the risk of a carotid injection and when doubt exists about the presence of a tumour this technique is a valuable first investigation and may be all that is required.

Duplex Doppler scanning may also be a useful non-invasive test.

The cranial nerves must be examined with care and indirect laryngoscopy must be a routine preliminary examination. The oropharynx should be inspected.

Carotid body tumours are rarely secretory but the routine examination for vanillylmandelic acid should prevent unexpected problems.

Large and particularly vascular tumours should be considered for preoperative embolization to reduce the technical problems in excising them. However, the evidence that this helps is anecdotal and the procedure carries some risk.

Position of patient

The patient is placed supine with the head of the table slightly elevated. A pad is placed longitudinally between the scapulae (a litre bag of i.v. fluid is suitable). The head, supported in a head ring, is extended and turned towards the opposite side. A bladder catheter may be inserted if a large tumour is to be removed.

Preoperative preparation

The usual preparations for major vascular surgery are undertaken and the blood pressure should be maintained at normal levels. Although hypotensive anaesthesia is an attractive theoretical prospect, it may increase the risk of stroke occurring during carotid manipulation. In addition to normal diathermy, the provision of a bipolar coagulator is valuable. A nerve stimulator may sometimes be helpful.

It is often helpful to palpate the oropharynx before starting the operation to assess the size of the tumour.

Nasal intubation in a high tumour may increase access.

The operation

Incision

2

The incision can be made exactly as in the previous chapter but the author prefers to make it along the anterior border of the sternomastoid muscle from the mastoid process to the lower part of the neck. The exact position depends on the level of the tumour.

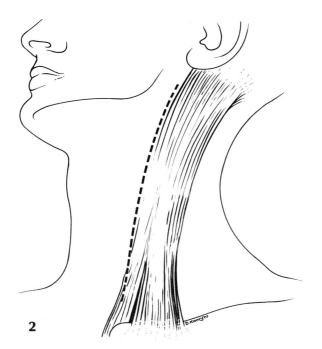

2

3

If the upper part of the tumour extends well above the angle of the mandible, the upper part of the incision may usefully be extended around the ear and anterior to the external auditory meatus, as in the routine approach to the parotid gland.

3

4

Cutaneous nerves cross the incision and are divided but the great auricular nerve is preserved.

The platysma is divided and the anterior border of the sternomastoid is exposed. Exposure is developed from the mastoid process to the lower limit of the wound by 'walking over' the muscle until the internal jugular vein comes into view. The muscle can then be mobilized and retracted with a self-retaining Travers retractor.

Great auricular nerve

Transverse cervical nerve

4

Internal jugular vein

5

The internal jugular vein is now dissected from the artery throughout its visible course, taking care not to injure the adjacent vagus nerve in the groove between artery and vein. The common facial vein and any other anterior tributaries are ligated and divided. The Travers retractor with its rounded 'teeth' can safely be used to retract the vein.

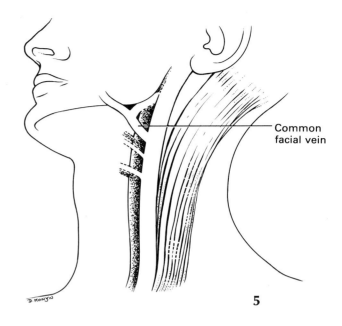

Common facial vein

5

6

The vagus nerve is carefully identified throughout its course in the neck. The hypoglossal nerve can usually be identified and preserved but sometimes its course is within the tumour and it can only be dissected out at a later stage. The ansa cervicalis is usually visible and, if possible, is preserved.

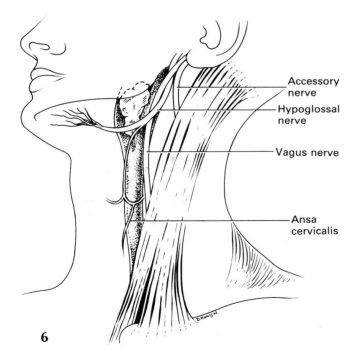

Accessory nerve

Hypoglossal nerve

Vagus nerve

Ansa cervicalis

6

7

Carotid arteries

In the common form of chemodectoma, the carotid body tumour, the tumour begins at the level of the carotid bifurcation and the internal and external carotids are splayed apart by it. In the simplest form the carotid vessels are clearly identifiable throughout, but in more complex tumours the arteries may be embedded in and surrounded by the tumour.

The internal and external carotids will come closer together again above the tumour and it is important to identify the internal carotid at that level, i.e. beyond the upper limits of the tumour, before commencing the dissection, in order to ensure its safety.

From then on the operation consists of the safe and meticulous dissection of the carotid vessels from the tumour. As most of the blood supply is derived from the external carotid the dissection is begun with that vessel.

The upper end of the dissection

When the carotid body tumour is confined to within the bifurcation which is at or below the angle of the mandible there is no need for this upper part of the operation. However, in the high and extensive tumours this is the most important and the most difficult part of the operation and these routine steps undertaken before exposure of the tumour will facilitate the excision.

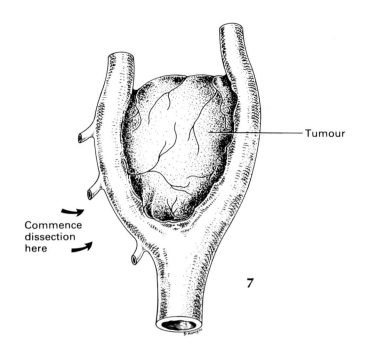

Tumour

Commence dissection here

7

8

First the facial nerve is identified by following up the sternomastoid until the posterior belly of the digastric is displayed and then dissection is carried out in the angle above this and between the posterior belly of the digastric and the mastoid process. There is usually no difficulty in recognizing the facial nerve but if any doubt exists the nerve stimulator can be valuable. The reason for displaying the facial nerve is simply to ensure its safety during the remainder of the dissection.

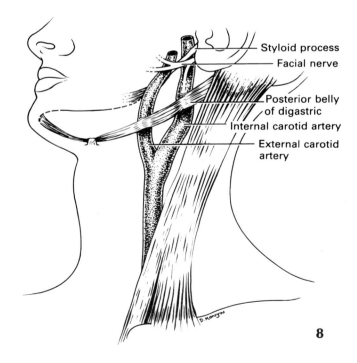

Styloid process
Facial nerve
Posterior belly of digastric
Internal carotid artery
External carotid artery

8

9

The posterior belly of the digastric can then be divided along with the stylohyoid. The occipital artery may have to be divided because it runs backwards along the inferior edge of the stylohyoid. The transverse process of the atlas can be palpated. It must remembered that deep to these muscles are the accessory nerve, the internal jugular vein and the carotid arteries. The styloid process is palpated in the depths between the mastoid process and the mandible. The styloid can then, if necessary, be fractured, allowing the space to open up further. Using this approach the author has never found it necessary to employ the alternative methods of anterior dislocation of the temporomandibular joint or osteotomy of the ramus of the mandible.

Styloid process

Internal jugular vein

Internal carotid artery

9

10

The dissection

10

Beginning with the external carotid side of the tumour, the plane between the tumour and vessel wall is identified and developed. The so-called white line of Gordon-Taylor in the adventitia can often be identified (as illustrated), but in other cases, when the tumour is particularly vascular, this is not apparent. Numerous small vessels will course between the vessel and the tumour and the diathermy is invaluable. The bipolar coagulator is very helpful for the numerous tiny vessels encountered. Larger feeding vessels are ligated and divided. Each such division renders the tumour less vascular but the vessels cannot be sought for and ligation must wait until the tumour is peeled off the carotid and they are exposed in the course of the dissection.

If the tumour completely surrounds the vessels it is usually necessary to divide the tumour in order to reach the correct plane of dissection. Again, any such dissection is best carried out on the external carotid side of the lesion. The dissection will then proceed over the external carotid to its anterior surface and similarly to its posterior surface. It is very important to avoid twisting the tumour, and hence the vessels, as this may result in cessation of flow up the internal carotid.

The lumen is most easily entered during the final stages of separation from the vessels in the 'crutch' between internal and external carotids. This is because the exact configuration of the vessels is unknown and because traction may be exerted on the tumour at this stage.

11

When the posterior surface of the tumour is being separated from the deep tissues it is very important to avoid injury to the glossopharyngeal nerve, which is in an immediate posterior relation in most moderate-sized tumours. It is not easy to identify and must be assumed to be in danger.

When the tumour has finally been separated from the vessels it will appear smaller and firmer. Most of the bleeding ceases at this stage although an occasional vessel in the tumour bed is diathermied using bipolar coagulation, ensuring first that the cranial nerves are not close by. The author employs suction drainage routinely.

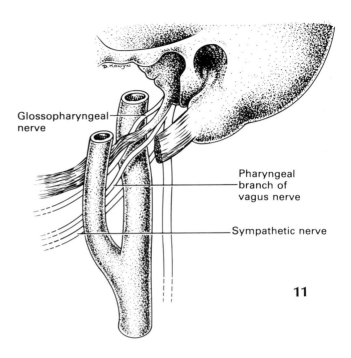

Glossopharyngeal nerve

Pharyngeal branch of vagus nerve

Sympathetic nerve

11

Internal carotid artery

External carotid artery

Shunt

A shunt, such as the Javid or Brenner shunt, should be available, so that if unexpected carotid injury occurs it can be inserted when prolonged clamping is envisaged.

12

Use of the shunt in order to reduce blood loss has also been advocated, although the author has no experience of this method. The shunt is inserted from the common carotid to the internal carotid, cutting off the orifice of the external carotid and hence the supply to the tumour. Consequently, the tumour is less vascular and the vessels safer.

Ligation of the external carotid to aid haemostasis has been suggested. However, the ligation would have to be at the origin of the external carotid and if this can be dissected out the operation is half completed; little would seem to be gained from ligation at that stage.

12

Complications

Stroke

Stroke is potentially the most worrying risk of the operation, but the author has had no experience of this. Reports would suggest two possible causes: injury to the internal carotid, and thrombosis as the result of stasis, which may be caused by twisting the vessels or by a haematoma in the vessel wall. In the older age group there is always the possibility of atheroma at the bifurcation and its embolization as the result of manipulation.

Cranial nerve injury

Three cranial nerves are anatomically closely related. Preoperative examination is essential as they may already be affected by tumour. The vagus nerve, except in chemodectomas arising from the vagus, can usually be easily identified and preserved. The hypoglossal is always seen crossing or entering the tumour and should be preserved, provided this does not prejudice the safety or completeness of the excision. The glossopharyngeal is the most difficult to identify and its injury can have serious effects on swallowing.

Arterial injury

If the vessel wall is entered accidentally it can usually be repaired with a 6/0 polypropylene suture. Arterial clamps must always be available. Invasion of the arterial wall by the tumour is rare, but when encountered it will require resection of the artery and vein graft replacement.

Haemorrhage

This can be steady and prolonged but rarely becomes a problem under the conditions of wide exposure, as advocated. Haemorrhage is only a serious problem when the tumour is an unexpected finding at attempted biopsy of a lump in the neck.

Haematoma

As there is a large dead space, suction drainage is necessary.

Conclusion

Carotid body tumours are slow growing and usually benign. They can be bilateral and may be associated with other tumours of APUD cells. Small tumours are easily removed, provided a preoperative diagnosis is made by angiography so that adequate wide exposure can be made. The necessary instruments for arterial repair should always be available but will rarely be required. A carotid shunt should also be available but the author has rarely used one and its use should not be regarded as routine.

Careful identification and preservation of the cranial nerves is a necesary part of the operation, but occasionally one or more of these nerves will already be involved in the tumour and have to be sacrificed.

Transperitoneal approach to the infrarenal abdominal aorta

Roger M. Greenhalgh MA, MD, MChir, FRCS
Professor of Surgery, Charing Cross and Westminster Medical School, London, UK

Introduction

The authors of the chapters in this section show a distinct preference for the transperitoneal approach to the infrarenal abdominal aorta, although reference is made to the alternative approach by the extraperitoneal route. The thoracoabdominal approach is necessary to repair thoracoabdominal aneurysms of the aorta and to expose the origins of the coeliac axis and superior mesenteric artery. The great majority of aortic aneurysms can be operated upon entirely from within the abdominal cavity and the majority of bypasses taken from the aorta for stenosing or occlusive arterial disease are taken from the infrarenal abdominal aorta.

This chapter introduces the approach to the aorta for end-to-side anastomosis and also comments on the principles of the siting of the distal limbs of aortic bifurcation graft surgery. Subsequent chapters detail the end-to-end aortic bifurcation surgical technique and the particular problem of juxtarenal aortic occlusion. For unilateral iliac disease, the femoro-femoral cross-over technique can be used when the donor iliac system is free from disease. This has proved to be a most useful method of reconstruction and is a relatively minor operative procedure.

Some surgeons prefer to use an oblique extraperitoneal approach for unilateral iliac disease, performing endarterectomy or taking a single tube graft of Dacron from the common iliac artery and bringing it down to the femoral artery. It is argued that this approach allows sympathectomy to be performed at the same time and it is also relatively atraumatic. In practice the vast majority of patients presenting with aortoiliac stenoses or occlusions have bilateral disease and, while an aortic bifurcation graft is a somewhat more extensive procedure, the results are durable and reoperation is less frequently required than when only one side of the iliac system is bypassed originally. Reoperation after unilateral iliac reconstruction involves consideration not only of the side operated upon but also of the untouched side where progression of disease may occur. In aortic bifurcation grafting it is important to sew the main trunk of the graft to the abdominal aorta well above the bifurcation and just below the left renal vein in order to avoid progression of arterial disease in the abdominal aortic stem between the renal arteries and the aortic bifurcation. Many of these concepts are from the teachings of Michael E. Debakey who contributes the next chapter.

The operation

The skin is covered with a large plastic drape. The incision can be either midline or transverse but the author prefers a full-length midline incision. This is a rapid and clean approach to the abdominal aorta and allows the easiest access at the upper end. It also facilitates anastomosis to the external iliac vessels should this be desirable. It is the quickest approach to the aorta in an emergency situation such as a leaking aneurysm. A laparotomy is performed and the intestinal contents are all carefully examined before the arteries are approached.

1

The posterior peritoneum fixes the fourth part of the duodenum and duodenojejunal flexure over the upper abdominal aorta and inferior vena cava and the dissection begins by dividing the peritoneum just to the left of the duodenum and passing through the ligament of the Treitz. The duodenum and small bowel can then be swept to the right to expose the aorta and vena cava. The incision in the posterior peritoneum begins somewhere at about the origin of the right common iliac artery towards the right of the aorta and is carried obliquely up the aorta, keeping clear of the inferior mesenteric artery. This frees the duodenum, divides the ligament of Treitz and allows the bowel to be freed and moved to the right. The bowel can then be retracted in a number of ways according to the surgeon's preference. Some prefer to pack it off within the abdominal cavity and use a self-retainer to squash the bowel under the right lobe of the liver. This can give a very satisfactory exposure but is thought by some to splint the diaphragm and lead to increased incidence of respiratory problems during the postoperative period. The author's preference is to allow some of the small bowel to extrude from the abdominal cavity and to cover it with moist large packs of turkish towels. A retractor can then be used to pull the bowel gently away from the aorta and vena cava without exerting very much pressure. In the author's experience, postoperatively this leads to a shorter period of ileus and fewer respiratory problems. It is important to dissect or open the peritoneum below the aortic bifurcation only as far as is necessary to allow application of angled Debakey forceps immediately at the origin of the common iliac arteries. Further dissection may damage the autonomic nerves, which cross the common iliac vessels, leading to failure to ejaculate in the male. An advantage of bypass over endarterectomy of the aortoiliac segment is that it avoids the possibility of dividing or disturbing the autonomic nerves.

As the abdominal aorta is approached, it is frequently crossed by the inferior mesenteric vein and this should be formally divided between clips and ligated to allow better access. The inferior mesenteric artery is carefully preserved

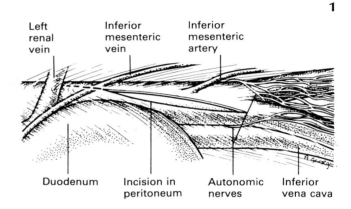

1

Left renal vein — Inferior mesenteric vein — Inferior mesenteric artery

Duodenum — Incision in peritoneum — Autonomic nerves — Inferior vena cava

and dissected sufficiently so that it can be easily controlled at a later stage with a bulldog clip. The left renal vein is seen crossing the aorta to the vena cava at the top of the operating field. Dissection should be continued just below this vein and a finger worked between the vena cava and the aorta and also close to the aorta on the left side to determine the position where the clamp will be placed. Inflammation is always greater in aneurysmal disease and dissection is much more difficult. In these circumstances it is preferable to put a straight clamp on the aorta rather than attempt to pass a sling around it, and it is essential to avoid going behind this vessel for fear of damage to lumbar veins. When an end-to-end anastomosis is envisaged, it is pointless to place a clamp around the aorta; a straight clamp is quite satisfactory but the lumbar vessels do not need to be clipped on the outside. However, if an end-to-side technique is used for a bifurcation graft for stenosing arterial disease, it is convenient to pass a Silastic sling around the aorta just below the left renal vein and another just above the aortic bifurcation. The aorta is then lifted and using careful blunt dissection with the finger the lumbar vessels can be felt and controlled with bulldog clamps before the aorta is opened.

2

Knitted Dacron grafts are generally easier to work with than woven Dacron grafts. They should be clotted at this stage, certainly before heparin is given systemically to the patient. The ends of the limbs of a knitted Dacron bifurcation graft are clamped with a cloth-covered clamp and the limbs and clamp are placed in a kidney dish. Using a 20-ml syringe, blood is taken from the inferior vena cava and squirted into the top of the bifurcation graft which is held up to receive the blood. Approximately 80–100 ml of blood is taken for the preclotting procedure. Blood pours through the knitted graft, is collected from the kidney dish with a 50-ml bladder syringe and syringed back into the main stem of the Dacron graft over and over again until the Dacron starts to hold the blood as it clots. The cloth-covered clamp is then removed and the blood is firmly squeezed from the graft between the finger and thumb.

2

3

3

An aortic clamp is passed around the back of the upper end of the aorta. The Debakey clamp illustrated has curved handles so that it will not be in the way of the operative field during the aortic anastomosis. Before clamping the author prefers to give approximately 5000 u of heparin intravenously and to wait for 3 min for the heparin to circulate. However, for aneurysmal disease the author does not use heparin and prefers to use woven Dacron.

The aortotomy is a cut of approximately 4–5 cm taken from just below the clamp which is situated just below the left renal vein. The aortotomy passes to the right of the inferior mesenteric artery and ends above the bifurcation of the aorta towards the right-hand side. The anastomosis is performed as described in the chapter on 'Techniques of anastomosis', and a decision must be taken at this stage as to which distal vessel the aortic limbs must be anastomosed.

4

If the disease is confined to the aorta and the origins of the common iliac vessels, and the external iliac, common femoral, superficial femoral and profunda femoris arteries are disease free, as shown on an arteriogram, the distal limb can be anastomosed to the external iliac artery provided this feels soft and free from disease at operation. The Dacron limbs are tunnelled immediately beneath the peritoneum and an end-to-side anastomosis is performed in the iliac fossae.

5

It is unwise to anastomose to the external iliac vessels if these are diseased and the Dacron limb must be tunnelled under the inguinal ligament to the top of the thigh. If the arteriogram has shown that the superficial femoral and profunda vessels are relatively free from disease, the easiest anastomosis in the groin is to the common femoral arteries. The author prefers to site such anastomoses just over the profunda origin to ensure a backbleed from both superficial femoral and profunda vessels independently.

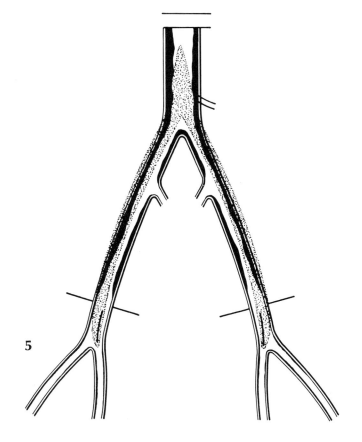

6

Where a superficial femoral artery is occluded the profunda femoris becomes the main run-off vessel and it is essential that the Dacron anastomosis is placed to guarantee a proper run-off into this important vessel. In these circumstances the author prefers to take the arteriotomy from the common femoral artery into the origin of the profunda so that the Dacron anastomosis produces a profundaplasty and widens the origin of the vessel. Details of the Dacron to groin anastomosis are given in the chapter on 'Techniques of anastomosis'.

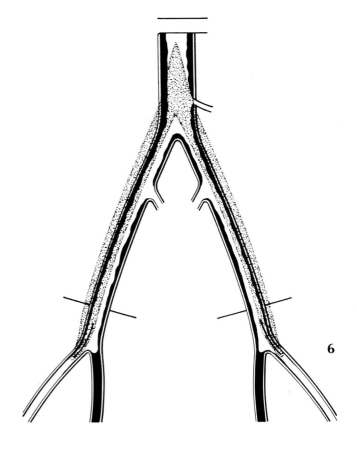

6

Complications

The immediate and most important complication is haemorrhage. Careful dissection and preclotting of knitted Dacron grafts can reduce the haemorrhage to an absolute minimum. When care is taken, no blood transfusion is required for the operations but it is possible to restore blood volume with 2 u of dextran. The other worrying complication is infection. Avoidance of infection and a clean technique is essential. The closure of groin incisions should be in three layers and haemostasis must be total. The closure of the abdominal wound should be with nylon. The author prefers a looped nylon suture and either this can be used as a mass closure of all the abdominal wall in one bite or the peritoneum can be sewn as one layer with looped chromic catgut and large bites of looped nylon can be taken to close the sheath layer.

Povidone-iodine spray reduces wound infection as has been described in the chapter on 'Operation planning'. Prophylactic antibiotics are always given before surgery begins. Aortoduodenal fistula seems to be a rarer complication following end-to-side than end-to-end aortic anastomosis. Theoretically, the suture line is more exposed to the bowel for end-to-side anastomosis and it is quite difficult in some cases to close the peritoneum over the Dacron. Nevertheless, the incidence of aortoduodenal fistula is extremely low following this procedure; it is certainly much greater following end-to-end anastomosis for aneurysmal disease.

Other important features of aortic bypass surgery are discussed in subsequent chapters.

Aortic bifurcation grafting for stenosing arterial disease

Michael E. DeBakey MD

Olga Keith Wiess Professor of Surgery and Chairman, Cora and Webb Mading Department of Surgery, and Chancellor, Baylor College of Medicine, Houston, Texas, USA

Introduction

Occlusive disease of the terminal abdominal aorta and common iliac arteries is usually well localized to this segment. The occlusive process may be complete or incomplete (stenosis) with the underlying pathologic lesion being arteriosclerotic or atherosclerotic. Whereas other diagnostic studies may be useful, arteriography is essential in order to obtain precise information regarding the site and extent of the disease, both proximally and distally, and is therefore important in planning the surgical procedure and in indentifying associated occlusive disease of the renal and visceral arteries and unsuspected aneurysmal disease. In our experience, about 30% of patients have secondary segmental occlusion of the distal arterial tree. Preoperative evaluation of the patient's condition should include studies for possible concomitant occlusive vascular disease in the extracranial carotid and coronary arteries. This is emphasized by the fact that about one-third of our patients were found to have significant disease in these arterial segments.

Several methods of surgical treatment or a combination of these methods are available: (1) bypass surgery, (2) thromboendarterectomy, (3) patch-graft angioplasty, and (4) excision with graft replacement. Selection of the appropriate method or combination of methods in an individual case depends upon a number of factors, including the extent and nature of the occlusive process and involvement of the aortic wall. In some occasional patients, for example, usually young women in whom the atheroma is extremely well localized to the abdominal aorta, thromboendarterectomy with patch-graft angioplasty may be employed. In other patients in whom the wall of the abdominal aorta is extensively diseased, as in the presence of periaortic fibrosis, intense inflammatory reaction, or aneurysmal formation, resection of this segment with graft replacement is required.

On the basis of our experience extending over a period of about 40 years, the bypass operation with certain variations according to the extent and nature of the disease, has become our procedure of choice because of its simplicity, avoidance of injury to adjacent structures, and its long-term good results. The technical application of the bypass principle and its modifications or combination with other procedures, depending upon certain factors influencing its use, will be described and illustrated in this presentation.

1a–o

In patients with complete occlusion of the abdominal aorta extending up to the origin of the renal arteries, the following procedure is employed. The peritoneal cavity is opened through a midline incision (*a*). The abdominal aorta is exposed by retraction of the small intestines to the right. A vertical incision is then made in the peritoneum overlying the aorta and separated from the aortic wall on each side, and the renal arteries are exposed. Occluding clamps are then placed on the renal arteries to prevent embolic debris into the renal arteries during the subsequent manoeuvres. The abdominal aorta immediately above the origin of the renal arteries is temporarily occluded manually, and a 4- to 5-cm vertical incision is made through the anterior aortic wall several centimetres below the origin of the arteries (*b*).

The fairly firm thromboatherosclerotic process is recognized, and thromboendarterectomy is performed after the proper cleavage plane in the aortic wall has been identified (*b*). The occlusive lesion is then dissected free proximally and removed. Intermittent release of pressure on the aorta permits flushing of any retained debris (*c*). Careful visualization of the ostia of the renal arteries is important to be certain that no debris is left in the renal arteries and that dissection of the ostia of the renal arteries has not occurred. An aortic clamp is then applied to the abdominal aorta just below the origin of the renal arteries. The clamps on the renal arteries are removed, and the temporary occlusion of the aorta above the renal arteries is released allowing restoration of renal artery perfusion (*d*). This is verified by palpation of good pulses in both renal arteries.

A suitable-sized DeBakey albumin-coated Dacron bifurcation graft is selected, and the aortic end of the graft is anastomosed end-to-side to the opening in the abdominal aorta (*d*). In some cases this may be done as an end-to-end anastomosis to the opening in the abdominal aorta just below the renal arteries. The site for the distal anastomosis is then determined on the basis of the arteriogram and observation and palpation of the distal arteries. If these findings suggest that the external iliac artery is suitable, the anastomosis (end-to-side) is done at this level within the abdominal cavity (*e*). If however, there is significant disease in the external iliac artery, the distal anastomosis must be performed in the common femoral artery in the groin (*o*).

The external iliac artery is exposed through an opening in the peritoneum overlying this artery in the pelvis. The appropriate limb of the previously inserted Dacron graft is passed retroperitoneally to the area of the external iliac artery. Occluding clamps are applied proximally and distally on the external iliac artery, a 1.5- to 2-cm vertical incision is made on the anterior wall of the external iliac artery, and the limb of the bifurcation is then cut at the appropriate length in a bevelled fashion and anastomosed by a continuous suture of 0000 Prolene to the opening in the artery (*e*). After completion of this anastomosis and just before closing to the final suture, the proximal and then the distal occluding clamps are temporarily released to flush the artery from any clot or debris (*f*). The occluding clamps are then reapplied to the external iliac artery, an occluding clamp is applied to the proximal part of this limb of the graft, and the aortic occluding clamp is released for one or two pulses to wash out any clot or debris in the graft (*g*). The end of a suction tube is then inserted into the open limb of the graft to remove any remaining clot or debris (*h*). The occluding clamps on the external iliac artery are then removed, an occluding clamp is applied to the proximal end of the open limb of the graft (*i*), and the occluding clamp in the aorta is removed, a manoeuvre that permits circulation through the anastomosed limb of the graft into that extremity (*j*). The remaining limb of the bifurcation graft is then brought retroperitoneally to the exposed portion of the external iliac artery and is anastomosed to an opening in this artery as previously described (*k*). Just before the suture of this anastomosis is closed, the occluding clamps on the external iliac arteries are temporarily released to flush the graft (*l*), and then the occluding clamp on the graft is temporarily released to flush the graft (*m*), following which the anastomotic suture is tied and all clamps are removed to permit restoration of circulation into this extremity (*n*). In patients in whom the limbs of the graft must be attached to the common femoral artery, this artery is exposed by a vertical incision in the groin, and the graft is tunnelled posterior to the inguinal ligament into the groin (*o*).

In patients in whom the distal limbs of the graft must be attached to the common femoral artery, it is important to determine that there is good outflow through the superficial femoral or profunda femoris or both arteries. This assumes great significance in regard to the profunda femoris when the superficial femoral artery is occluded. In such cases the profunda femoris may require profundaplasty.

1

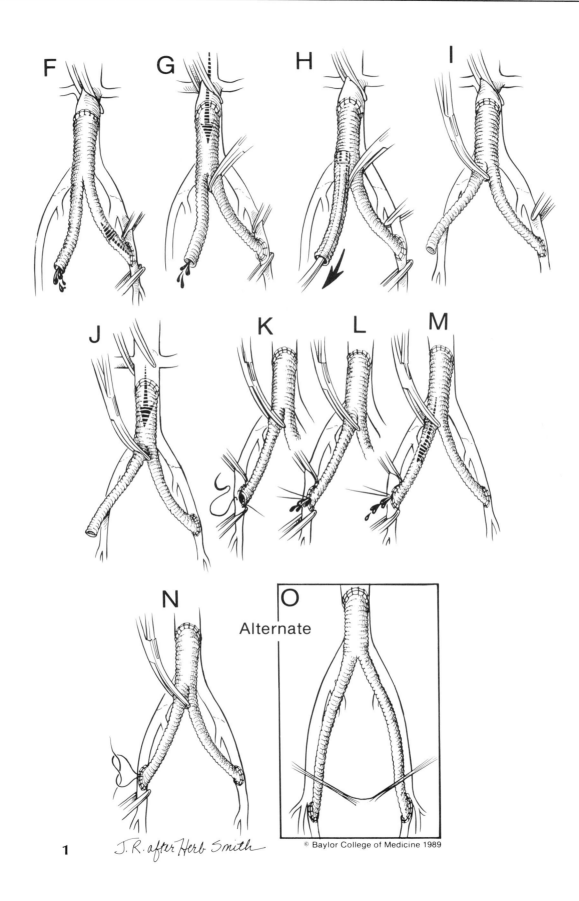

1   *J. R. after Herb Smith*

Alternate

© Baylor College of Medicine 1989

2a–j

In occasional patients in whom the occlusive or associated aneurysmal disease involves the abdominal aorta at or near the origin of the renal arteries, it may be necessary to occlude the aorta above the renal arteries using an aortic occluding clamp (*b*). The abdomen is entered through a midline incision (*a*), and the abdominal aorta is exposed by a vertical incision in the overlying peritoneal layer (*b, c*). In such cases, the renal arteries should be occluded as previously described (*d*). After the endarterectomy is performed and the ostia of the renal arteries are cleared of disease, there many not be a sufficient amount of aorta below the renal arteries to permit the placement of an occluding clamp below the renal arteries. Under these circumstances, after completion of the endarterectomy (*d*), the aorta is cirumferentially incised just below the ostia of the renal arteries, and the opening of the lumbar and inferior mesenteric arteries are oversewn (*e*). In order to prevent retrograde bleeding, occluding clamps are also placed upon the common iliac arteries (*e*).

The aortic limb of the graft is then sutured as an end-to-end anastomosis to the proximal opening in the aorta, care being taken to avoid compression of the ostia of the renal arteries (*f*). This may be assured by placing an appropriate sized dilator into the ostia of the renal arteries during the anastomosis. After completion of this anastomosis, the aortic clamp is temporarily opened to flush the aorta and remove any clots or debris, following which the occluding clamps on the renal arteries are similarly flushed. An occluding clamp is then applied to the Dacron graft just below the anastomosis, and the occluding clamps on the aorta and both renal arteries are removed to permit restoration of circulation to the kidneys (*h*). The attachments of the limbs of the bifurcation to the external iliac or common femoral arteries are then performed as previously described (*i, j*). The distal opening in the abdominal aorta just above the bifurcation is closed by suture (*f*) or the common iliac arteries are closed by suture (*g*) depending upon local circumstances.

Alternate

2

F

G

Alternate

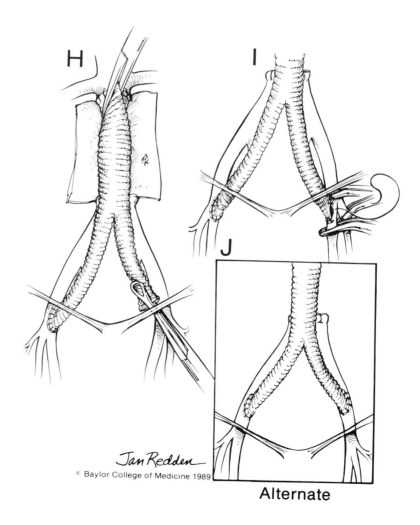

H

I

J

Jan Redden

Alternate

2

3a–b

In still other patients who have incomplete occlusion but significant stenosis, the bypass procedure is usually preferred. In such cases, the abdominal aorta just distal to the renal arteries may be relatively free of disease, and endarterectomy is thus not required. After an occluding clamp is applied to the abdominal aorta just below the origin of the renal arteries and to both common iliac arteries and inferior mesenteric arteries, an aortic occluding clamp is passed under the common iliac arteries to occlude the posterior wall of the abdominal aorta to prevent retrograde bleeding from the lumbar arteries (*a*). A longitudinal incision is then made in the abdominal aorta as close as possible to the proximal aortic occluding clamp (*b*). The aortic limb of the Dacron graft is attached to this opening by end-to-side anastomosis, and the two limbs of the graft are attached to the external iliac or common femoral arteries as previously described.

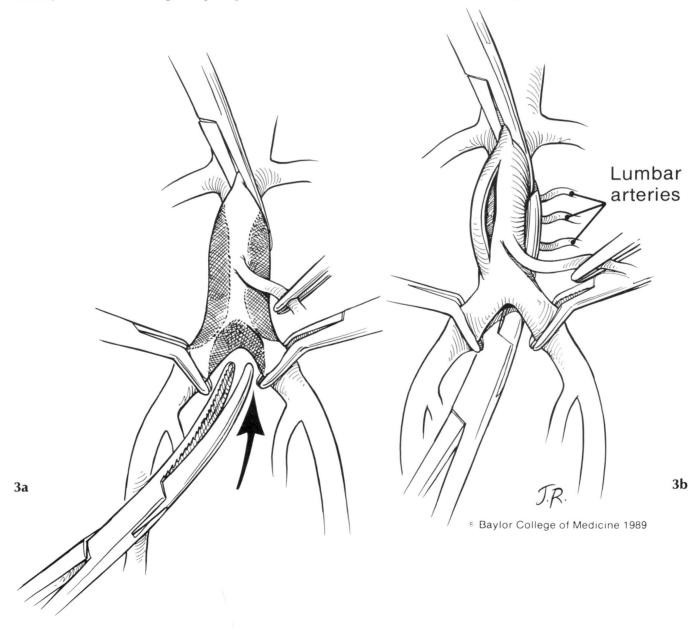

Lumbar
arteries

3a

3b

4a–d

There are still other more complicated cases, fortunately encountered only occasionally, that require a different approach. These may be exemplified by patients in whom the infrarenal aorta is densely adherent to surrounding structures owing to previous operation or is associated with intense inflammatory reaction or periaortic fibrosis, thus creating great difficulty or even jeopardy in dissection and exposure of the infrarenal abdominal aorta. In such cases, after the peritoneal cavity is opened through a midline incision (extending up to the xyphoid) (a), the abdominal aorta is exposed just below the diaphragm as it passes through the diaphragmatic hiatus by entering the lessor sac and retracting the left lobe of the liver (b). A partial occluding clamp is then applied to the aorta just above the celiac axis and a vertical incision is made in the anterior wall of the occluded portion of the aorta (c). An appropriate-sized (usually ranging between 10 and 16 mm in diameter) albumin-coated tubular DeBakey Dacron graft is attached to the opening in the aorta by end-to-side anastomosis (d).

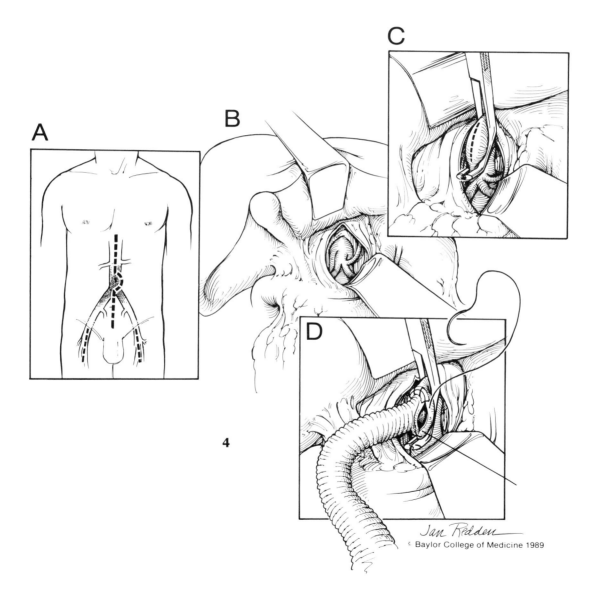

4

Jan Redden
© Baylor College of Medicine 1989

4e–h

After completion of this anastomosis, an occluding clamp is applied to the Dacron graft just distal to the anastomosis and the partial occluding clamp on the abdominal aorta is removed. An incision is then made in the peritoneum overlying the iliopsoas muscle to permit entrance into the retroperitoneal space (e), and by careful sharp and blunt dissection, a long sponge holder or other comparable clamp is inserted through this retroperitoneal space to the opening in the lessor sac at the site of the graft anastomosis to the aorta, and the distal end of this graft is brought out into the distal retroperitoneal opening (f). The left common femoral artery is exposed through a vertical incision, and the Dacron graft is then tunnelled under the inguinal ligament (g) and brought into the groin incision (h).

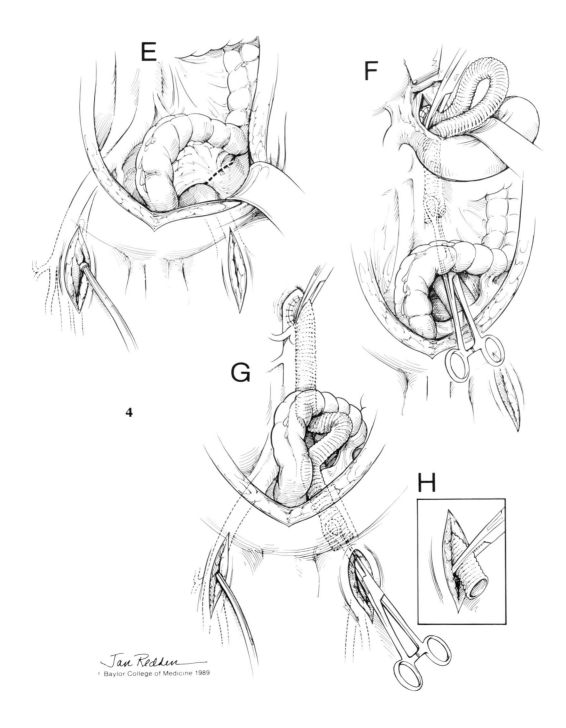

Jan Redden
© Baylor College of Medicine 1989

4i–l

Here, again, as previously noted, if the distal portion of the external iliac artery is relatively normal, it is preferable to the common femoral artery for anastomosis. Another appropriate-sized (approximately 8 to 10 mm) albumin-coated tubular DeBakey Dacron graft is then attached by end-to-side anastomosis to a vertical opening on the right side of the previously placed aorta to right femoral graft (*i*). This graft is then tunnelled retroperitoneally through an opening exposing the right common femoral artery (*j*). The distal end of the graft that is brought into the left groin incision is then attached to the left common femoral artery by end-to-side anastomosis (*k*). An occluding clamp is then applied to the Dacron graft going to the right groin just distal to its anastomosis to the main graft, and the occluding clamps on this main graft and the common femoral artery are sequentially temporarily released to flush any clots or debris, following which these clamps are removed and circulation is permitted to pass through the main graft into the legs (*k*). The right limb of the graft is then anastomosed to the right common femoral artery as previously described (*l*).

Jan Redden
© Baylor College of Medicine 1989

5

Occasionally in such cases as just described, it may be necessary to attach the proximal end of the graft to the lower part of the descending thoracic aorta rather than the abdominal aorta just below the diaphragm (*a*). A separate lower left intercostal incision is used to expose the lower descending thoracic aorta. A partial occluding clamp is then placed on the descending thoracic aorta and a vertical incision is made along the left lateral wall of the aorta to which the graft is attached by end-to-side anastomosis. The peritoneal cavity is opened through a separate midline incision, and the graft in the left pleural cavity is tunnelled retroperitoneally through an opening in the diaphragm along the left side of the aorta as it passes through the aortic diaphragmatic hiatus.

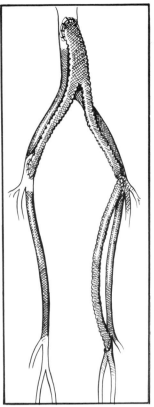

5

Juxtarenal aortic occlusion

R. Courbier
Professeur Agrégé à la Faculté de Medecine et Chef du Service de Chirurgie Cardio Vasculaire, Hôpital Saint Joseph, Marseille, France

J. M. Jausseran
Assistant du Service de Chirurgie Cardio Vasculaire, Hôpital Saint Joseph, Marseille, France

Introduction

In the Leriche syndrome, progressive atherosclerotic disease involves the origin of the inferior mesenteric artery. When this artery becomes completely occluded the clot proceeds up to the level of the renal arteries; this is known as a 'juxtarenal aortic occlusion'. Many reports have pointed to the technical problems involved in treating this (Courbier et al., 1974, 1979; Liddicoat et al., 1975; Starrett and Stoney, 1974; Traverso et al., 1978). A classic thromoendarterectomy (Vollmar, Gruss and Lauback, 1970) necessitates extensive exposure of the aorta and renal branches, which all have to be clamped.

A limited thromboendarterectomy is simpler and avoids extensive dissection, so that the aorta can be clamped at a lower level. Since 1963 we have used this technique in 85 cases (5.6% of cases of aortic reconstruction). Only in a few cases, when there is a high risk to the patient because of renal or respiratory insufficiency or when extensive disease of the visceral arteries cannot be treated, an extra-anatomical bypass is used.

Operative technique

The patient is placed in a supine position with the left arm raised, so that a left thoracotomy can be done in case of technical problems.

1

Incision

A vertical midline incision is made. Additional resection of the xyphoid increases the exposure of the upper part.

If it is not possible to expose the upper part or there is a wound in that area, a thoracoabdominal approach through the 8th intercostal space can be used.

1

2

Dissection of ligament of Treitz

After incision of the posterior peritoneum, the duodenum is retracted to the right and the ligament of Treitz is incised.

2

3

Limited exposure of the aorta

It is necessary to divide the inferior mesenteric vein, avoiding any arterial anastomotic branch.

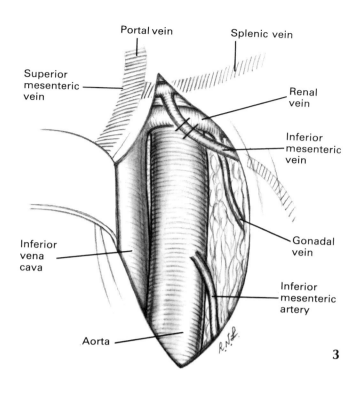

3

4

The left gonadal vein and capsular vein must also sometimes be divided.

4

5

Extended exposure of the aorta

This approach is used in case of arterial disease involving the origin of the renal arteries. The left renal vein is retracted and moved up or down so that a tape and a tourniquet can be placed on both renal arteries.

5

6

6

The left renal vein is divided between two arterial clamps and reconstructed later. The upper limit of the dissection is the origin of the superior mesenteric artery which does not need to be demonstrated. (With this extended dissection it is possible to perform endarterectomy of the aorta, and origins of the renal arteries. The clamp is placed across the aorta above the renal arteries. No clamp is required on the lower end.)

7

Illustration 7 shows the usual procedure where it is unnecessary to divide the left renal vein or to control the renal arteries with slings. The aorta is opened transversely, using scissors, 3 cm below the level of the renal arteries, without any posterior dissection. Clamping of the aorta is not necessary.

7

8

8

A small part of the clot is removed from the lower part of the aorta, and the artery is then occluded with a continuous suture.

Thrombectomy

9

This is performed on the upper part of the aorta. The surgeon's 2nd and 3rd left fingers are applied to the pulsating part of the aorta just beyond the upper limit of the thrombus.

Dissection is made with a dissector or with a thin sciscors. It is very important to avoid the plane of thromboendarterectomy, which is too near the exterior of the artery wall, but to use the plane of thrombectomy which leaves enough artery wall behind. Dissection begins anteriorly and posteriorly and continues upward.

9

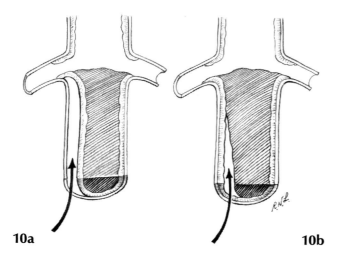

10a   10b

10a & b

The two different dissecting planes

The dissecting plane for thromboendarterectomy cannot be used in a retrograde manner because of the risk of a dissection on the origin of the renal arteries (*a*).

Thrombectomy can be done without any risk. The high flow after reconstruction allows a small part of the aorta to be left without risk of rethrombosis (*b*).

11

When bleeding occurs the two fingers create a temporary haemostasis and feel at the same time the tips of the dissecting scissors.

The total clot is removed *en bloc* with a forceps. The fingers' pressure is released to permit a flush of blood.

11

12

An aortic clamp is placed between the fingers and the origin of the renal arteries.

The operation can then be continued as for an ordinary aortic occlusion.

12

References

Courbier, R., Jausseran, J. M. and Reggi, M. (1974) Les thromboses aortiques juxta rénales. *Journal de Chirurgie* **107**, 281.

Courbier, R., Jausseran, J. M., Reggi, M., Schlama, G. and Monin, Ph. (1979). Traitement chirurgical des thromboses aortiques juxta-rénales – Résultats à long terme. *Journal de Chirurgie* **105**, 545.

Liddicoat, J., Bekassy, S., Dang, M. and De Bakey, M. (1975). Complet occlusion of the infrarenal abdominal aorta: Management and results in 64 patients, *Surgery* **77**, 467.

Starrett, R. and Stoney, R. (1974). Juxta renal aortic occlusion. *Surgery* **76**, 890.

Traverso, L. W., Backer, J. D., Dainko, E. A., Machleder, H. F. (1978). Infrarenal aortic occlusion. *Annals of Surgery* **187**, 397.

Vollmar, J., Gruss, J. and Lauback, K. (1970). Technique de la thromboendartériectomie. *Journal de Chirurgie* **100**, 67.

Surgical techniques for visceral artery revascularization

William K. Ehrenfeld MD
Professor of Surgery, University of California, San Francisco, California, USA

Peter G. Qvarfordt MD
Vascular Research Fellow, University of California, San Francisco, California, USA

Ronald J. Stoney MD
Professor of Surgery, University of California, San Francisco, California, USA

Introduction

Atherosclerotic visceral artery lesions may cause acute or chronic visceral ischaemia. The chronic form is also known as 'abdominal angina' (Dunphy, 1936; Mikkelsen, 1957). Acute occlusion of one or more visceral arteries due to thrombosis of an atherosclerotic artery or embolus from a proximal source may lead to bowel infarction. Bowel infarction is a surgical emergency requiring immediate removal of the affected bowel and possibly the offending clot or the atherosclerotic lesion. This is rarely technically feasible. Chronic mesenteric insufficiency with abdominal angina is a relatively rare condition. Extensive collateral vessels readily develop between the visceral aortic branches – celiac axis, superior mesenteric artery (SMA), inferior mesenteric artery (IMA) – and the hypogastric (internal iliac) arteries. These collateral pathways may be so efficient that very rarely gradual occlusion of all major aortic branches may actually occur without bowel infarction. Usually, involvement of two or more visceral branches cause symptoms. The main collateral circuits are: (1) the gastroduodenal and pancreaticoduodenal arteries between the celiac axis and the SMA; (2) the middle and left colic arteries between the SMA and the IMA ('meandering mesenteric artery', the arc of Riolan); and finally (3) the sigmoid and hemorrhoidal vessels between the IMA and the internal iliac arteries. Although at least two of the three major visceral arteries are severely narrowed or occluded in 85% of patients with abdominal angina, the symptoms are related more to the inadequacy of the collateral blood flow than to the actual number of obstructed primary arteries (Wylie, Stoney and Ehrenfeld, 1980). Occlusion of the celiac axis along with poor collateralization may occasionally cause bowel or organ ischaemia. Chronic occlusion of either the SMA or IMA only does not usually cause ischaemia.

The syndrome most typical of chronic intestinal ischaemia afflicts women between the ages of 50 and 70 years and includes: (1) epigastric postprandial cramping pain; (2) weight loss due to pain and/or fear of eating; (3) bowel motility disturbances (nausea, vomiting, diarrhoea and/or constipation) caused by bowel ischaemia. Malabsorption is seldom present, and there are no specific diagnostic laboratory tests. Evidence of atherosclerotic disease in other peripheral arteries is found in approximately 33% of the affected patients and an epigastric bruit is heard in 70%. The definitive diagnosis depends upon abdominal arteriography using both the anteroposterior projection, which best delineates collateral formation, and lateral or oblique projections, which best illustrate the degree of vessel obstruction. The stenotic lesions are usually seen at or near the vessel origins.

Unusual causes of visceral artery stenosis are fibromuscular dysplasia and median arcuate ligament compression of the celiac axis and occasionally includes the SMA. Cases of compression of these vessels by the celiac ganglionic nerve fibres have been reported. These cases are often atypical and are the subject of continuing surgical controversy.

During the past 25 years numerous methods for visceral artery revascularization have been evaluated including retrograde synthetic or autogenous grafts, transvisceral artery thromboendarterectomy and reimplantation. Two basic procedures are now preferred: transaortic thromboendarterectomy and antegrade synthetic graft bypass grafting.

Operative indications and preoperative preparations

Revascularization is indicated in patients with characteristic symptoms and significant stenosis of one or more visceral branches as seen by arteriography. The objectives are to relieve pain and prevent bowel infarction. Prophylactic visceral revascularization may also be indicated in coexisting aortoiliac and aortorenal vascular procedures (Stoney, Ehrenfeld and Wylie, 1977). Intra-abdominal disease of nonvascular origin must be thoroughly excluded before operation. Intravenous hyperalimentation is required in the catabolic patient with profound weight loss to restore an anabolic state. Antibiotics are administered prophylactically beginning 12 h before operation. When prosthetic grafts are used, antibiotics are given intraoperatively and during the next 48 h.

Antegrade prosthetic grafting

Atherosclerotic visceral artery lesions, in conjunction with lesions in the renal arteries, may be part of an unusually extensive atherosclerotic process of the abdominal aortic wall, which can make grafting at this level technically difficult. Antegrade prosthetic visceral bypass reconstructions may be desirable as the grafts will originate from the usually undiseased distal thoracic aorta. Antegrade graft placement is haemodynamically superior to retrograde placement which may predispose to early graft thrombosis. The antegrade route is shorter and usually requires shorter grafts. Retrograde bypass is particularly awkward for revascularization of the SMA since this artery arises from the aorta at an acute angle and is quite mobile, predisposing to kink and occlusion. Arterial autografts are ideal for revascularization procedures involving the renal arteries (Ehrenfeld, Stoney and Wylie, 1982). However, in visceral artery revascularization, synthetic grafts are preferred since the most common autografts, the hypogastric (internal iliac) arteries, constitute part of the visceral collateral system. The hypogastric artery autograft is generally too short for antegrade revascularization of the SMA. Venous autografts are not used, since it is thought that they frequently cause dilatation, stenosis and late occlusion (Stanley, Ernst and Fry, 1973). Flanged knitted Dacron

prostheses (5 or 6 mm) are preferred for single vessel bypass, and bifurcated grafts (10 × 5 mm or 12 × 6 mm) are used when both the celiac axis and the SMA are revascularized. Visceral erosion by these grafts has not occurred in our series. Revascularization of both the celiac axis and the superior mesenteric artery is preferred when indicated and feasible, since they supply 90% of splanchnic blood flow. This procedure is commonly used in patients with operative risk factors that preclude thoracoabdominal exposure. Despite temporary aortic occlusion of 20–30 min, the results with this procedure are excellent, with a long-term graft patency and durable relief of abdominal angina in over 90% of patients.

Operative technique

An upper midline incision extending from the xiphoid to the umbilicus is used. The celiac artery and the supraceliac aorta are reached by first dividing the gastrohepatic ligament. After division of the triangular ligament, the left lobe of the liver is retracted to the right and the oesophagus and the stomach to the left in order to expose the posterior fibres of the diaphragm.

1a–d

Illustration 1(a) shows the anterior approach to the celiac artery and supraceliac aorta. The inset depicts a typical celiac atherosclerotic lesion with contiguous aortic involvement. Isolated celiac disease is a more common cause of symptoms than isolated SMA disease. The arcuate ligament and diaphragmatic crura are divided in the midline to expose the distal thoracic aorta (*b*). The celiac ganglionic fibres are dissected and resected from around the artery. The aorta is temporarily occluded at a level 5 cm proximal to the celiac axis origin and also distal to the origin of the celiac axis, after intravenous administration of 2000–4000 i.u. of heparin. An elliptical disc of the aortic wall is cut out from the anterior surface of the aorta (*c*). A 6-mm flanged Dacron graft (made from 12 × 6 mm bifurcation graft) is anastomosed to the aortotomy site with a running 4/0 synthetic suture. Thereafter, the aortic clamps are released and a vascular clamp is applied on the proximal portion of the graft. The graft is then anastomosed end-to-end to the undiseased distal artery (*d*).

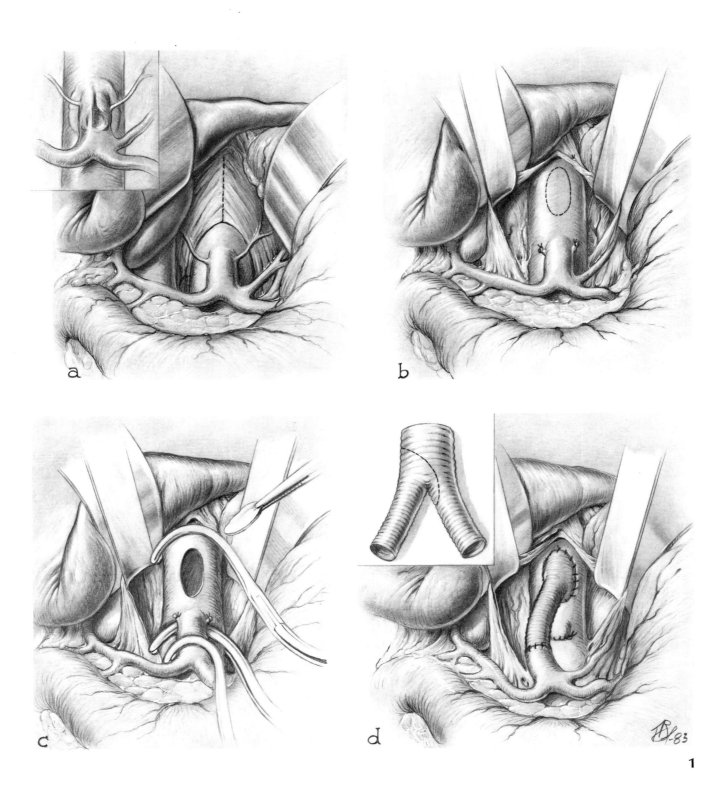

1

2a–c

If bypass to both the celiac and the SMA is planned, the SMA is also exposed by further dissection and resection of the celiac nerve fibres overlying the aorta. This manoeuvre frees the body of the pancreas which can then be elevated from the aorta with ease and retracted caudally, thus exposing the first 4–5 cm of the SMA. An elliptical aortotomy is made on the right anterolateral aspect of the aorta (a). With this technique, the two graft limbs will line up parallel to the celiac axis and the SMA, respectively, without kinking and buckling of the graft. A flanged tubular bifurcation graft (12 × 6 mm) is anastomosed between aortic clamps to the aorta using a 4/0 suture. The body of the graft is then clamped and aortic flow is restored. Thereafter the celiac axis is clamped, transected and the proximal end is oversewn. An end-to-end anastomosis is performed between the graft limb and the distal, nondiseased celiac artery using either interrupted or running 5/0 sutures. The clamp is then shifted to the right SMA limb and the same procedure is used for the SMA (b). The right (SMA) limb of the bifurcated graft lies behind the pancreas to parallel the course of the SMA (c). The full length of the retropancreatic course of the SMA limb is visualized in (c) by the artist's cutaway of a section of pancreas. The adequacy of the reconstruction may be assessed by electromagnetic flow probe measurement. Alternatively, intraoperative ultrasound B-mode imaging with Doppler flow velocity measurement can be used. Postoperative arteriography is also performed to verify the operative result.

a

b

c

Transaortic endarterectomy

The atherosclerotic lesion in the celiac axis is invariably limited to the very proximal portion of this short artery. Even when this vessel is occluded by atherosclerosis, the distal half of the artery maintains its patency as a result of collateral flow through its three terminal branches. SMA occlusion is generally more extended. When the orifice is occluded the clot usually progresses to the first major distal branch, 5–8 cm from the origin. The short lesion in celiac stenosis or occlusion is easily removed by a simple transaortic endarterectomy. The longer lesion in SMA occlusion may require an additional angioplasty. Transarterial endarterectomy through the diseased vessel only is no longer used because of the difficulty in removing the aortic intimal lesion surrounding the visceral artery orifice. The ventral course of the visceral arteries and the position of the SMA under the pancreas make access for endarterectomy of these arteries extremely difficult with the conventional transperitoneal approach. It is technically feasible, but exposure is not optimal. This problem has been solved by the use of the thoracoabdominal retroperitoneal approach which provides complete exposure of the aorta and its visceral and renal branches from the distal thoracic aorta to the aortic bifurcation (Stoney, Ehrenfeld and Wylie, 1977). This approach is particularly advantageous in the presence of coexistent distal aortic or aortorenal

atherosclerotic disease requiring additional surgical repair. Recently, we have used a new exposure that eliminates the need for thoracotomy and generally gives the same exposure as the thoracoabdominal incision and dissection. The exposure is provided by bilateral subcostal incisions with extra extension to the patient's left. By the same retroperitoneal dissection previously described, aortic exposure is readily obtained. This exposure allows for either visceral, renal and aortic endarterectomy, or antegrade aortovisceral, or aortorenal bypass. By avoiding thoracotomy, this exposure is much better tolerated by the patient.

Operative technique

The left chest is elevated 45° with the patient supine on the operating table. A posterolateral thoracic incision is made through the 8th interspace and is advanced across the costal margin to the midline where it can be extended to the pubis if necessary. Following retroperitoneal dissection the peritoneum with its contents is retracted to the patient's right. The left hemidiaphragm is transected circumferentially approximately 2–3 cm from the chest wall to try and avoid denervation of the diaphragm. The supraceliac aorta is exposed by dividing the crural fibres in the midline. After resection of the ganglionic fibres on the anterior surface of the aorta the body of pancreas can be lifted up slightly while dissection of the trunk of the SMA is completed.

3a, b & c

After application of proximal and distal aortic clamps as well as individual clamps on the visceral and renal arteries, excellent exposure of the celiac and the SMA orifices is provided by a 'trap door' aortotomy in the anterolateral aortic wall. The dissected renal vein is retracted caudally.

If the aortic atheroma is confined to the anterior aorta, the endarterectomy is limited to the undersurface of the 'trap door' as shown here. When advanced atheromatous disease involves the whole circumference of the aorta, a sleeve endarterectomy is performed. The aortic intima is transected to the cleavage plane in the outer media and the aortic endarterectomy is carried out.

3

a

b

c

3d, e & f

Removal of intimal lesions of the visceral artery orifice is then performed individually. Gentle traction is applied to the freed aortic intimal core while the media of the visceral artery is pushed away by a blunt dissection instrument (d). In the celiac artery this intimal core separates easily at the well demarcated atherosclerotic end-point under direct vision. In the SMA, the atherosclerotic lesion is usually longer and the distal end-point may not be reached by a transaortic endarterectomy alone if the occlusion extends distally. Therefore, the orifice lesion is first removed from the transaortic approach and, after closure of the aortotomy and restoration of renal and aortic blood flow, the SMA is clamped across its endarterectomized origin. A longitudinal aortotomy is made to a point just beyond the end of the occlusion. The thrombus is removed by thromboendarterectomy (e) and the arteriotomy is closed with a vein patch (f). When concomitant renal artery stenosis is present, the longitudinal portion of the aortotomy is extended to an infrarenal level to facilitate a transaortic renal endarterectomy.

As with the bypass grafting procedures, the adequacy of the endarterectomy is checked by electromagnetic flow probe measurement or ultrasound B-mode imaging with Doppler flow measurement. Intraoperative arteriography is rarely performed.

Transaortic visceral endarterectomy via the thoracoretroperitoneal approach is thus particularly useful in good risk patients for simultaneous correction of coexisting renal artery-lesions and aortic atherosclerotic disease (occlusive or aneurysmal). In poorer risk patients, the extended subcostal retroperitoneal is indicated. The mean aortic occlusion time has been approximately 26 min. Results have been excellent in over 90% of symptomatic patients and the operations have remained durable. In cases with acute visceral artery occlusion and bowel infarction, however, a transperitoneal approach is needed. Thrombectomy and endarterectomy are the necessary techniques, along with appropriate bowel resection. Synthetic grafts in this situation are contraindicated.

Postoperative care, complications and results

Intravenous infusion and nasogastric suction are maintained until the return of normal bowel movements. Prolonged supraceliac occlusion of the aorta may cause acute tubular necrosis (rare), and urinary output should therefore be monitored and kept at a high level. Traumatic pancreatitis may occur from excessive manipulation of the pancreas during its dissection and retraction (rare). In over 250 cases requiring supraceliac clamping other than for pararenal or thoracoabdominal aneurysmal disease, there have been no instances of paraplegia. Bowel infarction may occur due to graft occlusion or damage of pre-existing collaterals during the revascularization procedure, although this has not been experienced in this series.

Since 1959, over 150 cases of chronic visceral ischaemia have been treated. Of these, 128 patients were treated via transaortic thromboendarterectomy and 38 had aortovisceral bypass; 90 had endarterectomy and 38 had antegrade bypass. During late follow-up (mean 63 months), two patients from each group had recurrent symptoms of mesenteric ischaemia and all patients underwent successful reoperation. Four patients died in the perioperative period – three patients treated with endarterectomy and one with antegrade bypass. A total of 19% of the patients had perioperative cardiopulmonary complications which were primarily postoperative atelectasis and cardiac dysrhythmia. All other surviving patients have remained asymptomatic. We are not aware of a single case of enteric paraprosthetic fistula complicating an antegrade graft.

References

Dunphy, J. E. (1936). Abdominal pain of vascular origin. *American Journal of Medical Science* **192**, 102.

Ehrenfeld, W. K., Stoney, R. J. and Wylie, E. J. (1982). Autogenous arterial grafts. In *Biologic and Synthetic Vascular Prostheses*. Stanley, J. C., ed. New York: Grune and Stratton.

Mikkelson, W. P. (1957). Intestinal angina: Its surgical significance. *American Journal of Surgery* **94**, 262.

Rapp, J. H., Reilly, L. M., Qvarfordt, P. G., Goldstone, J., Ehrenfeld, W. K. and Stoney, R. J. (1985). Durability of endarterectomy and antegrade grafts in the treatment of chronic visceral ischemia. *Journal of Vascular Surgery* **3**, 799.

Stanley, J. C., Ernst, C. B. and Fry, W. J. (1973). Fate of 100 aortorenal vein grafts: Characteristics of late graft expansion, aneurysmal dilatation, and stenosis. *Surgery* **74**, 931.

Stoney, R. J. and Wylie, E. J. (1976). Surgery of the celiac and mesenteric arteries. In *Vascular Surgery: Principles and Techniques*, 2nd ed. Haimovici, H., ed. New York: McGraw-Hill.

Stoney, R. J., Ehrenfeld, W. K. and Wylie, E. J. (1977). Revascularization methods in chronic visceral ischemia caused by atherosclerosis. Annals of Surgery. **186**, 468.

Stoney, R. J., Reilly, L. M. and Ehrenfeld, W. K. (1984). Chronic mesenteric ischemia and surgery for chronic viseral ischemia. In *Vascular Surgery: Principles and Practice*. Wilson, S. E., Veith, F., Hobson, R. W. and Williams, R. A. (eds.) New York: McGraw-Hill.

Wylie, E. J., Stoney, R. J. and Ehrenfeld, W. K. (1980). *Manual of Vascular Surgery*, Vol. 1. New York: Springer-Verlag.

Surgical techniques for renal artery revascularization

William K. Ehrenfeld MD
Professor of Surgery, University of California, San Francisco, California, USA

Peter G. Qvarfordt MD
Vascular Research Fellow, University of California, San Francisco, California, USA

Ronald J. Stoney MD
Professor of Surgery, University of California, San Francisco, California, USA

Introduction

Renovascular hypertension is the most common indication for renal artery surgery. Extended surgical experience with renovascular hypertension has been acquired since Goldblatt *et al* (1934) discovered the impact of renal artery stenosis. Occlusive lesions of the renal artery are predominantly due to atherosclerosis and fibromuscular dysplasia. A number of operative techniques have been used with varying results including nephrectomy, segmental renal artery resection with reanastomosis or aortic reimplantation, and transrenal artery thromboendarterectomy with and without patching. Two basic operations are currently recommended: *transaortic thromboendarterectomy* and *aortorenal bypass*.

Although control of hypertension has been the primary indication for surgical management, prevention of renal failure or retrieval of renal function has become an increasingly important goal in recent years. This has been possible due to improved surgical and anaesthetic techniques, including better monitoring and more precise volume replacement. Other indications for renal artery surgery include aneurysm, renal artery injury, renal artery embolism, abdominal coarctation and von Recklinghausen's disease.

Renal autotransplantation, using a pulsatile perfusion *ex vivo* technique, facilitates reconstruction of multiple branch lesions in fibromuscular dysplasia and atherosclerosis, previously treated only by nephrectomy (Stoney, Silane and Salvatierra, 1978). Although percutaneous transluminal angioplasty (PTA) has been offered as alternative treatment to operative correction, the short-term benefits and potential complications (perforation, emboli) and the variety of lesions that are particularly resistant to dilatation limit the use of PTA to patients unfit for operation or to restore some renal function prior to operative treatment. The place of PTA is as yet undetermined.

Prophylactic renal artery reconstruction is indicated, together with aortic surgery, for abdominal aortic aneurysm or advanced aortoiliac occlusive disease involving the renal arteries. Nephrectomy is indicated only in cases with severe atrophy or infarction without renal artery stenosis.

The choice of operative treatment for renovascular hypertension is based primarily on the findings of renal arteriography. A hypertensive patient is a candidate for renal revascularization if significant obstructive lesions in one or more renal arteries are present. The intravenous pyelogram (IVP) is a moderately reliable screening procedure. It may show reduced kidney size, delayed excretion and late contrast density. Scan technique ([133]I Hippuran renogram) is a useful monitor of viable parenchymal tissue. Split renal function tests give information on the degree of functional changes in both kidneys but are painful and usually unnecessary. Renal-systemic renin indices as a means of prognostication for renal artery construction are useful when definitive assays are obtained. Intraoperative open renal biopsy to distinguish infarction from renal parenchymal ischaemia may be useful in deciding between nephrectomy and renal construction.

Preoperative arrangements

Fluid, electrolyte and blood pressure monitoring are cornerstones in the preoperative management of patients with renovascular hypertension. Hydration and mannitol-induced diuresis prior to aortic clamping reduces the vulnerability of the kidney to operative ischaemia.

Renovascular hypertension secondary to atherosclerosis

Transaortic renal endarterectomy

Endarterectomy is particularly suitable for renal artery stenosis caused by atherosclerosis (Wylie, 1975). Atherosclerotic renal artery stenosis or occlusion typically involves the renal artery ostium and extends 1–2 cm into the artery with a well-demaracted, easily palpable end-point. The aorta at the level of and below the renal arteries is nearly always affected by the atherosclerosis.

There is a cleavage plane in the outer part of the media in the atherosclerotic portion which readily permits removal of the lesion by endarterectomy. Approximately 60% of patients have bilateral atherosclerotic narrowing of the renal arteries. Accessory renal arteries, present in 20%, are also often involved in the atherosclerotic disease.

The typical localization of the aortorenal atherosclerotic lesions makes aortorenal bypass grafting potentially less suitable in most cases because of:

1. Technical problems with the proximal anastomosis to the thickened, calcified aorta.
2. Progression of aortic atherosclerosis which predisposes to closure of the proximal aortorenal anastomosis.
3. The necessity of bilateral grafts to the renal arteries in many cases.

Transrenal artery endarterectomy is no longer used because of difficulties in removing the aortic intima surrounding the renal artery orifice. Transaortic endarterectomy is our primary procedure for atherosclerotic renal artery stenosis. This technique facilitates simultaneous revascularization of bilateral and accessory renal arteries and repair of the diseased portion of the aorta at the level of the renal arteries, all within 10–15 min of renal ischaemia. Furthermore, with this technique no graft tissue is added. Immediate and long-term results for transaortic endarterectomy are excellent or good in more than 90%. Endarterectomy is not used when the aorta is ectatic or frankly aneurysmal.

Operative technique

A midline incision is made from the xiphoid to the pubis to expose the upper and middle abdominal aorta and the renal arteries. The standard renal incisions through the flank or back are unsatisfactory because of inadequate exposure of the adjacent aorta and the opposite renal artery. The small bowel, protected by a plastic bag, is displaced laterally to the right and outside the abdominal cavity. The posterior peritoneum over the aorta is incised and the aorta is freed between the origin of the celiac axis and superior mesenteric arteries. Mobilization of the suprarenal aorta is facilitated by the division of the crura of the diaphragm. The neural tissue on the anterior surface of the aorta between the celiac and superior mesenteric arteries is dissected free of the aorta. Blunt-finger dissection exposes the posterolateral aspects of the proximal abdominal aorta. The left renal vein is dissected free and mobilized completely in order to gain access to the suprarenal aorta and the left renal artery that lies under the renal vein. Sometimes the gonadal and/or adrenal vein must be divided to facilitate exposure. The right renal artery is exposed by incising the posterior peritoneum lateral to the duodenum and by reflecting the duodenum and head of the pancreas.

1a–d

The aorta is then occluded proximal to the superior mesenteric artery and distally immediately above the inferior mesenteric artery. Prior to aortic clamping, 3000–5000 i.u of heparin is given intravenously. Individual clamps are applied to the superior mesenteric artery and the renal arteries distal to the atherosclerotic lesions. The lumbar arteries are occluded by a straight aortic clamp posterior to the aorta. A midline anterior aortotomy, approximately 8–10 cm long, is made from just above the distal aortic clamp extending proximally between the renal arteries and ending in a curved fashion to the left of the superior mesenteric artery in order to facilitate exposure of the origins of the renal arteries (a). The aortic intima is transected distal to the cleavage plane in the outer media and a sleeve endarterectomy of the aorta is then performed proximally to the level distal to the origin of the superior mesenteric artery, where the aortic intimal sleeve is transected with scissors (b). Removal of the renal artery intimal lesions is the performed individually. Gentle traction is applied to the freed aortic intimal core while the media of the renal artery is pushed away with a blunt dissection instrument (c). This manoeuvre facilitates a limited eversion endarterectomy. The intimal core separates readily at the well-defined atherosclerotic end-point under direct vision (d). On rare occasions this separation does not occur and an intimal flap results. If this occurs, the intimal flap must be sutured down to the media to prevent thrombosis and occlusion. A distal flap may also be removed by a distal transverse renal arteriotomy. This has been necessary in less than 1% of patients. The whole area should be flushed with heparin-saline solution and any loose intimal fragments removed.

After allowing for backbleeding, the aortotomy is closed with a 4/0 continuous suture. The renal ischaemia time rarely exceeds 15–20 min. The adequacy of the renal endarterectomy is assessed by finger compression of the renal arteries and operative arteriography (to rule out any intimal flap or other operative defect). Recently, intraoperative ultrasound B-mode imaging with Doppler flow velocity measurement has been introduced as an alternative to intraoperative angiography. In cases with unilateral renal artery stenosis and/or an aorta that is mainly unaffected by atherosclerotic disease, only a disc of aortic intima surrounding the affected renal artery orifice is removed. A tapered renal artery orifice is obtained by cutting a disc with a diameter twice the external diameter of the renal artery.

If renal ischaemia time exceeds or is expected to exceed 15–20 min, the kidney is protected by the intermittent infusion of 120 ml cold (4°C) saline solution (1000 ml of Ringer's lactate with 2500 i.u. heparin and 15 ml sodium bicarbonate 8.4%) directly into the renal artery at 15-min intervals, permitting renal ischaemia for almost 50–60 min.

Aortorenal bypass

Renal endarterectomy is not suitable in patients with extensive aortic degenerative disease and/or aneurysm formation, and it is not feasible if these changes are present in the renal arteries. In these cases graft replacement of the infrarenal aorta is performed (Wylie, Stoney and Ehrenfeld, 1980). A side-arm prosthetic graft from the aortic prosthesis is anastomosed end-to-end to the transected renal artery. The aorta is clamped proximal to the celiac artery well above the level of intimal degeneration to avoid trauma to the intima and/or embolization. The infrarenal aorta is transected and the aortic prosthesis with the side-arm in place is anastomosed to the aortic stump. The aortic clamp is then removed to an infrarenal position while the distal iliac or femoral anastomosis is completed. The renal side-arm is made with a 5- or 6-mm graft with flange on the proximal end anastomosed proximally to an elliptical incision on the side of the aortic prosthesis. The side-arm may be placed prior to aortic graft placement. In order to minimize turbulence in blood flow and thrombosis, an end-to-end, rather than an end-to-side, anastomosis is preferred.

2a & b

It is important that the graft is cut to a length that allows it to assume a natural curve as it lines up to the outflow artery. This can be estimated by pinching the distal end of the uncut graft while the proximal clamp is released. The appropriate point for the anastomosis is thus determined before the graft is cut (*a*). Following completion of the distal anastomosis, the graft should be slightly curved and align itself with the outflow artery. The end-to-end anastomosis is performed with interrupted 6/0 synthetic sutures. Pulse palpation, angiography and/or B-mode ultrasound imaging is then performed to ensure the accuracy of the procedure.

2

Renovascular hypertension secondary to fibromuscular dysplasia

Autogenous aortorenal bypass

3

Fibromuscular dysplasia is the second most frequent cause of renal artery stenosis and is commonly bilateral. It is more frequent in young and middle-aged women but it may also occur much less commonly in males and children. The aetiology of the condition is unknown. It is typially localized in the mid- and distal portion of the main renal artery and has a characteristic appearance by angiography ('string of beads'). The inset shows intimal lesions of fibromuscular dysplasia. These lesions are not amenable to endarterectomy.

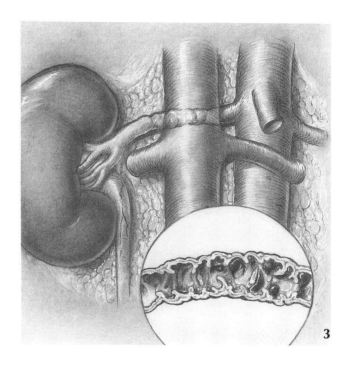

4a–d

Arterial autografts using the iliac or hypogastric artery (a–d) were introduced for aortorenal bypass of fibromuscular dysplasia in 1964 and have been used exclusively since that time for this disease (Stoney *et al.*, 1981). The arterial autograft is the ideal graft and is preferred to vein grafts since in general they do not stenose or become aneurysmal with time (Ehrenfeld, Stoney and Wylie, 1982).

The hypogastric artery is particularly suitable in children since it allows for growth and is expendable because of the rapid development of collateral circulation at the donor site. Excised internal iliac arteries, most frequently used as renal artery grafts, do not generally require replacement. Iliac artery donor sites are reconstructed with prosthetic grafts (b and c). The artery can be used in a branch configuration for replacement of the renal artery, including primary and secondary order branches (c and d).

The *ex vivo* technique is used to allow precise repair of branch lesions in arteries as small as 1 mm in diameter. Long-term assessment of 77 patients undergoing aortorenal arterial autograft reconstruction showed cure or improvement in 98% (Stoney *et al.*, 1981).

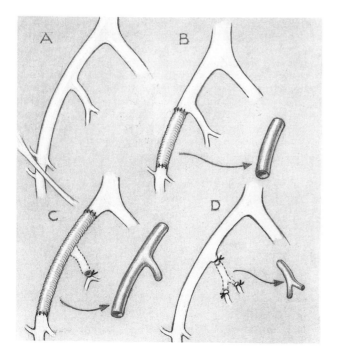

Operative technique

The operation is performed using a transabdominal approach. After exposure of the aorta and renal artery, the donor artery is mobilized circumferentially and excised. *Illustration 4* shows the harvesting sites of iliac artery autografts and the hypogastric artery autograft. After excision the autograft is preserved at normal temperature in heparinized saline.

5

In the presence of obliterating atherosclerosis, eversion endarterectomy is required prior to insertion. The arterial graft is anastomosed from the posterolateral side of the infrarenal abdominal aorta. The autograft is then anastomosed distally to the divided end of the main renal artery beyond the diseased segment, or at the level of the renal artery orifice if feasible. Placement at the latter level is rarely used as it may interfere with flow to the other kidney if present.

6

The hypogastric artery and its bifurcation branches can be used for the management of stenosing or aneurysmal lesions of the renal artery bifurcation. The illustration shows a branched hypogastric artery autograft anastomosed to the infrarenal aorta, positioned posterior to the vena cava, and anastomosed to the inferior polar artery in a patient with fibromuscular dysplasia of the distal renal artery. The superior polar artery is still being perfused by the main renal artery. A large aneurysm may involve multiple polar arteries. The common iliac artery with its external and internal artery segments can be used as an autograft for simultaneous bilateral renal artery reconstruction (*see Illustration 4c*). The proximal end of the harvested common iliac artery is then anastomosed to the anterior abdominal aorta or the thoracic aorta, and the external and internal iliac segments are anastomosed to reach each renal artery.

Postoperative care

Patients should be monitored closely with special attention to fluid and electrolyte management. Measurements of daily creatinine, BUN, CVP, body weight and hourly urinary output are determined to detect decreased renal function and to prevent over-hydration leading to cardiac failure and pulmonary oedema. Hypertension is common temporarily after operation and is treated with anti-hypertensive medication. Some degree of temporary tubular malfunction may occur and requires correction of the fluid and electrolyte losses. Renal failure caused by acute tubular necrosis is due to prolonged operative or postoperative ischaemia or hypotension secondary to hypovolaemia. These complications are preventable in the vast majority of cases by use of the techniques described.

References

Ehrenfeld, W. K., Stoney, R. J. and Wylie, E. J. (1982). Autogenous arterial grafts. In *Biologic and synthetic vascular prostheses*. Stanley, J. C., ed. London and San Diego: Grune and Stratton.

Goldblatt, H., Lynch, J., Hanzal, R. F., *et al.* (1934). Studies on experimental hypertension. I. The production of persistent elevation of systolic blood pressure by means of renal ischemia. *Journal of Experimental Medicine* 59, 347.

Stoney, R. J., Silane, M. and Salvatierra, O., Jr (1978). *Ex vivo* renal artery reconstruction. *Archives of Surgery* 113, 1272.

Stoney, R. J., DeLuccia, N., Ehrenfeld, W. K. and Wylie, E. J. (1981). Aortorenal arterial autografts – Long-term assessment. *Archives of Surgery* 116, 1416.

Wylie, E. J. (1975). Endarterectomy and autogenous arterial grafts in the surgical treatment of stenosing lesions of the renal artery. *Urologic Clinics of North America* 2, 351.

Wylie, E. J., Stoney, R. J. and Ehrenfeld, W. K. (1980). *Manual of Vascular Surgery*, Vol.I. New York: Springer-Verlag, p. 233.

Technical modifications in the repair of thoracoabdominal aortic aneurysms

Larry H. Hollier   MD, FACS, FACC
Chairman, Department of Surgery, Ochsner Clinic, New Orleans, Louisiana, USA

Introduction

Thoracoabdominal aortic aneurysms represent extensive deterioration of the aortic wall in patients who generally are elderly and often plagued with other degenerative diseases, especially hypertension and coronary artery disease. Failure to repair these aneurysms results in a 5-year survival rate of less than 20% (Bickerstaff *et al.*, 1982).

The advent of computerized tomography has aided greatly in the detection and delineation of the extent of thoracoabdominal aortic aneurysms. Additionally, simple suprarenal extension of abdominal aortic aneurysms are also being found with increasing frequency. In general, however, these latter aneurysms can be readily repaired by an abdominal approach and are not truly thoracoabdominal aneurysms. For purposes of this chapter, we limit the term thoracoabdominal aneurysm exclusively to mean aneurysms involving the origin of *all* the major visceral arteries. Clearly, these aneurysms require extensive technical reconstruction with revascularization of celiac, superior mesenteric and both renal arteries, as well as the spinal cord and the lower extremities.

144

1a, b & c

Using this criterion to delineate thoracoabdominal aneurysms, we find three clinical presentations: type I, which is essentially a thoracic aneurysm that extends inferiorly to the extent that it involves the visceral vessels; type II, the classic, diffuse thoracoabdominal aneurysm with extensive involvement of the aorta both above and below the visceral arteries; type III, a thoracoabdominal aneurysm in which the aorta above the visceral arteries is relatively normal.

The patterns are easily differentiated by computerized tomography, with type III aneurysms being identified most commonly in our experience. Although the type II thoracoabdominal aneurysm is best treated by the classic technique described by Crawford (1974), the other anatomical configurations allow for modifications in surgical approach so that operative time can be reduced and visceral revascularization can be facilitated. These technical modifications were actually suggested in Crawford's early publications (Crawford, 1974; Crawford et al., 1978), but their utility has not been appreciated by most surgeons.

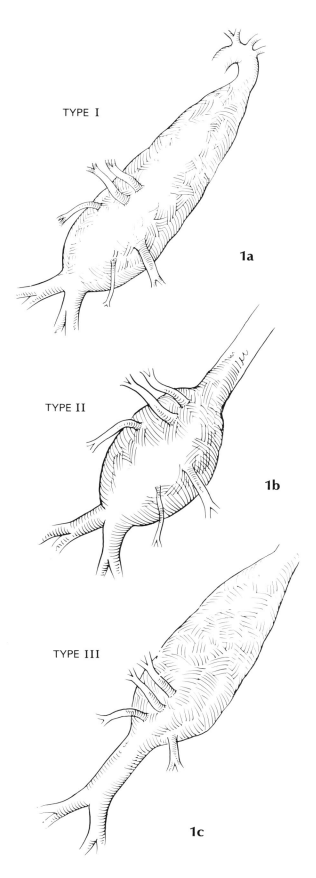

TYPE I

1a

TYPE II

1b

TYPE III

1c

Techniques

2a & b

For all cases of thoracoabdominal aneurysm repair, the patient is placed in a semilateral position, with the buttocks resting flat on the operating table, but with the chest and shoulders rotated approximately 45° anteriorly. The left arm is placed on an arm-rest rotated above and anterior to the patient's head.

The chest, abdomen and groins are scrubbed with povid-one-iodine solution, then covered with sterile drapes and an adhesive plastic skin barrier. The incision extends upward from the pubis to the umbilicus, then obliquely to the left up across the costal margin and through the appropriate intercostal space. If the aneurysm involves the abdominal aorta and the origin of the visceral vessels but terminates in normal or near-normal aorta near the diaphragm (type III), the thoracic portion of the incision is usually placed through the 9th or 10th intercostal space. If the mid- or upper thoracic aorta is involved with contiguous aneurysmal change (type I or II), the 4th or 5th intercostal space is incised.

Exposure of the infradiaphragmatic aortic may be accomplished either extraperitoneally or transperitoneally. However, if endarterectomy of the right renal, celiac or superior mesenteric artery is required, the transperitoneal approach allows more thorough inspection of the distal vessel beyond the site of endarterectomy. Except for type I thoraco-abdominal aneurysms, it is easier to reflect the left kidney along with spleen, pancreas and left colon, to expose the entire course of the aorta.

To complete exposure of the thoracoabdominal aorta, the diaphragm is divided in a circumferential rather than radial fashion, since this allows function of the left hemi-diaphragm to be preserved. We place alternating green and black marking sutures in the edges of the diaphragm as it is cut so that precise approximation can be achieved at the time of closure.

Prior to manipulation of the renal vessels, mannitol 25 g and lasix 10 mg are given intravenously. This places the kidneys in a diuretic state, thereby lessening the risk of acute tubular necrosis from renal ischaemia. Systemic heparin is not given, but the visceral vessels are irrigated with heparinized saline after opening the aorta later in the operation.

After exposure to the thoracoabdominal aorta, the extent of aneurysmal change in relation to the visceral vessels is assessed. As the greatest risk in thoracoabdominal aneurysm repair is myocardial infarction related to increased left ventricular afterload and subendocardial ischaemia, every effort should be made to minimize clamping time. Some surgeons have suggested the use of femorofemoral bypass or heparin-coated shunts to reduce ventricular strain, but additional complications have been noted as a direct result of these techniques. In our experience, intravenous nitroprusside has been a safe and useful means of pharmacologically off-loading the left ventricle and it avoids the problems of shunts and extracorporeal circulation. Despite vasodilatation techniques, however, prolonged cross-clamping of the thoracic aorta should be avoided, not only because of the cardiac risk, but also to lessen the risk of paraplegia.

2a

2b

Diffuse thoracoabdominal aneurysm

3

When widespread aneurysmal changes are noted throughout the aorta, we perform graft replacement in the manner popularized by Crawford. The entire aneurysm is exposed, proximal and distal occluding clamps are placed, and a vertical arteriotomy is made through the lateral wall along the entire length of the aneurysm. If the left kidney is left in place, the left renal vein is mobilized so that the graft may be passed beneath it without difficulty. After opening the aneurysm, a catheter is placed in the left renal artery and the kidney is perfused with iced heparinized saline to irrigate and cool it during ischaemia.

3

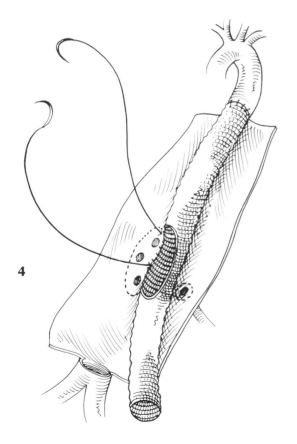

4

4

A low porosity woven graft is then sutured, end-to-end, to the partially transected proximal thoracic aorta using 0-polypropylene suture on a V-7 needle. Felt pledgets are commonly used to reinforce the anastomotic line. After the proximal anastomosis has been completed, any patent intercostal arteries are reimplanted into the graft after excising an elliptical section of the graft posteriorly. It is often possible to re-anastomose two or three pairs of intercostal arteries in one such anastomosis. Occasionally, a proximal intercostal artery can be revascularized by tailoring the proximal anastomosis obliquely to include these vessels. After intercostals have been reimplanted, the clamp is removed distally and flow is restored to the intercostal arteries. A button of graft is then excised opposite the orifices of the celiac, superior mesenteric and right renal arteries. The graft is then sutured side-to-side to the aorta with 0-polypropylene suture, encompassing the origins of all three vessels as a single anastomosis.

5

Flow is then restored to these vessels. The total occlusion time thus far is usually no more than 30 min. Because flow through these vessels is generally more than 2000 ml per min, its early restoration provides excellent off-loading of the left ventricle. The distal anastomosis to the aortic bifurcation is then performed and flow is cautiously restored to the lower extremities. If significant iliac disease is present, a woven bifurcation graft may be used instead of the straight graft.

After lower extremity flow has been restored, the left renal artery may be implanted into the graft directly.

5

6

6

If stenosis of the left renal artery is noted, we use a short-segment (6 or 8 mm) Dacron graft to revascularize the left kidney. After completion of all anastomoses, the sac of the aneurysm is closed tightly around the graft for added haemostasis.

Vessels are examined for adequacy of pulses, and flows are measured in the revascularized arteries. The abdominal viscera are then restored to their normal anatomical position and the diaphragm is closed with interrupted horizontal mattress sutures of 2/0 braided Dacron. Two chest tubes are placed through separate stab incisions to drain the left chest, and the chest and abdominal incisions are closed in layers in standard fashion.

Low thoracoabdominal aneurysm

With increasing frequency, we see patients who have thoracoabdominal aneurysms which involve the entire abdominal aorta, including the site of origin of the visceral vessels, but in whom the aorta is relatively normal from the diaphragm upwards. In this situation we find that slight technical modifications can significantly reduce the time of increased afterload on the left ventricle.

7

A low thoracoabdominal approach is utilized (see *Illustration 2a*), and the aorta is dissected as previously described, although only the lower third of the thoracic aorta need be exposed in these cases. Because of the proximity of normal aorta to the visceral vessels, clamp time can be minimized by including a tongue of aorta bearing the orifices of these vessels in an oblique proximal anastomosis.

8

The woven low-porosity Dacron graft is trimmed as shown and an anastomosis is fashioned to provide revascularization of the celiac, superior mesenteric and right renal arteries in conjunction with the proximal anastomosis. The proximal clamp can then be repositioned on to the graft below the right renal artery and visceral flow can be restored. Total occlusion time to this stage of the procedure is usually 15 min.

7

8

9

9

The distal anastomosis and left renal revascularization are then performed as previously described, and the sac of the aneurysm is closed over the graft with a running suture of 3/0 polypropylene.

10, 11 & 12

Thoracic aneurysm with abdominal extension

Some patients present with thoracoabdominal aneurysms that are primarily thoracic aneurysms, but the aneurysmal changes extend down below the diaphragm and involve the aorta at the site of origin of the visceral vessels. In such cases, operative time may be reduced by incorporating the visceral revascularization with the distal anastomosis. Total aortic occlusion time in these cases is generally no more than 30 min.

In all variations of revascularization procedures described here, the visceral and spinal artery anastomoses are performed in a side-to-side fashion; that is, the aortic wall is not incised in 'button' fashion around the orifices, but the reimplantations are done by suturing into the inside of the intact aortic wall. This is most clearly shown in *Illustration 4*.

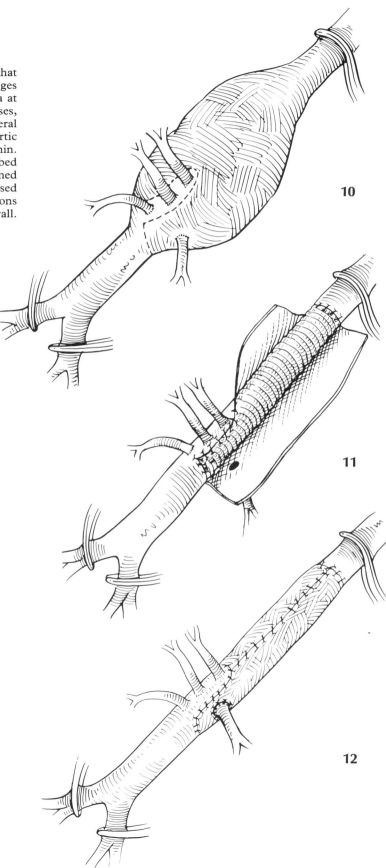

10

11

12

Prevention of paraplegia

Despite the use of evoked potential monitoring, heparin-bonded shunts, femorofemoral or atriofemoral bypass, or routine intercostal reimplantation, paraplegia still occurs. Obviously, when technically feasible, use of shunts or bypass can reduce the risk of paraplegia if clamp time is expected to be prolonged, but they are often ineffective, especially in type II aneurysms.

Recent experimental and clinical experience with spinal fluid drainage has suggested that this technique may improve spinal cord perfusion and may increase the safe clamp time. This may allow a longer safe interval in which to reimplant the intercostal arteries to revascularize the spinal cord.

After endotracheal anaesthesia is instituted, the patient is placed on his right side and an 18 gauge spinal needle is introduced intrathecally between the 4th and 5th lumbar vertebrae and a silastic catheter is introduced. A total of 10–15 dl of spinal fluid is withdrawn and the needle is withdrawn, leaving the intrathecal catheter in place; the catheter is then connected to a pressure transducer for continuous monitoring. If the spinal fluid pressure rises during the case, additional spinal fluid is withdrawn to keep the spinal pressure below 10 mmHg.

It is important to remember that spinal fluid drainage alone does not prevent paraplegia and is not a substitute for intercostal artery reimplantation which is mandatory in some patients. Additionally, it seems unlikely that it will reduce the incidence of paraplegia that sometimes occurs several days after otherwise successful repair of thoracoabdominal aneurysms.

Complications and results

Use of the techniques mentioned above has resulted in expeditious repair of thoracoabdominal aneurysms with acceptable morbidity and mortality. We have recently reported a series of 101 patients who underwent repair of non-dissecting thoracoabdominal aneurysms. Of these, 55 underwent elective thoracoabdominal aneurysm repair by this author without the use of shunts or bypass; the overall mortality was 2% and none of these patients required dialysis, although transient creatinine elevation was seen with some

frequency. The most common complication encountered was pulmonary, particularly the need for prolonged ventilation. Paraplegia or paraparesis occurred in 6% of patients. In two of the three patients done early in the series, intercostal reimplantation had not been done; the third patient developed paraplegia despite reimplantation of the single pair of patent intercostal arteries. Spinal drainage had not been used in any of the patients in that series. Since then, however, routine spinal fluid drainage has been instituted and we have not yet seen paraplegia occur when intercostal arteries have been reimplanted. A single patient with contained rupture of a type II thoracoabdominal aneurysm had spinal drainage but did not have any intercostal artery reimplantation performed – despite normal neurologic function after surgery, she did develop sudden paraparesis on the 5th postoperative day.

Continuing experience and the relaxation of surgical indications will undoubtedly increase the mortality and morbidity of any series. None the less, careful preoperative evaluation and preparation, careful and expeditious surgical technique, and meticulous attention to postoperative management, will improve salvage in patients with thoracoabdominal aortic aneurysms.

References

Bickerstaff, L. K., Pairolero, P. C., Hollier, L. H., et al. (1982). Thoracic aortic aneurysms: A population-based study. Surgery 92(6), 1103

Bower, T. C., Murray, M. J., Gloviczki, P., et al. (in press). The effects of thoracic aortic occlusion and cerebrospinal fluid drainage on regional spinal cord blood flow in dogs: Correlation with neurologic outcome. Journal of Vascular Surgery.

Crawford, E.S. (1974). Thoracoabdominal and abdominal aortic aneurysms involving renal, superior mesenteric, and celiac arteries. Annals of Surgery 179(5), 763.

Crawford, E. S., Snyder, D. M., Cho, G. C., et al. (1978). Progress in treatment of thoracoabdominal and abdominal aortic aneurysms involving celiac, superior mesenteric and renal arteries. Annals of Surgery 188(4), 404.

Hollier, L. H. (1987). Protecting the brain and spinal cord. Journal of Vascular Surgery 5(3), 524.

Hollier, L. H., Symmonds, J. B., Pairolero, P. C., Cherry, K. J., et al. (1988). Thoracoabdominal aortic aneurysm repair: Analysis of postoperative morbidity. Archives of Surgery 123, 871.

McCullogh, J. L., Hollier, L. H. and Nugent, M. (1988). Paraplegia after thoracic aortic occlusion: Influence of cerebrospinal fluid drainage. Journal of Vascular Surgery 7(1), 153.

Abdominal aortic aneurysms

John A. Mannick MD
Moseley Professor of Surgery, Harvard Medical School;
Surgeon-in-Chief, Brigham and Women's Hospital, Boston, Massachusetts, USA

Anthony D. Whittemore MD
Assistant Professor of Surgery, Harvard Medical School;
Surgeon, Brigham and Women's Hospital, Boston, Massachusetts, USA

Introduction

The indication for repair of an abdominal aortic aneurysm is the presence of an aneurysm of significant size in a patient of any age who does not have another non-correctable, life-threatening condition. It is generally conceded that aneurysms which have reached 6 cm in diameter are in danger of rupturing and surgery for such aneurysms is clearly indicated. There is some debate as to whether aneurysms of smaller diameter than 6 cm are likely to rupture. Our own practice has been to operate electively on aneurysms greater than 5 cm in diameter. We seldom operate on aneurysms smaller than this. Patients with tender aneurysms or with symptoms of back pain or abdominal pain suggesting recent expansion in aneurysm require urgent surgery. Obviously, a patient with the diagnosis of a ruptured abdominal aortic aneurysm should be taken to the operating room immediately.

In addition to standard preoperative preparation, it has been our practice for the past decade to study every patient undergoing elective or urgent aneurysm repair by inserting a Swan-Ganz catheter preoperatively (Whittemore *et al.*, 1980). Several points on the ventricular performance curve are then determined for each individual so that a pulmonary capillary wedge pressure can be selected which will result in a desirable cardiac index on the upslope of the individual's ventricular performance curve. Volume replacement during surgery can be regulated to maintain this optimal pulmonary capillary wedge pressure and thus ensure adequate tissue perfusion throughout the operation. Declamping hypotension can also be minimized with this technique.

We routinely perform preoperative aortography using the retrograde Seldinger technique in order to define the upper extent of the aneurysm better in relation to the renal arteries and to ensure that there are no anomalous renal arteries arising from the aneurysm itself. We obtain biplane views to ensure patency of the superior mesenteric artery and celiac axis since aneurysm repair will involve ligation of the origin of the inferior mesenteric artery.

We believe that it is helpful to recover shed blood during the course of aneurysm surgery by the use of a Cell Saver. Since we began using this device 7 years ago, approximately 30% of patients undergoing elective abdominal aneurysm repair have not required banked blood transfusions.

The operation

The technique of aneurysm repair employed by our service is a modification of the graft inclusion technique previously described by Creech (1966) and Javid *et al.* (1982).

1

The abdomen is opened and explored through a midline incision extending from the pubis to the xiphoid. The small bowel is lifted superiorly and to the right, and is packed outside the abdominal cavity in a Lahey bag. The peritoneum is incised with scissors along the inferior border of the third and fourth portions of the duodenum, and the duodenum is retracted superiorly. The peritoneum and areolar tissue overlying the aorta are opened longitudinally, exposing the anterior surface of the aneurysm.

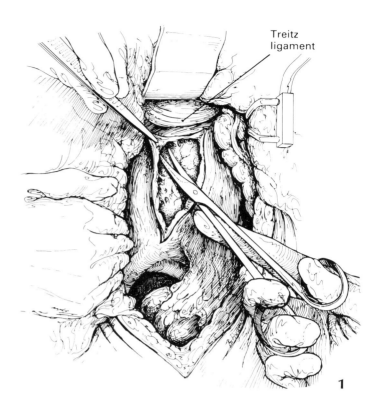

Treitz ligament

1

2

The incision is carried superiorly to the level of the left renal vein and inferiorly 2.5-5 cm beyond the aortic bifurcation. The aorta just above the aneurysm and below the left renal vein is freed from its surrounding tissues by sharp dissection anteriorly and laterally. No attempt is made to dissect behind the aorta at this level, nor is the neck of the aneurysm encircled with tape. However, the dissection along each lateral wall of the aorta is continued far enough posteriorly so that the neck of the aneurysm can be compressed easily by an occluding clamp which will be applied at this level.

Inferiorly, the anterior and lateral walls of both common iliac arteries are freed by sharp dissection in a similar fashion without separating these vessels from their attachments to the common iliac veins posteriorly. If it is convenient at this point, the inferior mesenteric artery is temporarily controlled with a bulldog clamp near its origin from the aorta as illustrated. In most instances, the origin of the inferior mesenteric artery is ligated from inside the aneurysm at a later stage. Ligation and division of the inferior mesenteric artery away from its origin is avoided for fear of damage to vital collateral branches which feed the sigmoid colon. Dissection of the lateral walls of the aneurysm is kept to a minimum to eliminate the necessity for ligating multiple small vessels that traverse the surrounding lymphatic and areolar tissue. Dissection of the aneurysm wall from the inferior vena cava is particularly avoided to reduce the risk of injury to that structure.

Heparin is administered to the patient systemically intravenously, 4000–5000 u in an average adult. While it is possible to repair many, if not most, abdominal aortic aneurysms successfully without the use of heparin, it is advisable to heparinize the patient partially when the aorta and iliac arteries are clamped; otherwise, extensive distal thrombosis can occur in patients who have severe distal arterial occlusive disease and in those instances where mural thrombus or arteriosclerotic debris from the aneurysm is inadvertently embolized distally. It has been our experience that retrograde thrombosis is kept to a minimum in such instances before the embolic debris is retrieved if the patient has been prophylactically heparinzied.

2

3

After heparinization, large straight Fogarty vascular clamps are applied to both common iliac arteries and a deBakey reverse-angle aortic clamp is applied to the aorta above the aneurysm. The aneurysm is then opened longitudinally with a knife.

3

4

The incision in the aneurysm is completed with Mayo scissors.

4

5

All mural thrombus and loose arteriosclerotic debris is
evacuated from the lumen of the aneurysm.

5

6

The origins of bleeding lumbar arteries are oversewn with
figure-of-eight sutures of 3/0 polypropylene. The origin of
the inferior mesenteric artery is similarly sutured if this vessel
is still patent and the bulldog clamp removed.

6

155

7

In patients with no significant iliac aneurysms, a tube graft of woven Dacron is preferred for aneurysm replacement. This graft will be sutured distally to the aortic bifurcation which usually remains of reasonably normal size even when the aneurysm involves the entire infrarenal abdominal aorta. Cuffs may be cut proximally and distally extending partially down each side of the aorta at the neck of the aneurysm above and at the aortic bifurcation below. However, in large aneurysms, we have found it just as convenient to avoid this step and simply to suture the graft to the ring of normal vessel superiorly and inferiorly.

8

The posterior wall of the aorta is not divided either proximally or distally. The posterior aortic wall is often a rather tenuous structure and we prefer to add strength to the posterior suture line by including the surrounding fascial tissue in the posterior stitches of the anastomosis. A woven Dacron tube graft of appropriate size is sewn with a double-armed polypropylene suture to the posterior wall of the aorta at the neck of the aneurysm. A double-thickness of aortic wall is included in each bite posteriorly.

7

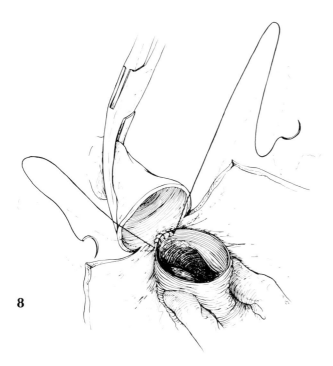

8

9

The suture is carried around each side of the neck of the aneurysm and tied anteriorly.

9

156

10

The proximal anastomosis is then tested for leaks by clamping the tube graft and releasing the aortic clamp briefly. This also serves to preclot the graft despite the partial heparinization of the patient by filling the interstices of the Dacron mesh with platelets and fibrin. If any leaks are noted in the anastomosis they are repaired with simple or figure-of-eight sutures of 3/0 polypropylene. The aortic clamp may then be reapplied or, if preferred, the graft may be clamped just distal to the proximal anastomosis.

10

11

After being evacuated of all blood with a sucker, the graft is placed under slight tension and cut to the appropriate length for anastomosis with the aortic bifurcation.

11

12

The lower anastomosis is performed using a double-armed suture of 3/0 polypropylene.

All vessels are flushed before completion of this suture line. If there is adequate backbleeding from both iliac systems no attempt is made to pass Fogarty catheters distally to retrieve possible emboli. The suture line is then completed and tied anteriorly as for the proximal anastomosis. The iliac clamps are released and the lower anastomosis is inspected for leaks which are repaired as for the proximal anastomosis. The proximal aortic clamp is then gradually released while the anaesthetist carefully monitors the patient's blood pressure and infuses extra volume intravenously if needed. If the patient has been maintained with an optimal pulmonary capillary wedge pressure, declamping hypotension is ordinarily not observed. After release of clamps the iliac arteries are inspected for adequate pulsations and the presence of good femoral pulses in the groin is determined by palpation. The heparin is then neutralized with protamine sulphate.

12

13

13

After reversal of the heparin any residual bleeding points in the aneurysm wall are sutured, ligated or electrocoagulated and the aneurysm wall is sutured back over the prosthesis with a running stitch of polypropylene. This manoeuvre ordinarily covers both the proximal and distal suture line with residual aneurysm wall.

If the wall is too large to fit conveniently around the prosthesis it may be overlapped in vest-over-pants fashion as a double suture line. We have found that this is usually more convenient than trimming the wall, since trimming often produces further bleeding which must then be controlled. The periaortic tissues are then approximated over the aorta and, if possible, over the resutured aneurysm wall by a second running suture of polyglycolate in order to provide further retroperitoneal haemostasis. This also has the advantage of placing yet another layer between the prosthesis and the posterior wall of the duodenum. The posterior peritoneum is then closed over the aorta and resutured aneurysm wall with a second running suture of polyglycolate. It is ordinarily possible to interpose the peritoneum as an additional layer between the posterior wall of the duodenum and the aorta. The abdomen is then closed using the mass closure technique with continuous strong polypropylene.

14

Iliac aneurysms

If common iliac aneurysms are present, a similar operative procedure is followed. However, the iliac clamps are applied to the iliac bifurcations, taking care to avoid injury to the ureters which usually cross the common iliac arteries distally. Iliac aneurysms are opened longitudinally. A bifurcation graft of woven Dacron is used and the upper anastomosis is performed as described. The iliac limbs are sutured on either side to the distal common iliac arteries, again from inside the iliac aneurysms. The aneurysm walls may also be sutured back over the graft limbs to provide an extra layer of host tissue between the graft and the abdominal viscera.

14

Proximally extended abdominal aortic aneurysms

In cases where the abdominal aortic aneurysm extends more proximally than usual and there is little or no neck of normal aorta between the aneurysm and the renal arteries, it is helpful to place the aortic clamp at the level of the diaphragm while the proximal anastomosis is performed.

15

The aorta at the level of the diaphragm can be exposed by incising the attachments of the left lobe of the liver to the diaphragm and retracting the liver to the right. The lesser sac is entered and the aorta is exposed as it passes underneath the crus of the diaphragm.

15

16 & 17

With finger dissection, the crus can be stretched and split enough so that a clamp can be applied to the aorta at the hiatus, where this vessel is usually of normal calibre and free of branches.

Backbleeding from the celiac axis and superior mesenteric artery can be controlled with an intra-aortic balloon catheter inserted from below, and the graft can be anastomosed proximally with excellent visibility from inside the aneurysm into the normal aorta just distal to the renal artery orifices. After completion of the proximal anastomosis, the aortic clamp is released and the prosthesis is clamped, restoring flow to the viscera and to the renal arteries. We believe that this manoeuvre is much less hazardous to the kidneys than attempts to clamp the aorta close to the renal artery orifices which may result in arteriosclerotic embolization to one or both kidneys.

The retroperitoneal approach

In some patients the retroperitoneal approach (Williams *et al.*, 1980) to abdominal aortic aneurysms is preferable. We believe this approach is especially indicated in patients who have had prior abdominal surgery in order to avoid the lysis of adhesions which would be necessary in the transabdominal approach. We believe the retroperitoneal approach is also indicated in those rare individuals with a horseshoe kidney and an abdominal aneurysm, and is probably the preferred approach in patients with inflammatory aneurysms since the attachment of the duodenum to the inflammatory aneurysm is not an issue with this approach. We have also found that the thick inflammatory aneurysm wall is usually thinner posteriorly than anteriorly. We now prefer the retroperitoneal approach in many patients with juxtarenal abdominal aneurysms since the crus of the diaphragm is readily visualized by this approach and can be divided with ease for application of a clamp to the supraceliac aorta.

18

For the retroperitoneal approach, the patient is placed in the left lateral thoracotomy position with the hips rotated back toward the supine position. The positioning of the patient is greatly aided through the use of a 'bean bag' moulded by suction. The incision is placed in the left flank beginning at the lateral border of the rectus muscle just below the umbilicus and extending out into the 11th interspace. The abdominal muscles are cut in the line of the incision and the peritoneum and left kidney are retracted medially and to the right. This allows easy visualization of the left posterolateral wall of the aorta, the left common iliac artery, and the origin of the left renal artery.

16

17

18

19, 20 & 21

The neck of the aneurysm can be exposed without difficulty below the left renal artery for application of a clamp. In those instances where aneurysmal disease extends to the region of the renal vessels, this approach can be ideal. It enables easy suprarenal control and the Dacron is tailored to enable a single oblique suture line to incorporate the origins of the renal arteries as shown. Exposure of the right common iliac artery is sometimes difficult with this approach and control of this vessel with a balloon catheter after the aneurysm has been opened is sometimes preferable. The operation is otherwise conducted as in the anterior transperitoneal approach. The aneurysm wall is closed back over the prosthesis at the completion of the procedure. Obviously, no closure of the periaortic tissues or the parietal peritoneum is possible or necessary.

We have not found retroperitoneal exposure to reduce operative time, operative blood loss or postoperative hospital stay, as has been claimed by some authors. In fact, postoperative discomfort, in our experience, is greater with this incision than with the midline abdominal incision. However, bowel function does appear to return earlier in the postoperative period with this approach.

We believe the retroperitoneal approach is relatively contraindicated in patients with right iliac aneurysms. These aneurysms would otherwise need to be dealt with through a separate right lower quadrant transperitoneal or retroperitoneal incision. We also believe that adequate exposure with this approach is difficult to achieve in patients with a high narrow costal arch in whom the distance from the incision to the diaphragm is great, mandating that the operation take place almost entirely underneath the shelf of the rib cage.

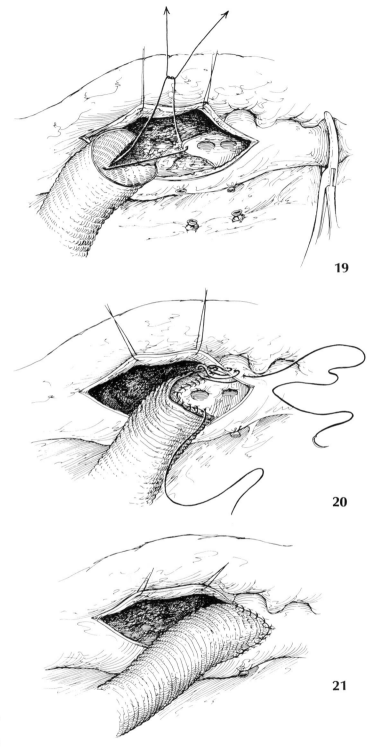

19

20

21

References

Creech, O., Jr (1966). Endo-aneurysmorrhaphy and treatment of aortic aneurysm. *Annals of Surgery* **164**, 935.

Javid, H., Julian, O. C., Dye, W. S., *et al.* (1982). Complications of abdominal aortic grafts. *Archives of Surgery* **85**, 650.

Whittemore, A. D., Clowes, A. W., Hechtman, H. B. and Mannick, J. A. (1980). Aortic aneurysm repair. Reduced operative mortality associated with maintenance of optimal cardiac performance. *Annals of Surgery* **192**, 414.

Williams, G. M., Ricotta, J., Zinner, M. and Burdick, J. (1980). The extended retroperitoneal approach for treatment of extensive atherosclerosis of the aorta and renal vessels. *Surgery* **88**, 846.

Surgical management of aorto-enteric fistulae

Roger N. Baird   ChM, FRCS
Consultant Surgeon, The Royal Infirmary, Bristol, UK

Introduction

Anaemia from gastrointestinal blood loss, whether of clinically silent onset, or following haematemesis or melaena, in a patient with an intra-abdominal arterial prosthesis, is caused by an aorto-enteric fistula until proved otherwise. This truth is self-evident to all vascular surgeons, but not, it seems, to those whose lack of awareness leads to numerous expensive and usually fruitless investigations, delaying the diagnosis and causing more than necessary blood loss and subsequent replacement (Thomas and Baird, 1986). Upper G.I. endoscopy detected only two-thirds (8 of 12) of fistulae in a recent series (Tilanus *et al.*, 1988), and arteriography will show extravasation of contrast into the duodenum only if bleeding is brisk when the investigation is being done. The decision to do a laparotomy is usually taken on clinical grounds.

Pathophysiology

1

Most fistulae arise between an aortic/Dacron anastomosis and the fourth part of the duodenum. Occasionally, the abnormal communication is between an iliac/Dacron anastomosis and the small bowel or the appendix or colon, and from the suture line of an aorto-iliac endarterectomy. Isolated examples have been reported in which a length of prosthesis remote from anastomoses erodes through the bowel wall, described as 'cannibalization' (Monson *et al.*, 1985) or 'paraprosthetic-enteric sinus' (Williams, Charlesworth and Jones, 1987).

The overall incidence of aorto-enteric fistulae following Dacron aortic bypass is low (0.5–2.5%) and gastrointestinal blood loss occurs without warning 6 months to 5 years or more after the original operation. The pathogenesis is unknown, but the routine use of antibiotic prophylaxis and the substitution of prolene for silk as the suture material have been associated with fewer reported cases.

Experimental studies suggest that close apposition alone is an inadequate cause without an added infective challenge (Busuttil *et al.*, 1979). Of course, efforts are needed to ensure that prosthetic tubes remain retroperitoneal to avoid loops of small bowel being trapped and causing intestinal obstruction.

1

2

At laparotomy, three separate categories can be recognized from the operative findings. First, a rupture of a false aneurysm into the bowel and, secondly, a simple fistula between the anastomosis and the duodenum. In both instances, there is no pus around the prosthesis, which remains well incorporated. In the third category, the infective process is advanced and the prosthesis lies slackly and unincorporated in a bed of pus throughout its length.

AORTO-ENTERIC FISTULAE

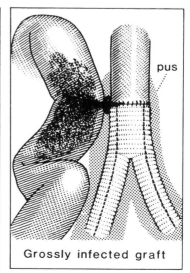

2

False aneurysm   Simple fistula   Grossly infected graft

pus

No gross graft sepsis

The operation

3

Full cardiovascular monitoring including arterial and central venous lines are mandatory. Wide bore venous access for rapid blood replacement is needed and at least 6 u of blood should be available. The abdomen is opened under antibiotic cover with a combination such as cefuroxine, metronidazole and gentamicin, and the fistula is disconnected.

3

4

The duodenal defect is repaired using two layers of catgut or vicryl. Attention is then turned to the aortic prosthesis and suture line. Provided that the aortic wall is not discoloured the prosthesis is well incorporated, and no obvious pus is present, the fistula is likely to be caused by mechanical weakness of the aortic wall.

4

5

Consideration is then given to a local repair, either by inserting 2–3 prolene sutures to close the defect, or by inserting a short Dacron tube to link the prosthesis to a more proximal aortic suture line without tension (Thomas and Baird, 1986; Eastcott, 1982).

5

6

If, on the other hand, the prosthesis is unincorporated and lies in a bag of pus encased by fibrous tissue, then it should be removed. Usually, the aortic stump is oversewn and an axillobifemoral bypass performed.

7

Added measures can help to reduce the risk of aortic stump blowout. These include double layers of sutures covering the closure with a flap of the anterior spinous ligament, and covering by omentum. However, Walker *et al.* (1987) has reported an alternative – placing a new prosthesis in the same location by primary exchange similar to the replacement of an infected heart valve.

The advocates of extra-anatomical bypass typically acknowledge a high operative mortality of 49% and an amputation rate of 27% resulting from this approach (O'Hara *et al.*, 1986). In an attempt to reduce the magnitude of the undertaking, staged operations for patients not actively bleeding are proposed. The axillobifemoral bypass is inserted first, and the infected prosthesis is removed later (Reilly *et al.*, 1987). The results have gradually improved in the last 20 years (Bouhoutsos *et al.*, 1974; Umpleby, Britton and Turnbull, 1987). Whichever procedure is done, the duodenum and aorta should be separated as far apart as possible to minimize the risk of a further aortoduodenal fistula. The omentum, mobilized if necessary, is used to wrap the aortic anastomosis or stump. Such is the anxiety about further gastrointestinal bleeding that there is even speculation that the duodenum might be transected and relocated in an antecolic position.

Less frequently, the fistula occurs between the distal anastomosis to the iliac arteries and the small bowel, appendix or colon or the mid-portion of the prosthesis erodes into the gut without anastomotic involvement. In these circumstances a local repair is usually done.

Conclusions

The general risks of treating aorto-enteric fistulae are those of major vascular surgery in arteriopaths rendered weak from blood loss. The likelihood of perioperative death and limb loss is increased if operation is precipitated by a major gastrointestinal bleed or if infection is a problem. Specifically, rupture of the aortic stump and infection of the axillofemoral bypass by cross-contamination are unsolved problems, as is recurrence of the aorto-enteric fistula leading to further haemastemesis and malaena. Further thrombosis without premonitory symptoms after months or years is a frequent problem with axillofemoral bypass and the patient should not stray too far from access to skilled hospital care, since urgent embolectomy may be required.

References

Bouhoutsos, J., Chavatzas, D., Martin, P. and Morris, T. (1974). Infected synthetic arterial grafts. *British Journal of Surgery* **61**, 108.

Busuttil, R. W., Rees, W., Baker, J. D. and Wilson, S. E. (1979). Pathogenesis of aortoduodenal fistula: Experimental and clinical correlates. *Surgery* **85**, 1.

Eastcott, H. H. G. (1982). Aorto-enteric fistula: Possibilities for direct repair. In *Extra-anatomic and Secondary Arterial Reconstruction.* Greenhalgh, R. M. ed. London: Pitman.

Monson, J. R. T., Courtney, D. G., Jones, N. A. G. and Kester, R. C. (1985). Cannabilization of a Goretex aortohepatic graft by the duodenum. *British Journal of Surgery* **72**, 101.

O'Hara, P. J., Hertzer, N. R. Beven, E. G. and Krajewski, L. P. (1986). Surgical management of infected abdominal aortic grafts: Review of a 25 year experience. *Journal of Vascular Surgery* **3**, 725.

Reilly, L. M., Stoney, R. J., Goldstone, J. and Ehrenfeld, W. K. (1987). Improved management of aortic graft infection: The influence of operation sequence and staging. *Journal of Vascular Surgery* **5**, 421.

Thomas, W. E. G., Baird, R. N. (1986). Secondary aortic-enteric fistulae: Towards a more conservative approach. *British Journal of Surgery* **73**, 875.

Tilanus, H. W., Terpstra, O. T., de Smit, P., van Urk, H. and Veen, H. F. (1988). Diagnosis and management of graft-enteric fistulae. *British Journal of Surgery* **75**, 915.

Umpleby, H. C., Britton, D. C. and Turnbull, A. R. (1987). Secondary arterio-enteric fistulae: A surgical challenge. *British Journal of Surgery* **74**, 256.

Walker, W. E., Cooley, D. A., Duncan, J. M., Hallman, G. L., Ott, D. A. and Reul, G. J. (1987). The management of aortoduodenal fistula by *in situ* replacement of the infected aortic graft. *Annals of Surgery* **205**, 727.

Williams, G. T., Charlesworth, and Jones, D. L. (1987). Entrovesical fistula due to a Dacron aortic graft. *British Journal of Surgery* **74**, 645.

Surgery for vasculogenic impotence

Ralph G. DePalma MD

Chairman, Department of Surgery, George Washington University Medical Center, Washington, D.C., USA

Michael J. Olding MD

Department of Surgery, George Washington University Medical Center, Washington, D.C., USA

Introduction

Operations for vasculogenic impotence are performed on large arteries: aortoiliac to distal branching of the internal iliacs, small arteries including the internal pudendal, proper penile arteries, and upon the venous penile drainage. The physiological basis for erection depends on adequate arterial inflow combined with closure of cavernous veins, both mediated by an intact neural mechanism. In selecting candidates for operation, an accurate diagnosis of a physiological defect is essential. Only 10–15% of impotent men are candidates for vascular interventions. Vascular impotence can be purely arteriogenic, purely venogenic, or combined arterial and venogenic. It has recently been shown that arterial inflow mediates cavernosal closure of venous outflow. During normal erection, intracavernosal pressure increases to levels approximating 80 mmHg, with little or no cavernosal venous outflow. Preoperative physiological testing for surgery outlined by DePalma *et al.*, (1987) and Michal (1985) is described.

Preoperative considerations

Penile brachial pressure indices (PBPI)

Reappearance of Doppler signals are detected distal to a pressure cuff placed at the base of the penis. The pressure is noted and expressed as a ratio between pressure in the distal branches of dorsal arteries over systemic pressure. A ratio above 0.75 in the flaccid state suggests that no major obstacle exists to blood flow in the aortoiliac system. PBPI may not detect lesions of the pudendal or penile arteries, which do not become evident until demand is placed on these vessels by the erectile process.

Penile pulse volume recording

Using an air plethysmographic cuff with a transducer contained, penile expansion in response to flow is recorded in the flaccid state. The variables characterizing pulse wave are crest time, waveform and the presence or absence of dicrotic notch. The waveform reflects the pulsatility, i.e. the contribution of all the arterial elements of penile expansion. It more sensitively separates impotent from potent patients in whom borderline PBPIs range from 0.6 to 0.75 (Stauffer and DePalma, 1983). It also detects small vessel disease when PBPIs are normal.

Artificial erection, cavernosal artery closing pressure and cavernosometry

These tests require injection of a pharmacological agent (e.g. papaverine) to produce an artificial erection. Two 19-gauge needles are inserted into the cavernous bodies, one for pressure recording and one for calibrated infusion of warm heparinized saline. Infusion rates to obtain and maintain erection are measured. These rates are compared before and after papaverine injection. A maintenance rate of less than 40–80 ml suggests absence of cavernosal leak or venogenic impotence. During artificial erection, Doppler flow probes placed at the base of the penis and directed toward each cavernosal body respectively can detect disappearance of deep cavernosal flow. The values obtained indicate pressure available for erection through each of the deep cavernosal arteries. The usual pressure obtained on cavernosometry during erection is 80 mmHg; higher pressures are produced during contraction of the muscles of the pelvic floor.

Duplex scanning

Using duplex scanning, both deep cavernosal arteries are examined at intervals before and after papaverine injection. Observation of these arteries and knowledge of the flow diameter and velocity detected by Doppler ultrasound signals provide estimates of total flow. Further experience in duplex scanning is needed to relate abnormalities to sites of vascular obstruction. Failure of cavernosal vessels to dilate can be due to proximal or distal obstruction.

Physiological examinations to provide quantitative data on impaired erectile haemodynamics are essential for proper patient selection. Comprehensive physiological study for surgical candidates cannot be totally non-invasive. Cavernosometry quantitates cavernosal leakage and angiographic studies are needed to display abnormal anatomy.

Preoperative angiographic studies

Cavernosograms obtained during cavernosometry and artificial erection delineate sites of venous leakage. Conventional arteriogrpahy demonstrates large vessel occlusive disease and is selected when PBPI is grossly abnormal. Highly selective internal pudendal arteriograhy using artificial erection is required to display pudendal and penile arterial anatomy.

Neural studies

To ensure intact nervous mechanisms, measurement of bulbocavernous reflex amplitude and time and pudendal-evoked potentials are used. These rule out neurogenic impotence which contraindicates a vascular operation.

Hormonal studies

Abnormalities can be found in serum prolactin and testosterone levels. Most commonly, blood glucose levels are abnormal. Thyroid and renal function tests should be obtained preoperatively.

Operative considerations

This chapter considers procedures for impotence on the internal illiac artery, small arteries (i.e. dorsal penile) and deep dorsal vein arterialization for mixed impotence. Venous ablation for cavernosal leak syndrome use a variety of approaches depending on demonstrated sites of venous leakage. These approaches are still evolutionary and will only be outlined. The candidate for vascular surgical correction of impotence must exhibit an identifiable physiological and anatomic vascular defect in the absence of neurogenic or hormonal causes of impotence.

Operations on large arteries

Operative steps in aortoiliac surgery to prevent sexual dysfunction and restore potency have been described (DePalma, 1985; DePalma *et al.*, 1988). These operations provide flow to the interal ililac arteries and avoid disruption of neural arcs. Operations for impotence *per se* on the large arteries involve mainly those done in isolated internal iliac artery disease.

Internal iliac endarterectomy or bypass

1

With the patient in the supine position, an incision is made just through the fascial layers at the lateral border of the rectus sheath. The peritoneum remains intact and is reflected medially. This method provides a wider exposure than the previously described muscle-splitting incision (DePalma, 1985). The exposure obtained allows proximal control of the origin of the internal iliac and the common and external iliac arteries. The lateral as opposed to a medial approach enhances internal iliac exposure. Distal control of the internal iliac is obtained at its division into anterior and posterior branches as the superior gluteal exits through the greater sciatic foramen.

1

2

After systemic heparinization, endarterectomy is carried out and the artery closed with 4/0 or 5/0 prolene.

2

3

In cases of diffuse disease, a vein bypass from the external iliac to the branching of the internal iliac can be employed. After bypass heparinization is reversed.

The extraperitoneal incision is closed with 0 polydioxanone (PDS) in the confluence of the layers comprising the edge of the rectus sheath and the combined abdominal layers.

3

Revascularization of dorsal penile arteries

4 & 5

Revascularization of dorsal penile arteries requires adequate retrograde flow into the deep cavernosal artery or the presence of accessory deep cavernosal branches connecting the dorsal penile and cavernosal systems so that antegrade perfusion occurs. The vessel diameter distal to an occlusion site is small, i.e. less than 1.5 mm; however, in most cases it is adequate for anastomosis using standard microvascular techniques. Heparin is not used; the patient is given aspirin 320 mg preoperatively.

Penile arteriographic findings suitable for dorsal bypass must be obtained. These studies are obtained using artificial erection. Intraoperative visual assessment is often quite helpful.

4

5

6

The inferior epigastric artery is the usual vessel of choice. The length required extends from its origin from the external iliac to 25 mm above the umbilicus. Small vein grafts originating from the common femoral artery or the inferior epigastric artery can be used when this vessel is insufficient. This has not occurred in the senior author's experience. A paramedian incision just medial to the lateral edge of the rectus sheath is used for exposure. The incision extends to at least 25 mm above the umbilicus. A midline incision can also be used to mobilize both inferior epigastric arteries; here exposure is slightly more difficult as more retraction of the recti is needed. Side branches are ligated with fine silk suture and fine vessels closed using bipolar cautery.

6

7

7

Bipolar cautery and loupe magnification are essential in penile dissection for precise haemostatic control and to avoid neural damage. Final preparation and anastomosis of the donor and recipient vessel ends are performed with the aid of an operating microscope using standard microsurgical techniques and interrupted 10/0 nylon on a BV 75 μ or BV 50 μ needle. An end-to-side anastomosis is preferred whenever possible, i.e. between, for example, the donor inferior epigastric and one of the laterally placed dorsal penile arteries. This obviates the need to rely on an accessory corpus vessel. Anastomotic patency is assessed using the strip patency test.

The rectus sheath is closed with interrupted 0 PDS. An aperture in the inferior fascial portion is created so that the inferior epigastric graft pedicle passes without fascial impediment to the dorsal penile artery.

Deep dorsal vein arterialization for mixed vasculogenic impotence

8

These operations are used for mixed vasculogenic impotence, i.e. arteriogenic and venous. The usual abnormalities are aplasia or hypoplasia of dorsal penile arteries, distal penile occlusive disease, and venous leakage.

Variations in this technique have been describrd by Virag *et al.* (1983). Their technique is depicted showing the donor artery anastomosed end-to-side to the centrally situated deep dorsal vein of the penis, with distal vein ligation.

8

9

Other variations include abandoning venocavernostomy. An important pitfall has been found to be the occurrence of glans hyperemia. This now contraindicates valve ablation and suggests wider application of distal vein ligation. The proximal vein is usually ligated.

10

Hauri's (1985) variation is shown, where an arteriovenous fistula is fashioned between a dorsal artery and the dorsal vein for joint anastomosis of these to the end of the donor artery.

9

10

11

Postoperative arteriography at 1 year shows a patent epigastric artery to dorsal vein fistula with run-off via the circumflex penile veins. This patient continued to be potent but later required transluminal angioplasty. Dorsal vein arterialization and its variants are still evolutionary operations, while large vessel interventions such as internal iliac artery interventions are more securely based.

11

Venous interruption for cavernosal leak

These operations are also in a developmental stage (Wespes and Schulman, 1985; Lewis and Puyau, 1986). The dorsal penile vein is first resected from the penile hilum to the sulcus behind the glans. Exposure of the deep dorsal vein and its proximal ligation at the hilum of the penis are facilitated by division of the suspensory ligament. For this procedure, either a transverse or a lateral pen-scrotal incision is used. The latter avoids section of lymphatics and produces much less oedema. Ligation of the periprostatic venous plexus in the space of Retzius using an extraperitoneal incision and crural plication using a perineal incision have also been performed. To assess efficacy of venous interruption, the senior author uses intraoperative cavernosometry and cavernosography. This assures as complete an interruption of abnormal cavernous drainage as possible and documents increased postoperative intracavernous pressure.

References

DePalma, R. G. (1985). Prevention of sexual dysfunction in aortoiliac surgery. In *Current Operative Surgery–Vascular Surgery*. Jamieson, C. W. ed. London: Baillière Tindall.

DePalma, R. G., Emsellem, H. A., Edwards, C. M., Druy, E. M., Schultz, S. W., Miller, H. C. and Bergsrud, D. (1987). A screening sequence for vasculogenic impotence. *Journal of Vascular Surgery* **5**, 228.

DePalma, R. G., Edwards, C. M., Schwab, F. J. and Steinberg, D. L. (1988). Modern management of impotence associated with aortic surgery. In *Arterial Surgery: New Diagnostic and Operative Techniques*. Bergan, J. J. and Yao, J. S. T., eds. London and San Diego: Grune and Stratton.

Hauri, D. (1985). Operative Moglichkeiten bei der vaskular bedingten Impotenz. *Angio Archiv* **8**, 25.

Lewis, R. W. and Puyau, F. A. (1986). Procedures for decreasing venous drainage. *Sem. Urology* **IV**, 263.

Michal, V. (1985). Arteriogenic impotence. *Angio Archiv* **8**, 4.

Stauffer, D. and DePalma, R. G. (1983). A comparison of penile–brachial index and penile pulse volume recordings. *Bruit* **17**, 29.

Virag, R., Frydman, D., Legman, H., *et al.* (1983). Possibilities chirurgicales dans l'impuissance vasculaire. *Gaz. Med. France* **90**, 2031.

Wespes, E. and Schulman, C. C. (1985). Venous leakage: Surgical treatment of a curable cause of impotence. *Journal of Urology* **133**, 796.

Axillofemoral bypass

Sven-Erik Bergentz MD

Department of Surgery, Lund University, Malmö General Hospital, Malmö, Sweden

Introduction

Axillofemoral bypass was first performed in 1962 by Blaisdell and Hall (1963) in the USA and by Louw (1963) in South Africa. The former operation was performed for an occluded abdominal aortic aneurysm, the latter for arteriosclerotic occlusive disease.

The technique for this operation should be known by all vascular surgeons, but it should not be used very often. The most important indication is when a standard aortic reconstruction is precluded due to aortic graft infection, an aortoenteric fistula, or intra-abdominal sepsis (Bergqvist *et al.*, 1987). The operation may also be used when there is a colostomy-ileostomy, or other types of enterocutaneous fistula. Another indication is dense abdominal adhesions, following previous surgery or irradiation. Threatening limb loss in high-risk patients due to severe cardiac or pulmonary disease is a rare indication in our institution. A rare and controversial use of axillofemoral bypass is for non-resective treatment of an abdominal aortic aneurysm after induction of acute thrombosis of the aneurysm by bilateral iliac artery ligation (Schwartz, Nichols and Silver, 1986).

Axillofemoral bypass is contraindicated in extensive subclavian or axillary artery occlusive disease. As outflow vessel, a patent deep femoral artery, and/or superficial femoral artery, is mandatory.

Preoperative evaluation

With regard to the inflow vessels, preoperative blood pressure measurements in both arms and auscultation over subclavian and axillary arteries are important. The right axillary artery is usually preferred as inflow vessel since stenotic lesions in the subclavian artery are three to four times more common on the left than on the right side. If, however, the blood pressure is more than about 20 mm Hg higher on the left side, this side should be preferred. If the blood pressure is low bilaterally, or if there are murmurs to be heard over the subclavian and axillary arteries, arteriography of the aortic arch and its branches should be performed.

If an axillofemoral graft is indicated, there is usually a need to vascularize both legs. Originally, this was done by performing one axillofemoral bypass on each side, but now we prefer to use axillofemoral bypass on one side, and add a cross-over graft to the contralateral groin ('axillobifemoral bypass'). This will increase the flow in the long axillofemoral graft, which decreases the risk of occlusion.

The operation

1

Anaesthesia, positioning and draping

Axillofemoral bypass may be performed under local anaesthesia, but light general anaesthesia is preferable. This gives better airway control and ventilation and is usually well tolerated even by debilitated patients.

The patient lies in a supine position with the arm on the ipsilateral side placed on an armboard, at right angles to the body. This arm is draped free and is mobile during the operation. Abduction of the arm moves the clavicle upwards, facilitating access to the first part of the axillary artery. Chest, neck, upper arm, abdomen, both groins, and upper parts of the thighs should be draped. The contralateral arm is used for blood pressure recording, sampling and infusions.

It is sometimes recommended to use two teams to speed up the operation. We prefer using one team, although the dissection of the axillary and femoral vessels may sometimes be carried out simultaneously by two surgeons.

1

2

Axillary artery dissection

The axillary artery lies behind and slightly above the axillary vein. It is divided into three parts, in relation to its relation to the pectoralis minor muscle. The first is located medial to, the second behind and the third lateral to this muscle. The axillary artery is crossed by the lateral and medial anterior thoracic (pectoral) nerves, innervating the pectoralis major muscle. The first part of the axillary artery gives off one branch, the highest thoracic artery. The second part, behind the pectoralis minor, usually gives off two branches. The first and, to some extent, the second part of the artery should be used for the anastomosis, since this is the fulcrum when the arm is abducted. Therefore, traction of the axillary artery by the graft is minimized.

If at least one of the common, deep or superficial femoral arteries are known to be patent, the operation starts by exploring the axillary artery. An incision is made about 2 cm below and parallel to the clavicle. Its length should be about 8 cm. The transversely running fibres of the pectoralis major muscle are split between its clavicular and sternal heads. The pectoralis minor muscle is identified behind the costoclavicular fascia. This muscle might be divided close to the clavicle, but sometimes it is possible to retract at least part of it laterally. The axillary vein is now exposed, lying anterior and inferior to the artery.

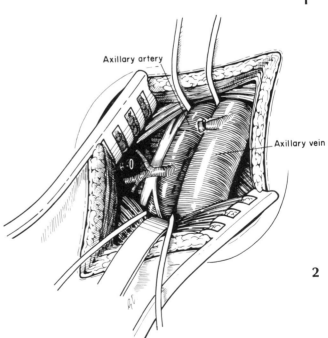

Axillary artery

Axillary vein

2

Ligation of branches to the vein, particularly those crossing in front of the axillary artery, is necessary for the mobilization. The middle part of the axillary artery now emerges below the clavicle. There are usually two branches from this part, and one from the first part of the artery which should be divided. Polyethylene tubing around the artery facilitates its mobilization. About 5–6 cm of the axillary artery should be mobilized.

3

Femoral artery dissection

The femoral artery is now dissected via a longitudinal incision over the common femoral artery. If it is not known that the common femoral artery or at least one of its branches is patent, the operation should start with a groin dissection. The common, superficial and deep femoral arteries are mobilized. A part of the inguinal ligament may be divided to facilitate a proximal dissection of the common femoral artery if necessary. In the relatively uncommon situation, when it is known from a good angiography that both the superficial and deep femoral arteries are patent and without stenosis in the beginning, the anastomosis may be performed to the common femoral artery. Usually, the superficial femoral artery is occluded and the deep femoral artery is often stenotic at its beginning. In these situations the deep femoral artery must be dissected to, or even beyond, its first muscular branches, thereby also dividing the lateral circumflex vein.

If the groin has been used for previous anastomosis, or is infected, the deep femoral arteries may be approached by incisions a few centimetres lateral and distal to the original groin incision. The sartorius muscle is drawn medially, exposing the deep femoral artery, which can be mobilized to a length of several centimetres.

3

4

4

Axillofemoral tunnel

The tunnel for the graft starts from the axillary incision deep to the pectoralis major muscle. In the beginning it should go in a lateral-caudal direction, the angle to the axillary artery being between 30 and 40°. When the tunnel reaches the midaxillary line (where an incision might be necessary to facilitate the formation of the tunnel), it should be directed caudal to the anterior superior iliac spine, and from there it should continue to the groin. It is important to avoid having the prosthesis anteriorly. This may result in compression of the prosthesis to the costal margin, or kinking when the patient bends.

Selection, preparation and placement of graft

We prefer an 8–10-mm knitted Dacron graft. Careful preclotting is important to avoid haematoma formation in the long tunnel. At least 50 ml of blood is necessary for this long graft. A graft with external support might be of value to avoid compression. This point is, however, still controversial. A non-porous prosthesis, such as PTFE, has the advantage of precluding preclotting, but the disadvantage of being non-elastic. It remains an open question whether or not this might contribute to a disruption of the axillary anastomosis when the patient raises his arm.

5a & b

When a *bilateral* axillofemoral bypass is indicated, a femorofemoral graft is anastomosed to the (main) axillofemoral graft. The femorofemoral graft should be 2 mm narrower than the main graft. The origin of the femorofemoral graft from the axillofemoral graft should be as close as possible to the femoral anastomosis, and the graft-to-graft anastomosis should be oblique.

Specially prepared, commercially available axillobifemoral grafts may be used. In most of them, the femorofemoral branch originates from the axillofemoral branch at a right angle, which makes it necessary to place the branching of the axillofemoral graft a few centimetres up from the femoral anastomosis of the axillofemoral graft.

5a

5b

The proximal anastomosis

6

The axillary artery is elevated into the field by traction of the slings encircling the artery. A 2-cm long arteriotomy is made in the anterior and inferior aspect of the axillary artery as far medially as possible. The graft is bevelled at an angle of 30–40°. A 5/0 synthetic double-armed vascular suture is used. The prosthesis is placed anterior to the axillary vein. The sutures are started at the lateral and at the medial ends of the arteriotomy. The back wall of the graft is sutured to the inferior part of the artery from the inside, using one end of the lateral and one end of the medial suture. These two ends are tied together at the midpoint of the back wall.

The other ends of the two sutures, the lateral and the medial, are then used to complete the anterior part of the anastomosis and meet at its midpoint. The clamps on the axillary artery are released. The graft is occluded close to the anastomosis, using a hydrogrip Fogarthy clamp before the clamps on the axillary artery are released.

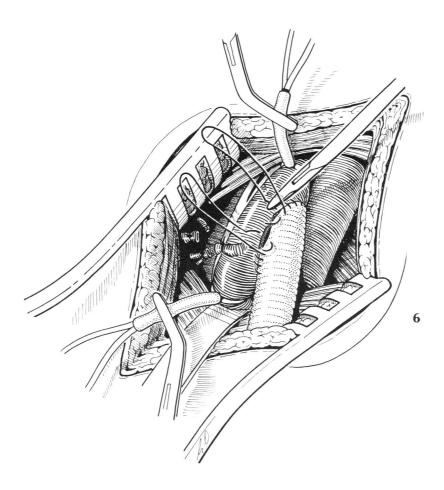

6

7

The distal anastomosis

The prosthesis is drawn from the groin incision, care being taken to avoid any twists and kinks. It is also important to avoid too much tension on the graft, which may draw the axillary artery into a Y configuration. This may result in a thrombosis of the axillary artery, or even disruption of the anastomosis, or a formation of a pseudoaneurysm.

The anastomosis between the graft and the (ipsilateral) femoral artery is made according to the principles described for aortofemoral grafting . If the common femoral artery and the superficial and/or deep femoral arteries are widely patent and without stenosis, the anastomosis is made to the common femoral artery. Very often, however, the superficial femoral artery in these patients is severely diseased or even occluded. The deep femoral artery is often stenotic at its origin. In these cases the arteriotomy of the common femoral artery is carried down 1–2 cm or even further into the deep femoral artery. The graft is formed as an onlay patch in the deep femoral artery. Endarterectomy should be avoided if possible. It it has to be done, it is important to prevent a distal flap development by using several intima-tacking sutures. Several interrupted sutures should be used to prevent purse string constriction when suturing the distal end of the patch on to the rather delicate deep femoral artery.

After completion of the distal anastomosis, the Fogarthy clamp on the proximal part of the graft is released. The clamp on the proximal part of the common femoral artery is then removed, forcing the initial blood flow, with any remaining thrombotic material, debris and air bubbles, in the proximal direction. After a few pulses, the superficial and deep femoral artery clamps are removed. If a graft-to-graft anastomosis has been prepared to a femorofemoral graft, this can be used for flushing the axillofemoral graft. After that, a Fogarthy clamp is placed on the cross-over graft close to the graft-to-graft anastomosis.

The anastomosis between the cross-over graft and the (contralateral) femoral artery is then performed, following the principles just described.

Wound closure

Before closing the wounds, the feet should be inspected. It is usually not possible to feel any ankle pulses, but the colour and the vein-filling in the feet can give some preliminary information about the limb perfusion.

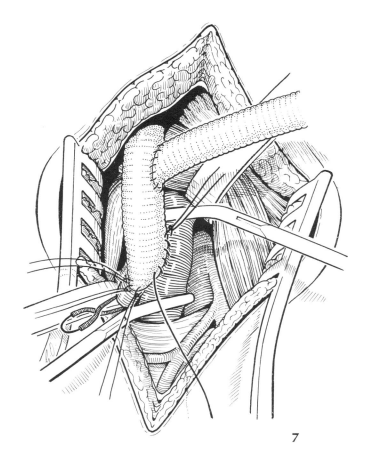

7

Arteriography is considered if there is any question of distal perfusion. A total of 30 ml of contrast medium is injected through a catheter threaded into the prosthesis proximal to the graft-to-graft anastomosis.

The axillary incisions are closed in two deep layers, approximating the fascia of the pectoralis major muscle, and the subcutaneous tissue. We prefer 3/0 synthetic absorbable suture material. The groin wounds are similarly closed in two layers of subcutaneous synthetic absorbable material. The skin is closed with interrupted 3/0 synthetic suture material.

Intra- and postoperative care

Antibiotics

Prophylactic broad spectrum antibiotics, active against staphylococci, is started before surgery and continued for 48 h.

Anticoagulation

We do not use systematic heparinization during these operations. Before occluding a vessel, we irrigate carefully with heparinized saline, and inject 20–40 ml of the solution peripherally. Furthermore, we give dextran 40 in a 10% solution continuously during the operation. The dose is 500 ml during surgery, 500 ml after surgery on the day of surgery, and 500 ml a day for the first 3 postoperative days. We strongly advise the patient to stop smoking. We see no reason to recommend aspirin since it has not been shown to decrease the risk of graft occlusion.

Graft compression

It is not quite clear whether or not compression of the graft plays a role in occlusion. Nevertheless, the patient should be encouraged to avoid constricting clothing and, if possible, lying on the graft. If the patient can cooperate, he may be encouraged to palpate the pulse daily to detect graft occlusion early, which otherwise may be difficult.

Postoperative care and complications

The life-span of an axillofemoral graft can be prolonged by careful monitoring, and early intervention in the case of occlusion. Declotting of an occluded graft is usually a simple procedure, which can be performed under local anaesthesia. An intraoperative angiogram may facilitate complete removal of thrombotic material. Thromboembolic occlusion of the axillobrachial arteries may occur when the graft occludes.

Disruption of the proximal anastomosis, or formation of an anastomotic aneurysm, may occur if this anastomosis is placed too far laterally, and under too much tension.

References

Bergqvist, D., Alm, A., Claes, G., *et al.* (1987). Secondary aortoenteric fistulas – an analysis of 42 cases. *European Journal of Vascular Surgery* 1, 11.

Blaisdell, F. W. and Hall, A. D. (1963). Axillary-femoral bypass for lower extremity ischemia. *Surgery* 54, 563.

Louw, J. H. (1963). Splenic-to-femoral and axillary-to-femoral bypass grafts in diffuse atherosclerotic occlusive disease. *Lancet* 1, 1401.

Schwartz, R. A., Nichols, K. W. and Silver, D. (1986). Is thrombosis of infrarenal abdominal aortic aneurysm an acceptable alternative? *Journal of Vascular Surgery* 3, 448.

Femorofemoral bypass

P. Fiorani MD
Professor of Surgery, University Hospital of Rome, Rome, Italy

V. Faraglia MD
M. Taurino MD
F. Speziale MD
M. Colonna MD
Department of Vascular Surgery, University Hospital of Rome, Rome, Italy

Introduction

Cross-over femorofemoral bypass was first proposed in clinical practice by Vetto in 1966 for the treatment of unilateral iliac obstructive lesions. Its indications were subsequently extended to an increasing number of patients with unilateral iliac lesions, obtaining satisfactory immediate and long-term results.

Clinically, there seems to be no doubt about the indications, while special attention should be paid to the haemodynamic assessment of the donor iliofemoral axis due to its involvement with immediate patency and long-term evolution.

Indications

The clinical indications for revascularization by cross-over femorofemoral bypass include unilateral stenotic-obstructive lesions of the iliac axis with claudication of limited autonomy or with rest ischaemia, showing general or local contra-indications for conventional revascularization (Eugene, Goldstone and Moore, 1977; Whittemore *et al.*, 1980).

General contraindications are represented by advanced age, severe cardiorespiratory failure, or of other systems, the presence of metabolic imbalance or limited life-expectancy (Vijayanager, Bogudo and Eckstein, 1982). This procedure is extra-abdominal, feasible under local anaesthesia, requires a short operative time and involves only a minor surgical trauma. Local contraindications are represented by the presence, near the aorta, of an infected area or marked sclerosis due to previous surgery, retroperitoneal fibrosis or possible onset of septic foci because of iatrogenic lesions from abdominal surgery as well as from possible peripheral trophic lesions. The presence of extensive lesions of the host femoral axis which may affect the immediate result in terms of patency, can be considered a further local contraindication for major abdominal surgery. Moreover, cross-over femorofemoral bypass is indicated for acute thrombosis of the iliac axis and for occlusion of the branch of a previous aortofemoral bypass (Rutherford, Patt and Pearce, 1987).

Special indications for this procedure include the need to preserve the erectile function by preventing iatrogenic lesions of the pelvic splanchnic nerves of the preaortic plexus, in patients affected by morbid obesity (De Laurentis *et al.*, 1978) or previously treated with radiation therapy at the level of the pelvis or retroperitoneum. Together with clinical indications, problems related to haemodynamic peformance should also be considered. They concern both the host and donor limbs. The host artery frequently shows a femoro-popliteal lesion, and thus it should be assessed whether the deep femoral artery is able to ensure adequate perfusion of the limb or not (Nelelsteen *et al.*, 1980; Martinez, Hertzer and Beven, 1980). As for the donor limb, the problem is more complex because obstructive lesions present at this level can be the cause of flow diversion which leads to distal ischaemia (the steal phenomenon).

The steal phenomenon

In 1968, based on observations of patients treated with a cross-over femorofemoral bypass for unilateral iliac obstructive lesions, and who developed ischaemia of the donor limb, explained by a diversion of blood flow between the lower limbs (i.e. the steal phenomenon), and based on other evidence (Harper *et al.*, 1967), Ehrenfeld carried out a canine experiment to try to understand the problem more fully. By modifying the inflow pressure of the donor axis and the peripheral resistance by the creation of an aortovenous fistula, Ehrenfeld was able to demonstrate that lesion-free iliac arteries are able to increase their flow ten fold, allowing them to perfuse proximally as well as contralaterally.

When an iliac artery is significantly stenosed, the flow required by both limbs cannot be satisfied. If distal to the donor axis the peripheral resistance is higher than in the contralateral axis due to femoropopliteal lesions, a femoro-femoral revascularization would result in ischaemic symptoms in the donor limb. Therefore, it is important to determine whether a stenotic lesion is present or not. However, even in the presence of a 50% stenosis, this procedure can still be indicated for elderly and non-ambulatory patients. On the other hand, 30% stenosis is considered the limit for young patients with patent infrainguinal arteries who are likely to experience vasodilatation during exercise, and who therefore require an additional blood flow (Hill, Lord and Tracy, 1982).

However, in some cases postoperative ischaemia of the donor limb can be ascribed to a faulty surgical technique (stenosed anastomosis or embolization) or to a progressive distal atherosclerosis.

Preoperative assessment

The integrity of the donor iliac axis is mandatory to ensure perfusion of both limbs. Therefore, clinical, morphological and haemodynamic testing is proposed, both while the patient is at rest and while exercising the lower limbs.

Clinical testing is based on a normal femoral pulse and the absence of bruits both in the iliac artery and iliac fossa, an indication of the integrity of the donor iliac artery, especially when associated with an obstructive lesion of the ipsilateral femoral bifurcation.

The Doppler system is used to detect and assess possible pressure gradients, to examine the iliac vessels and any lesions, and to measure directly the pressure in the iliac and femoral arteries. The criteria proposed are that the Doppler thigh pressure should be equal to but not greater than the brachial pressure, and that the Doppler ankle pressure should be equal to or no more than 15 mmHg below the brachial pressure (McDonald et al., 1978). The iliac axis is considered normal when the pressure in the femoral artery is not more than 10 mmHg below the brachial pressure. A further non-invasive procedure is to study waveform using a Doppler zero-crossing detector.

Nicolaides and Angelides (1981) modified the wave peak of a haemodynamically effective proximal stenosis to deter-mine the pulsatility index. However, in the presence of a diffuse lesion, this procedure is not totally reliable. In the presence of a mildly stenosed lesion which might result in the steal phenomenon after maximal peripheral dilatation, active-passive or intra-arterial papaverine-induced hyperaemia tests have been proposed to stimulate this response (Flanigan et al., 1984).

Angiography is considered the best form of assessment which, when adequately performed, is able to detect with lateral and oblique projections the presence of iliac stenoses not shown up by standard anteroposterior angiography, due to frequent posterior atherosclerotic plaque. Moreover, lesions at this level of the aortic and iliac bifurcation, i.e. where overlapping bone segments can block the view, can also be detected by these projections.

Surgical techniques

1 & 2

The patient is placed in the supine position and general, local or spinal anaesthesia is administered. Most surgeons make an inguinal incision along the projection of the host femoral vessels, preparing and locating with loops the common femoral, superficial and deep femoral arteries, from the orifice to the lateral femoral circumflex vein, which is ligated to expose a portion of healthy artery suitable for the anastomosis or profundaplasty (De Laurentis et al., 1978; Wylie et al., 1980). The donor femoral artery is then prepared using a similar incision, but more limited downwards and more extended upwards to allow the best possible exposure of the common femoral artery.

1

2

3, 4, & 5

The patient is heparinized and preclotted knitted Dacron is used as the prosthesis. PTFE or autologous saphenous vein can also be used, provided that their calibre is not less than 6 mm. In particular instances, it should be possible to use an autologous artery such as an endarterectomized superficial femoral artery (Blaisdell *et al.*, 1970).

Arteriotomies should be performed on the anteromedial aspect of the host vessels to avoid kinking and twisting of the graft. An oblique inflow orifice is also advisable to prevent inflow stenosis (Tyson and Reichle, 1972).

After completion of the donor anastomosis, the prosthesis is canalized bluntly up to the contralateral groin following a subcutaneous course. This is then reversed to form a 'U'-shaped subcutaneous bypass.

3

4

5

6

Other surgeons prefer a deeper positioning of the prosthesis and improved bypass haemodynamics (Courbier *et al.*, 1982). Donor vessels are prepared using an oblique incision parallel to the inguinal ligament, approximately 2–3 cm proximally to permit proximal anastomosis to the external iliac artery. The prosthesis is canalized more deeply behind the rectal muscle in the space of Retzius and below the inguinal ligament, resulting in a 'S'-shaped bypass.

With this procedure, the prosthesis is better protected against external compression, though there is a greater risk of bleeding due to the presence of a rich venous plexus. This cross-over iliofemoral bypass is thus very different from the simple cross-over femorofemoral bypass.

Iliofemoral bypass allows the prosthesis to be positioned outside the donor inguinal region, with its consequent lower risk of bacterial contamination from the the contralateral groin. Canalization in the space of Retzius, which lies at a deeper level than the inguinal ligament, involves the section of the fibrous layer of the ligament. This avoids compression of the prosthesis and traction on the suture line, which is frequently responsible for the formation of anastomotic aneurysms.

In the case of an infected groin, cross-over transperineal bypass can be carried out. This entails a subcutaneous route at the level of the inguino-scrotal folds close to the spongy body, from the common femoral artery to the contralateral superficial or deep femoral artery, far from the site of infection. Autologous saphenous vein is the prosthesis of choice, otherwise PTFE.

Anastomoses are usually performed end-to-side, but with extended lesions of the host deep femoral artery requiring endarterectomy, at this level the anastomosis can be performed end-to-end. The suture material is usually 5/0 or 6/0 monofilament. After completion of the anastomoses with flush to prevent possible distal embolizations, the clamps are released and the pulsatility of the prosthesis and the proximal and contralateral vessels is controlled. Immediate postoperative control is performed by Doppler evaluation of the ankle pressure index (Winsor index) and by intraoperative angiography to evidence possible technical errors, e.g. torsion of the prosthesis or the intimal flap, which can be repaired immediately. After tubular drainage of the area, the groins are sutured by reconstruction of the fascia and section planes. Postoperatively, the antibiotic prophylaxis of infection plays a major role, especially in patients who show trophic lesions.

Contraindications

If adequate haemodynamic testing is carried out, there are no absolute contraindications for cross-over femorofemoral bypass, though particular attention should be paid to the prophylaxis of infection, because the areas involved with the prosthesis are rich in lymphatic vessels and lymph-node stations, and are thus at risk.

In conclusion, femorofemoral bypass should be considered the procedure of choice in the treatment of unilateral iliac occlusion in high-risk patients. An accurate preoperative and haemodynamic assessment provides useful information for obtaining good long-term patency and haemodynamic function.

6

References

Blaisdell, R. W., Hall, A. D., Lim, R. C. Jr and Moore, W. C. (1970). Aortoiliac arterial subcutaneous grafts. *Annals of Surgery* **172**, 775.

Courbier, R., Larranaga, J., Ferdani, M., Jausseran, J. M., Reggi, M. and Bergeron, P. (1982). Le faux anévrismes sur prothèse artérielle. *Chirurgie* **108**, 459.

De Laurentis, D. A., Sala, L. E., Russell, E. and McCombs, P. R. (1978). A twelve years experience with axillofemoral and femorofemoral bypass operations. *Surgery, Gynecology, and Obstetrics* **147**, 881.

Eugene, J., Goldstone, J. and Moore, W. S. (1977). Fifteen years experience with subcutaneous bypass grafts for lower extremity ischemia. *Annals of Surgery* **186**, 177.

Flanigan, P. D., Ryan, T. J., Williams, L. R., Schwatrz, J. A., Gray, B. and Shuler, J. J. (1984). Aortofemoral or femoropopliteal revascularization? A prospective evaluation of the papaverine test. *Journal of Vascular Surgery* **1**, 215.

Harper, S. A., Goldin, A. L., Mazzei, E. A. and Cannon, S. A. (1967). An experimental hemodynamic study of the subclavian steal syndrome. *Surgery, Gynecology and Obstetrics* **124**, 1212.

Hill, D. A., Lord, R. S. A. and Tracy, G. D. (1982). Haemodynamic consequences of cross femoral bypass. In *Extra-anatomic and Secondary Arterial Reconstruction*. Greenhalgh, R. M. ed. London: Pitman.

Kalman, P. G., Hosang, M., Johnston, K. W. and Walker, P. M. (1987). The current role for femorofemoral bypass. *Journal of Vascular Surgery* **6**, 71.

McDonald, P. T., Rich, N. M., Collins, J. G., Anderson, A. C. and Kozloff, L. (1978). Femorofemoral grafts: The role of concomitant extended profundaplasty. *American Journal of Surgery* **136**, 622.

Martinez, B. B., Hertzer, N. R. and Bevan, E. G. (1980). Influence of distal arterial occlusive disease on prognosis following aortobi-femoral bypass. *Surgery* **88**, 795.

Nelelsteen, A., Suiw, R., Daeneen, W., Boel, A. and Stalpeert, G. (1980). Aortofemoral grafting: Factors influencing late result. *Surgery* **88**, 342.

Nicolaides, A. N. and Angelides, N. S. (1981). Waveform index and resistance factor using directional Doppler ultrasound and zero-crossing detector. In Nicolaides, A. N., Yao, J. S. T., eds. New York: Churchill Livingstone.

Rutherford, R. B., Patt, A. and Pearce, W. H. (1987). Extra-anatomic bypass: A closer view. *Journal of Vascular Surgery*, **6**, 437.

Tyson, R. R. and Reichle, F. A. (1972). Retropubic femorofemoral bypass: A new route through the space of Retzius. *Surgery* **72**, 401.

Vijayanagar, R., Bogudo, D. A. and Eckstein, P. F. (1982). Extra-anatomic bypass operation for aorto-iliac disease in poor risk cardiopulmonary patients. *Angiology* **33**, 69.

Whittemore, K. E., Billig, P. M., Pavlides, C. and Matsumoto, T. (1980). Special considerations in the revascularization for aorto-iliac occlusive disease: Anatomic and extra-anatomic bypass. *Annals of Surgery* **46**, 279.

Wylie, E. J., Stoney, R. J., Ehrenfeld, W. K. and Effeney, D. S. (1980). In *Manual of Vascular Surgery*. Egdahl, R. E. ed.

Obturator canal bypass

G. Kretschmer MD
B. Niederle MD
M. Wunderlich MD

1st Clinic of Surgery, University of Vienna, Vienna, Austria

Introduction

Since obturator canal bypass was introduced by Shaw and Baue in 1963, its indications and techniques have been precisely defined. Today the method is an established standard procedure in vascular surgery, with the results of 250 patients being published. In general, more or less anecdotal reports are available; the largest series comprise 13 and 27 patients, respectively (Van Det and Brands, 1981; Niederle *et al.*, 1988). Guidelines and conclusions are drawn from these reports and our own experience (Van Det and Brands, 1981; Prenner and Rendl, 1982; Buchardt-Hansen, Holstein and Krogh-Christofferson, 1982; Cotton, 1982; Geroulakos, Parvin and Bell, 1988; Niederle *et al.*, 1988).

1

Concept

The basic principle is to create an extensive extra-anatomical bypass from the pelvic to the distal femoral or infra-genicular arteries, the site of distal anastomosis depending on the respective morphological conditions.

Graft-conduction through the foramen obturatum, dorsal to hip-joint and adductor muscle group, avoids the femoral triangle so as to prevent any contamination. Accordingly, the procedure allows thorough separation of the graft from the obviously or potentially infected inguinal area through an uncompromised barrier of normal tissue.

Principally, any vascular substitute of adequate dimensions may be acceptable and most have been tested. As would be expected, autologous saphenous vein has been employed in 16% of patients. Although autologous grafts give the most satisfying long-term results, the limited diameter of these conduits often precludes their use. In the remaining patients, the greater distance to be bridged usually requires the use of fabric grafts.

We have found PTFE prostheses (21 out of 27 cases) to have been most satisfactory. Our initial experience with externally reinforced grafts has been promising, due to their greater resistance against kinking and compression.

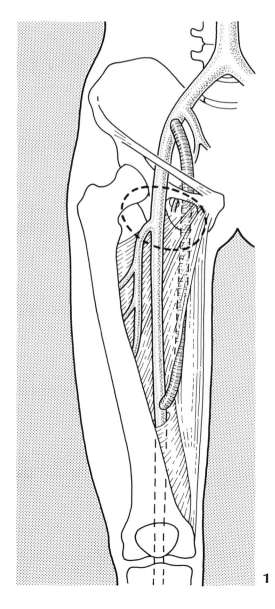

1

Indications

Throughout the literature there is unanimous agreement that the most frequent indication (58%) is unilateral deep infection, strictly confined to the groin (type III according to Szilagyi *et al.*, 1972) as a sequel of vascular surgery of any kind (Brücke and Piza, 1968; Prenner and Rendl, 1982). Less frequent indications are rather evenly distributed between infections subsequent to vascular access surgery (12%; Prenner and Rendl, 1982), inguinal skin and subcutaneous tissue defects after extensive tumour surgery and/or therapeutic irradiation (17%; Niederle *et al.*, 1988) and, finally, complicated (non-arteriosclerotic) aneurysms and severe inguinal scarring (13%; Buchardt-Hansen *et al.*, 1982; Cotton, 1982).

Angiography

The value of preoperative arteriography to identify suitable areas for proximal and distal anastomoses is undisputed. However, in the case of massive bleeding as an emergency indication, valuable time can be wasted waiting for preoperative information. The site of distal anastomosis may then be chosen on grounds of radiology, obtained prior to the primary procedure, or by distal exploration, if necessary with adjunctive on-table angiography during the present bypass procedure.

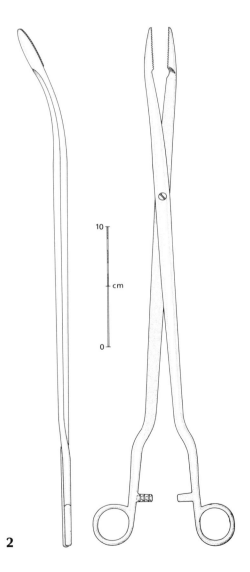

2

2

Instrumentation

In addition to the standard instruments for vascular surgery, we use a slim, long-bladed grasping-forceps, 65 cm in length and with a slight bend of 20° for boring the tunnel and guiding the graft into place. Sponges and dressing clamps are used according to Sims–Maier (Brücke and Piza, 1968). Of course, any other forceps of adequate length with long blunt jaws will be adequate.

3

Positioning and preparation of the patient

With the patient in the prone position, the spine and hip-joints are slightly over-extended to allow the grasping-forceps to be directed through the obturator canal behind the superior branch of the pubic bone without impediment from the abdominal wall – an obstacle most likely to be met in obese patients.

The entire abdomen and the limb concerned are disinfected and draped in such a way as to permit good access to the abdominal and distal incisions at the medial aspect of thigh and calf. Our practice is to use incisive drapes covering the skin, paying particular regard to the crucial femoral triangle so as to avoid any contamination therefrom.

Anaesthetic management

Surgery is performed under general anaesthesia, with the use of at least one or two major i.v. lines, preferably a central venous catheter. A urinary catheter is essential (see *Illustration 3*). The operative strain on the patient can be estimated by using a mean duration of anaesthesia of $3\frac{1}{2}$ h and a mean quantity of blood loss corresponding to 3 units (Kretschmer *et al.*, in press).

3

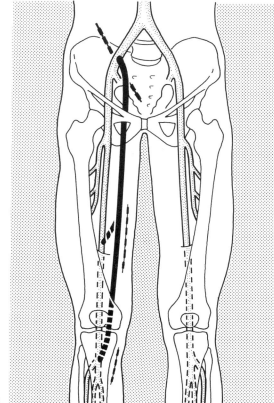

4

Surgical procedure

4

Standard approaches are used for extraperitoneal exposure of the pelvic arteries as well as for medial exposure of the femoral, popliteal or even crural vessels (Leitz, 1981). As a rule, we prefer the extraperitoneal ($n = 17$) to the trans-peritoneal ($n = 10$) approach, the latter being reserved for redo-surgery.

5 & 6

Gentle sweeping of the peritoneal sac, ureter and bladder to the midline gives access to the foramen obturatum. In male and obese patients in particular, the foramen is often better identified by mere digital palpation of its sharp fascial circumference than by actually viewing it during deep pelvic dissection (Brücke and Piza, 1968). It is our practice to penetrate the membrana obturatoria from the proximal distally, and then bore the tunnel and place the graft, taking care to leave the obturator vessels and the nerve unharmed. In order to avoid blind tunnelling in a heparinized patient, systemic heparin (100 i.u./kg body weight) is administered after graft placement only. Alternative sites for the anas-

tomosis are shown in *Illustration 6*. The proximal anastomosis is constructed by using the side-to-end-technique. Cross-clamping of externally supported grafts is not advisable. The distal end of the graft is cut to shape during full extension of the knee joint. After completion of the distal anastomosis, the vascular clamps are released.

If possible, the external iliac artery should not undergo preliminary ligation from within the pelvis in order to preserve a maximum of collateral circulation to the leg. Suction drains are left in place for 2 days.

Some authors prefer boring the tunnel from the distal proximally (Pearce *et al.*, 1983; Prenner and Rendl, 1982), suggesting that lesions of the obturator artery and vein are better avoided; however, we cannot confirm this.

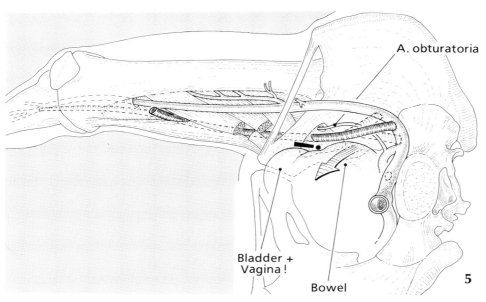

A. obturatoria

Bladder + Vagina!

Bowel

5

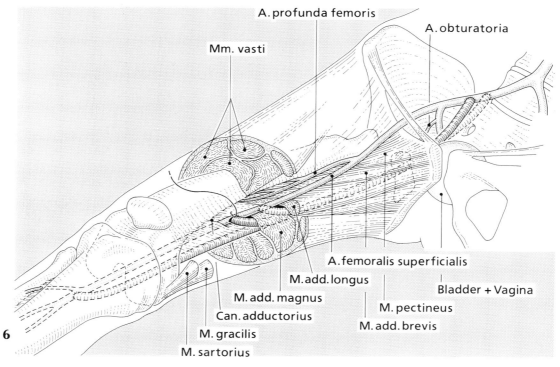

A. profunda femoris

Mm. vasti

A. obturatoria

A. femoralis superficialis

M. add. longus

M. add. magnus

Can. adductorius

M. gracilis

M. sartorius

M. pectineus

M. add. brevis

Bladder + Vagina

6

7

If it is felt necessary, the bypass procedure is followed by debridement of the inguinal wound by removing the remaining alloplastic material and local suturing of vascular defects, so as to secure haemostasis. At the same time, swabs are taken so as to prescribe antibiotic therapy accordingly.

Complications

The usual complications following implantation of long-distance fabric grafts are encountered. In the absence of underlying arteriosclerotic disease, long-term graft performance is excellent. However, patency rates cannot be reliably derived from the literature, as most reports do not distinguish if lesions requiring obturator canal bypass have originally been related to chronic occlusive vascular disease or not.

As circulation along the deep femoral artery has to be sacrificed, or is at least severely compromised, graft occlusion will inevitably threaten the entire extremity. Unless prompt surgical correction is feasible, the ischaemic syndrome will necessitate major, it not above-knee, amputation. Therefore, thrombectomy should be attempted without delay, the long-term performance of the graft depending on the availability of the more favourable distal anastomotic site above the knee, the peripheral run-off conditions and the progression of the underlying disease.

The preservation of the collateral circulation in the inguinal area may become of vital importance. If the collateral blood supply is insufficient following preliminary ligation of the external iliac artery, eradication of the common femoral and the superficial and deep femoral at the origin will lead to necrosis of the thigh musculature, the graft remaining obviously patent (Rudich, Gutierrez and Gage, 1979).

If a combination of infection plus haemorrhage demands an extra-anatomical bypass, the procedure will reliably eradicate the danger of exsanguinating haemorrhage while preserving the limb's blood supply (Kretschmer *et al.*, in press). However, in our series, this combination of events caused two fatalities, the patients with viable limbs having finally succumbed to irreversible sepsis (Kretschmer *et al.*, in press). Topographical misplacement of the graft was observed, leading to perforation of the bladder or vagina (Szilagyi *et al.*, 1972) with subsequent infection and ultimate loss of limb.

Obturator canal bypass may be considered as a valuable addition to the armamentarium of vascular surgery, designed as it is for the treatment of isolated lesions concerning the femoral triangle. The procedure permits generous bypassing of the inguinal risk area and warrants surgery within operative fields as yet untouched. However, it is not devoid of the disadvantage of alloplastic grafts over long distances, with an increased risk of infection.

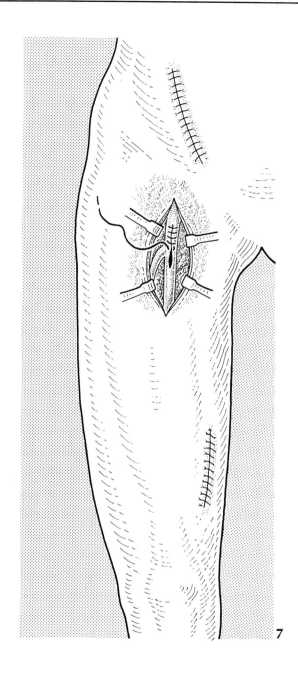

7

Acknowledgement

We would like to thank Mrs Ursula Schattaeur for her secretarial assistance.

References

Brücke, P. and Piza, F. (1968). Zur Indikation des Obturator-Bypass. *Zbl. Chir.* **93**, 489.

Buchardt-Hansen, H. J., Holstein, P. and Krogh-Christoffersen, J. (1982). Obturator canal bypass to avoid an infected or scarred groin. In *Extraanatomic and Secondary Arterial Reconstruction.* Greenhalgh, R. M., ed. London: Pitman.

Cotton, L. T. (1982). Obturator canal bypass for aneurysms in the thigh. In *Extraanatomic and Secondary Arterial Reconstruction.* Greenhalgh, R. M. ed. London: Pitman.

Geroulakos, G., Parvin, S. D. and Bell, P. R. F. (1988). Obturator foramen bypass, the alternative route for sepsis in the femoral triangle. *Acta Chir. Scan.* **154**, 111.

Kretschmer, G., Niederle, B., Huk, I., Karner, J., Piza, H., Polterauer, P. and Walzer, L. R. (in press). Groin infections following vascular surgery: Obturator bypass (BYP) versus biologic coverage (TRP) – a comparative evaluation. *European Journal of Vascular Surgery.*

Leitz, K. H. (1981). *Zugangswege in der Gefäßchirurgie.* Heidelberg: Springer.

Niederle, B., Polterauer, P., Kretschmer, G. and Piza, F. (1988). Der Obturatorbypass – Indikation und Ergebnisse bei 27 Patienten. *Angio Arch.* **16**, 90.

Pearce, W. H., Ricco, J. P., Yao, J. S. T., Flinn, W. R. and Bergan, J. J. (1983). Modified technique of obturator bypass in failed or infected grafts. *Annals of Surgery* **197**, 344.

Prenner, K. V. and Rendl, K. H. (1982). Indications and technique of obturator bypass. In *Extraanatomic and Secondary Arterial Reconstruction.* Greenhalgh, R. M., ed. London: Pitman.

Rudich, M., Gutierrez, I. Z. and Gage, A. A. (1979). Obturator foramen bypass in the management of infected vascular prosthesis. *American Journal of Surgery* **137**, 657.

Shaw, R. S. and Baue, A. E. (1963). Management of sepsis complicating arterial reconstructive surgery. *Surgery* **53**, 57.

Sheiner, N. M., Sigman, H. and Stilman, A. (1969). An unusual complication of obturator foramen arterial bypass. *Journal of Cardiovascular Surgery* **10**, 324.

Szilagyi, D. E., Smith, R. F., Elliott, J. P. and Vrandecic, M. P. (1972). Infection in arterial reconstruction with synthetic grafts *Annals of Surgery* **176**, 321.

Van Det, R. J. and Brands, L. C. (1981). The obturator foramen bypass: An alternative procedure in iliofemoral artery revascularization. *Surgery* **89**, 543.

Cervical sympathectomy

Giorgio M. Biasi MD
Professor, Institute of General and Cardiovascular Surgery, University of Milan, Milan, Italy
Sergio Miani MD
Professor, Institute of General and Cardiovascular Surgery, University of Milan, Milan, Italy
Ugo Ruberti MD
Professor and Chief, Institute of General and Cardiovascular Surgery, University of Milan, Milan, Italy

Introduction

Although it is a term in common usage, 'cervical sympathectomy' is a misnomer. Access, to facilitate division of the thoracic sympathetic chain, can be gained by a supraclavicular approach (described here), an axillary approach or by the posterior approach of Smithwick (1940).

The principal indications for this procedure have altered in recent years. At one time the operation was performed for many ischaemic conditions of the upper limbs caused by vasospasm, obliterative disease or arterial injuries. It continues to have an important role in the treatment of Raynaud's phenomenon, when it is resilient to sympatholitic drugs and not associated with collagenopathy, and is excellent for hyperhidrosis of the hands (Greenhalgh, Rosengarten and Martin, 1971). Other indications include trophic subungual lesions and causalgic-type pain following costal resections for thoracic outlet syndrome.

For all of these pathological conditions radiographs of the cervical vertebrae are studied before surgery in order to determine the presence of transverse mega-apophysis or of supranumerary ribs which can be the underlying cause of an outlet syndrome. In the case of trophic subungual lesions, it is wise to carry out an arteriogram of the distal arteries.

Using this approach it is possible to reach down to the third thoracic ganglion quite easily, but for more extensive sympathectomy, the axillary approach is recommended. This route, proposed by Jonnesco (1923), Bruning (1923), Royle (1924), and Leriche and Fontaine (1933), has been well documented and described by Gask and Ross (1937).

The operation

1

The operation is performed under general anaesthesia with tracheal intubation, because accidental opening of the pleural dome can cause a pneumothorax. With the patient's head turned away from the side of the incision and with the neck slightly hyperextended, a horizontal incision is made 1 cm above the superior border of the clavicle, 1–2 cm lateral to the jugular fossa on the anterior face of the clavicular head of the sternocleidomastoid muscle. An incision of 5–6 cm is sufficient to facilitate division of the clavicular head of the sternomastoid. The incision passes through the platysma muscle and the external jugular vein may have to be divided.

1

2

The clavicular head of the sternocleidomastoid muscle is then divided, leaving sufficient muscle below for the reconstruc- tion. The omohyoid muscle crosses the operative field obliquely and occasionally it may have to be divided.

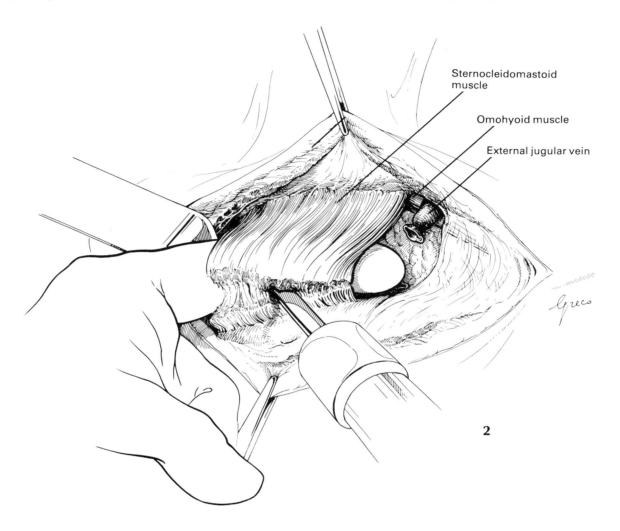

Sternocleidomastoid
muscle

Omohyoid muscle

External jugular vein

2

3

The internal jugular vein is identified and preserved. The scalene pad of fat with lymph nodes is situated in the centre of the field; this is displaced upwards and must sometimes be divided between clips. The scalenus anterior muscle is now visible. The phrenic nerve, attached to the muscle by fascia, can be seen running from lateral to medial on the muscle from above downwards. The nerve must be dissected free and isolated. Using extreme delicacy it is retracted medially with a small retractor or, preferably, with a Silastic loop. The scalenus anterior muscle is then divided very near its insertion into the first rib. Immediately behind the scalene muscle lies the subclavian artery and from it the vertebral artery branches and runs upward. It is vital, therefore, when dissecting the scalene muscle, to avoid damage to these deep vascular structures. For this reason some surgeons first pass an instrument behind the muscle before dissecting it. However, we prefer not to perform this potentially dangerous manoeuvre, and instead cautiously dissect the muscle with an electroknife, eventually inserting the index finger of the left hand behind the remaining bundles of the muscle. The muscle fibres retract as the dissection proceeds and, when only a few layers remain, the transparent sheath of the subclavian artery can be seen. The last muscle fibres are then cut with dissecting scissors.

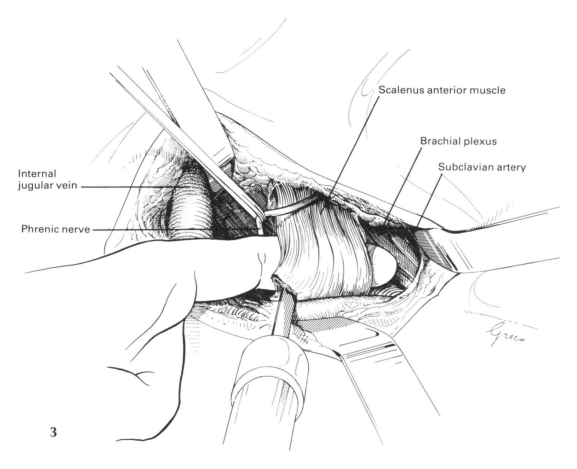

Internal jugular vein

Phrenic nerve

Scalenus anterior muscle

Brachial plexus

Subclavian artery

3

4

The subclavian arch is thus isolated from the internal jugular vein and under it lies the vertebral artery. Distally the thyrocervical trunk, which may be tied, originates from the subclavian artery. Whenever a *left* sympathectomy is performed one should be aware of the presence of the thoracic duct that emerges from the mediastinum and enters the subclavian vein lateral to its confluence with the internal jugular vein. At this point, the subclavian arch is retracted upward to display the apex of the lung, the pleural dome and the suprapleural membrane (Sibson's fascia). Sibson's fascia is bluntly dissected from the rib, thus allowing entry to the retropleural space. It begins to strip more easily below on the medial side. Once the stripping beings a swab is gently pushed into the enlarging space with the index finger until the lung is fully depressed without injury to the pleura.

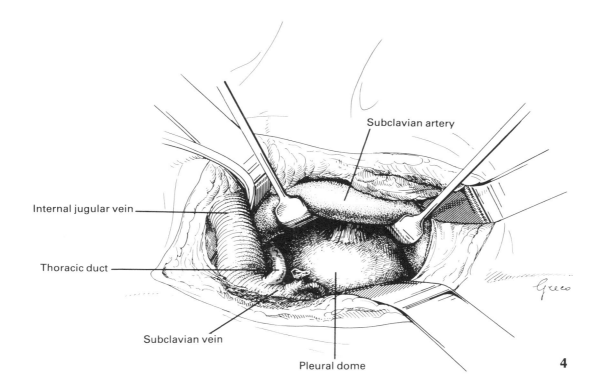

Subclavian artery

Internal jugular vein

Thoracic duct

Subclavian vein

Pleural dome

4

5 & 6

The sympathetic chain can now be seen but it is more important that the surgeon's hand be guided by a sense of touch in this deep space. The chain is like a thick corded structure that passes across the neck of the first rib. The intercostal artery and vein must be carefully avoided (the first intercostal artery is a branch of the subclavian costocervical trunk). The chain is palpated with the finger and an illuminated lighted retractor is used to view it. A hook is then used to lift the sympathetic chain which is traced as far as possible.

Usually, it is easy to reach the third thoracic ganglion and below this the chain is divided and delivered upwards. All of the rami communicantes are divided between neurosurgical metal clips, but the stellate ganglion is not mobilized for fear of producing a Horner's syndrome. Some surgeons divide the chain and take the lower part of the stellate ganglion, but it has been shown that embedding the cut chain into the scalenus anterior muscle with a transfixion stitch is sufficient. *Illustration 6* shows the anatomy of the chain and its relations.

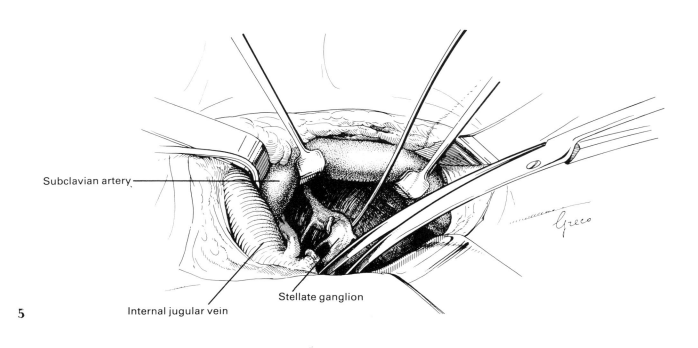

Subclavian artery

Internal jugular vein

Stellate ganglion

5

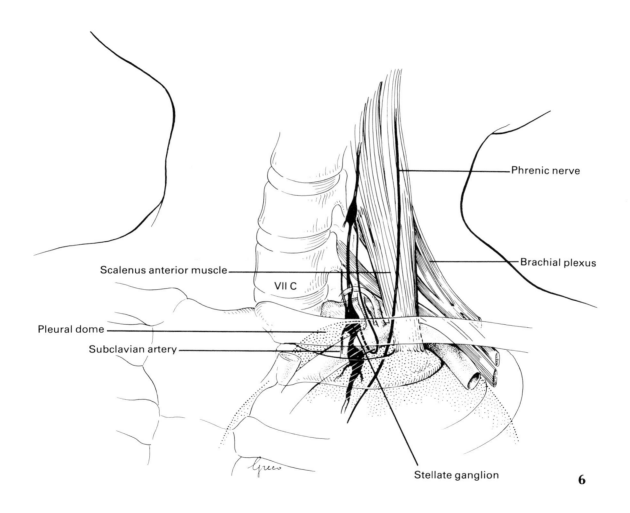

Phrenic nerve

Brachial plexus

Scalenus anterior muscle

VII C

Pleural dome

Subclavian artery

Stellate ganglion

6

7 & 8

Once haemostasis has been secured the incision is closed without drainage. (However, if damage to the pleural dome is suspected, it is advisable to place a slender catheter in the extrapleural space.) The edges of the clavicular head of the sternocleidomastoid muscle are brought together, followed by the platysma muscle, with fine catgut sutures. Finally, the skin is closed, either with Michelle clips or very fine nylon sutures. If a drain is used a Redivac suction drain is usually ideal.

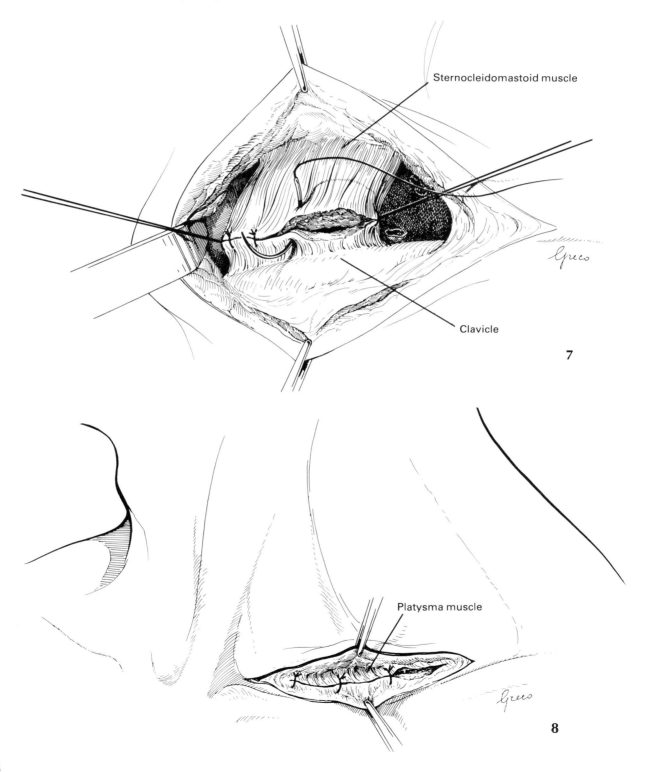

Sternocleidomastoid muscle

Clavicle

7

Platysma muscle

8

Complications

Horner's syndrome, pneumothorax and damage to the brachial plexus, phrenic nerve or internal jugular vein, are all possible. Careful technique and a thorough apprenticeship with this procedure are essential – it is not an operation for the occasional surgeon.

References

Bruning, F. (1923). Weitere Erfahrungen uber den Sympathicus. *Klinische Wochenschrift* **2**, 1872.

Gask, G. E. (1933). The surgery of the sympathetic nervous system. *British Journal of Surgery* **21**, 113.

Gask, G. E. and Ross, J. P. (1937). *The Surgery of the Sympathetic Nervous System,* 2nd ed. Baltimore: William Wood and Company

Greenhalgh, R. M., Rosengarten, D. S. and Martin, P. (1971). Role of sympathectomy for hyperhidrosis. *British Medical Journal* **1**, 1332.

Jonnesco, T. (1923). *Le Sympatique Cervico-thoracique.* Paris: Masson et Cie

Leriche, R. and Fontaine, R. (1933). Technique de l'ablation du ganglion étoilé. *Journal de Chirurgie* **41**, 353.

Royle, N. D. (1924). The treatment of spastic paralysis by sympathetic ramisection. Experimental basis and clinical results. *Surgery, Gynecology and Obstetrics* **39**, 701.

Smithwick, R. H. (1940). The rationale of sympathectomy for the relief of vascular spasm of the extremities. *New England Journal of Medicine* **222**, 699.

Transthoracic sympathectomy

Harold Ellis   CBE, DM, MCh, FRCS

Professor of Surgery, Charing Cross and Westminster Medical School, London, UK

Preoperative

Indications

Excision of the upper portion of the thoracic part of the sympathetic chain has, as its main indication, the treatment of severe idiopathic hyperhidrosis of the hands. This has an equal sex distribution, although women with this condition are more likely to complain of the excessive associated axillary sweating. Symptoms usually commence at the time of puberty but may be seen in childhood (Law and Ellis, in press). All four limbs may be affected but individual patients may complain that the sweating of the axillae, the hands or the feet is the principal nuisance. There is often little difference during summer or winter and the sweating is not usually aggravated by exercise. It is precipitated by emotional or mental stress and ceases during sleep. There is often an associated Raynaud's phenomenon, with the hands and feet being cold and blue as well as sweating.

The cause of this condition is unknown. The sweat glands in the involved areas are normal, both histologically and numerically. Histochemical and electron microscopic changes cannot be detected. The clinical effects of severe hyperhidrosis are most distressing; slippery objects drop out of wet hands, it may be impossible to use a pen and the patient avoids social contact.

Upper thoracic sympathectomy is also indicated in severe examples of Raynaud's phenomenon which do not respond to conservative measures. However, unlike the permanent results of sympathectomy for hyperhidrosis, there is a tendency to progressive relapse following the operation so that only some 50% of patients show persistent improvement when assessed several years postoperatively.

Advantages and disadvantages of the transthoracic approach

The advantages of the transthoracic approach are the almost invisible scar, which lies hidden in the axilla, the avoidance of Horner's syndrome in the great majority of cases, provided that the stellate ganglion is carefully preserved, and the simplicity of the anatomical approach to the chain compared with the transcervical technique.

The disadvantages of the operation are that most surgeons, including the author, consider that it is only safe to perform one side at a time. I usually leave at least a month between the two operations in bilateral cases. Some surgeons, however, have practised synchronous bilateral thoracotomy successfully. The operation is also contraindicated if there has been previous intrathoracic infection, e.g. quiescent pulmonary tuberculosis, with resultant pleural adhesions. In such cases (and I have only encountered one example of this) the transcervical approach becomes mandatory.

Surgical anatomy

1

In planning excision of the upper thoracic sympathetic chain for sympathetic denervation of the upper limb and axilla, the surgeon needs to know how much of the chain to remove in order to effect satisfactory denervation and how to prevent a Horner's syndrome. The thoracic portion of the chain continues downwards from the cervical sympathetic chain and lies anterior to the heads of the ribs. It lies immediately external to the parietal pleura, almost invariably immediately anterior to the intercostal vessels. However, the chain lies uncomfortably close to the intercostal veins, which may occasionally cross in front of it. Each ganglion is situated fairly consistently in front of the corresponding rib head. The first thoracic ganglion may be independent or, more usually, is fused to the inferior cervical ganglion to constitute the stellate ganglion. Occasionally, the second thoracic ganglion may be fused into this ganglionic conglomeration. Each ganglion lies below the level of the corresponding intercostal nerve to which it is connected by the white ramus communicans of preganglionic fibres and the grey (postganglionic) ramus. The grey ramus usually lies medially to the white ramus but occasionally these are combined into a single trunk and at times there may be more than two rami.

The fibres in the white ramus communicans of the first thoracic nerve ascend in the chain to the superior cervical ganglion in order to supply sympathetic fibres to the face. Interruption of the sympathetic chain at or above this first thoracic ganglion level will thus result in Horner's syndrome, comprising ptosis, pupillary constriction, flushing of the face and facial anhidrosis on the affected side.

The second thoracic nerve is the highest one to contain preganglionic fibres to the upper limb. There is much more variability to the lower limit and fibres as low as the seventh thoracic nerve may contribute fibres to the upper limb. Although there is this widespread origin of preganglionic fibres to the upper limb, division of the thoracic sympathetic chain immediately below the first ganglion will usually interrupt all fibres that traverse the sympathetic chain to reach the upper limb by distribution through the brachial plexus. In practice, removal of the thoracic sympathetic chain to include the second, third and fourth ganglia, which means removing the chain from the head of the second to the head of the fourth rib, is found to produce effective sympathetic denervation of the upper limb and axilla.

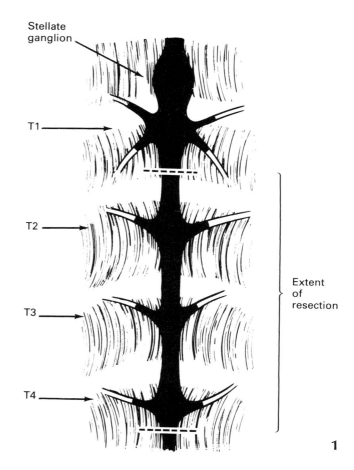

Stellate ganglion

T1

T2

T3

T4

Extent of resection

1

Surgical technique

2

The transaxillary approach was first described by Sir Hedley Atkins in 1949. Endotracheal general anaesthesia is used. The patient is placed in the lateral position with the arm abducted to 90°. A suitable right-angled arm support is used. It is convenient to tilt the patient in the head-up position at about 20° to allow adequate illumination of the depths of the wound. It is useful to have a malleable light on a probe to improve illumination if necessary, particularly in an obese patient.

2

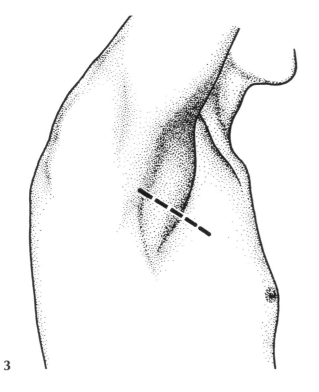

3

3

The incision is made along the line of the second intercostal space from pectoralis major in front to latissimus dorsi posteriorly. The obliquity of this incision varies quite considerably from one subject to another. Because the area is quite vascular, bleeding is controlled by preliminary infiltration of the subcutaneous tissues with a 1:200 000 solution of adrenaline in normal saline and by the use of the diathermy cutting needle. The incision is made through the axillary fat down to the serratus anterior. The nerve to this muscle (the long thoracic nerve of Bell) is identified at the posterior limit of the incision and is carefully preserved. Injury to this nerve will produce winging of the scapula.

The second intercostal space is now palpated and the serratus divided with diathermy over the space. The dissection is then continued through the intercostal muscles down to the pleura. By staying immediately superior to the second rib, damage to the intercostal bundle can be avoided. The pleura is opened, the lung collapses and the intercostal space is opened for the full length of the wound. The ribs are then retracted by means of a Price-Thomas self-retaining retractor which is slowly opened to its full extent. A wet pack is placed over the collapsed lung, which is retracted downwards by means of a suitably bent malleable copper retractor.

4

The sympathetic chain can now be easily identified as it lies beneath the parietal pleura on the heads of the upper ribs. On the right side, the azygos vein is seen lying medially to the chain, whereas on the left side, the aorta and left subclavian artery can be seen.

It is important to identify the sympathetic chain quite precisely before the parietal pleura is opened, otherwise oozing of blood may obscure the anatomy. The line of the chain is indicated on the pleura by two or three scalpel nicks and 2 or 3 ml of the dilute adrenaline solution is then injected via a fine needle beneath the pleura to free it from the underlying ribs.

4

5

5

The parietal pleura is now divided longitudinally along the line of the sympathetic chain using a fine scalpel blade on a long handle. The pleura is pushed aside from the chain by means of small gauze pledgets held in long artery forceps.

The chain is caught up on a nerve hook and carefully removed from below upwards from the level of the fourth rib to just below the stellate ganglion, thus removing the fourth, third and second ganglia.

6

Bleeding may be encountered from branches of the intercostal vessels, particularly the veins, and haemostasis is effected by means of diathermy coagulation, Cushing's silver clips or a combination of the two.

It is my practice to mark the upper and lower extremities of the chain resection by means of Cushing's clips so that subsequent radiology can confirm the extent of the resection.

A check is made to ensure complete haemostasis before the anaesthetist is asked to inflate the lung.

A plastic intercostal tube is inserted through the second space and brought out through a small stab wound. The wound is closed in layers using catgut, the skin sutured and the intercostal drain connected with an underwater seal. Meanwhile, the anaesthetist continues to ensure that the lung is completely inflated in order to obliterate the pneumothorax.

The patient is transferred to the recovery room and, when conscious, a check X-ray of the chest is carried out. If this confirms that complete expansion of the lung has occurred, the chest tube can be removed in the recovery room before the patient is returned to the ward.

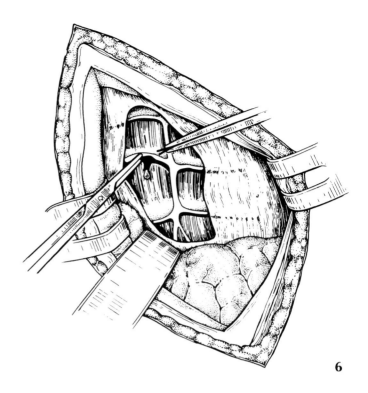

6

Postoperative care

The patient requires vigorous postoperative chest physiotherapy and a repeat chest X-ray the day following operation ensures the absence of a pneumothorax or pleural effusion. The great majority of patients can leave hospital 3 or 4 days postoperatively.

References

Atkins, H. J. B. (1949). Per axillary approach to the stellate and upper thoracic sympathetic ganglia. *Lancet* **2**, 1152.
Ellis, H. (1979). Transaxillary sympathectomy in the treatment of hyperhidrosis of the upper limb. *American Surgeon* **45**, 546.
Law, N. and Ellis, H. (in press). Transthoracic sympathectomy for hyperhidrosis in children under the age of 16. *Annals of the Royal College of Surgeons* **70**.

Embolectomy for acute lower-limb ischaemia

Hans O. Myhre   MD, PhD
Professor and Chairman, Department of Surgery, Trondheim University Clinic, Trondheim, Norway
Ola D. Saether   MD
Senior Registrar, Department of Surgery, Trondheim University Clinic, Trondheim, Norway

Introduction

In the Scandinavian countries, embolectomies for acute limb ischaemia have increased about 50% during the last 10 years. Approximately 50% of the procedures are performed by junior staff. The reasons for the increasing incidence of embolism may be due to an increase in the elderly population and the fact that more patients survive major cardiac disease.

In acute limb ischaemia the differential diagnosis between emboli and acute arterial thrombosis is important, because the treatment must be selected accordingly. Thus, an aggressive surgical approach is justified in most cases with emboli, whereas initial conservative treatment may be preferred following acute arterial thrombosis provided the limb is viable (Dale, 1984).

1

The diagnosis of embolism is based on the presence of a potential source and the sudden onset of symptoms. The location of the arterial obstruction may also indicate the source. Thus, an embolus leading to ischaemia of an isolated toe usually arises from atherosclerotic changes in the aorta or the iliac arteries, whereas an embolus in the aortic bifurcation most likely has a cardiac origin. An embolus usually lodges where the artery divides and its calibre reduces.

In arterial thrombosis the onset of symptoms is gradual, often with a previous history of intermittent claudication without signs of cardiac disease. In addition, the pulses may be absent on the contralateral limb.

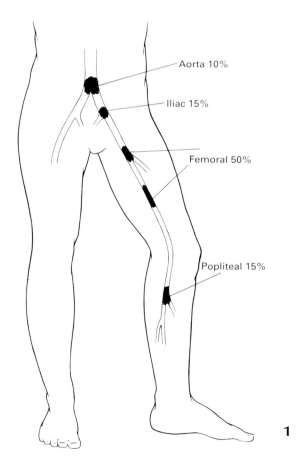

Aorta 10%

Iliac 15%

Femoral 50%

Popliteal 15%

1

Preoperative considerations

Critical ischaemia is indicated by loss of sensitivity, discolouration that blanches with pressure, decreased skin temperature and moderate rigour of the calf muscles. It is generally agreed that embolectomy is indicated even in these patients (Tawes *et al.*, 1985). Although early diagnosis and treatment is important, the time from onset of symptoms to admission is of less importance than the clinical status of the limb. Thus, the time factor does not contraindicate embolectomy by itself.

In irreversible ischaemia there is blotchy cyanotic discolouration which is not influenced by digital pressure. The calf muscle has a firm consistency and, in addition, there is anaesthesia and paralysis of the extremity. The treatment of choice for patients with irreversible ischaemic changes is primary amputation.

Patients with a clear-cut history of emboli are not referred to preoperative angiography. Angiography should, however, always be done when there is doubt about the diagnosis or when acute arterial thrombosis is suspected.

If present, cardiac insufficiency and dehydration should be corrected preoperatively, but the operation should not be delayed by lengthy evaluations.

Heparin is given intravenously as a bolus of 100–150 i.u. per kg bodyweight, taking into consideration that heparin may influence the selection of anaesthesia. Blood is typed and cross-matched and the patient is transferred to the operating room.

In general, the patient is prepared from the nipples to the toes of both feet, keeping in mind that more extensive surgery can become necessary and that multiple emboli often occur. For unilateral femoropopliteal embolectomy when the femoral pulse is palpable, some surgeons prepare the groin and limb only.

Anaesthesia technique and monitoring

Local anaesthesia with lidocaine 0.5–1% is recommended when the embolectomy can be completed via the common femoral artery. Local anaesthetics with adrenaline must be used with care in patients with severe coronary heart disease. Should clinical signs or angiography indicate that additional proximal or distal surgery becomes necessary, local anaesthesia may be a disadvantage. Epidural anaesthesia is contraindicated if the patient is already heparinized, but spinal anaesthesia by a thin needle can be used in these patients without risk of intraspinal bleeding. However, most surgeons prefer general anaesthesia when the operation cannot be completed with local anaesthesia.

Since there is a high incidence of concomitant cardiovascular disease, close monitoring is necessary, especially to detect the systemic effects of revascularization. Monitoring of central venous pressure, systemic arterial pressure and urine output is recommended. In patients with advanced ischaemia, monitoring of central haemodynamics by a Swan–Ganz catheter is justified. Prior to re-establishment of blood flow in such patients, a high urinary output should be obtained by volume therapy and osmotic diuretics. The acid–base status should be closely monitored and sodium bicarbonate added in case of acidosis (Tawes *et al.*, 1985).

The operation

Femoropopliteal embolectomy

2

The advantage of the Fogarty balloon catheter is that emboli can be removed from the aorta as well as the leg arteries via a local arterteriotomy in the common femoral artery. Most femoropopliteal embolectomies can be performed by this approach.

2

3a & b

A vertical incision in the groin is used (*a*), and the common, superficial and the deep femoral arteries are dissected (*b*). Elastic vascular tapes are applied to these arteries for vessel occlusion rather than vascular clamps, so as to minimize blood loss during repeated introductions of the embolectomy catheter. Furthermore, vascular clamps may break the embolic material making it more difficult to remove.

A small incision in the common femoral artery is performed using a No. 11 scalpel blade. A longitudinal arteriotomy of about 1.5 cm is made using fine-angled scissors just proximal to the orifice of the profunda femoris artery. Stay-sutures are applied to the edges of the arteriotomy to facilitate repeated introductions of the Fogarty catheter without damage to the edges of the arteriotomy, which should not be handled by forceps (*b*).

The stylet of the embolectomy catheter is removed and the patency of the balloon is tested by inflation of saline as recommended for each catheter size. A 1-ml tuberculine syringe is useful for the inflation of a No. 4 embolectomy catheter. Various modifications of the balloon embolectomy catheter have been presented. A channel at the end of the catheter can be used for intraoperative angiography and for irrigation with heparin saline solution. Side-ports central to the balloon may be advantageous for the removal of adherent embolic material and will probably minimize intimal damage. Resterilized catheters should not be used.

The end of a deflated No. 3 or 4 Fogarty catheter is dipped in heparin saline solution or blood and then introduced into the superficial femoral artery (*b*). In patients without atherosclerosis, the catheter can usually be advanced to the foot. The catheter is withdrawn 0.5–1 cm and the balloon is then inflated while moving the catheter to prevent excessive shear forces (Dobrin and Jorgensen, 1985). The grade of inflation must be varied according to the calibre of the artery. Extra caution is necessary during embolectomy of small arteries to avoid overdistention of the balloon. The catheter should be inflated and pulled back by the same surgeon.

3a

3b

3c, d & e

The embolic material is now removed through the arteriotomy (c). The procedure is repeated until no residual embolic material is found, keeping in mind that several withdrawals with a high shear force can induce subsequent intimal hyperplasia (Bowles *et al.*, 1988; Schwarcz *et al.*, 1988). Coagulated blood and debris must be cleaned off the catheter between each introduction. Brisk backbleeding from the distal arterial tree can now be expected, but is not synonymous with a complete embolectomy.

Embolectomy of the profunda femoris artery is now performed. It is extremely important that this artery is free of embolic material. The catheter can usually be advanced about 20 cm from the orifice of the artery. The arteries are flushed with heparine saline solution (1000 i.u. in 100 ml saline) and blood flow from the proximal arteries is tested before the arteriotomy is closed. Provided the artery is unaffected by atherosclerosis and of good calibre, the arteriotomy can be closed by direct suture using 5/0 or 6/0 monofilament suture material (d). A patch graft angioplasty is preferred to avoid stenosis during closure of narrow arteries or when there are atherosclerotic changes in the arterial wall (e). The saphenous vein is harvested at the ankle and used for patch graft material.

Completion angiography is mandatory following femoropopliteal embolectomy, since incomplete embolectomy has been found in 25–40% of the cases when judged by backbleeding only.

3c

3d

3e

4a, b & c

The peroneal and posterial tibial arteries may be embolectomized through the common femoral artery by bending the tip of the catheter. However, not all types of catheters can be manipulated in this way (Gwynn, Shearman and Simms, 1987). The anterior tibial artery is not readily accessible by this approach. When the popliteal pulse is palpable preoperatively, we explore the popliteal artery below the knee (*a,b*). Following arteriotomy, a No. 3 embolectomy catheter can then be introduced into the different leg arteries. The arteriotomy is closed by patch graft angioplasty (*c*) (Abbott *et al.*, 1984).

In all cases, embolic material should be investigated by microscopy for verification of the aetiology.

4a

4b

4c

5a & b

Aortoiliac 'saddle' embolectomy

Patients with emboli at the aortic bifurcation or the iliac arteries have a more serious prognosis than patients with femoropopliteal embolism (Busuttil *et al.*, 1983). The abdomen and the lower extremities are prepared as previously described. Vertical incisions are made in both groins and the femoral arteries dissected as described for femoropopliteal embolectomy, preferably by two surgeons working simultaneously (*a*).

A deflated No. 5 or 6 Fogarty catheter is introduced into the aorta through the arteriotomy of the common femoral artery. The balloon is distended and the catheter withdrawn, thereby removing embolic material. The risk of losing embolic material into the contralateral limb can be reduced by compressing the common femoral artery, thereby reducing the

blood flow of the contralateral iliac system. When sufficient blood flow from the iliac artery on the embolectomized side is obtained, the embolectomy is repeated on the contralateral side (*b*).

A No. 3 or 4 catheter is then introduced into the superficial femoral and profunda femoris arteries on both sides to remove possible embolic material. The arteriotomies are closed as previously described. A suction drain is routinely left close to each arteriotomy and can usually be removed on the following day.

A similar approach as described for the removal of saddle embolus is used for iliac embolectomy. It is usually sufficient to expose the arteries of one groin only, but great care is taken not to push embolic material into the opposite leg.

5a

5b

Percutaneous aspiration thromboembolectomy (PAT)

PAT is performed through a specially designed catheter–sheath system for clot extraction. The advantage is that it can be used at the time of diagnostic angiography. It is not within the scope of this presentation to describe the technical details of PAT, which is preferably used for removal of smaller emboli from the distal arterial tree. (Starck *et al.*, 1985).

Handling of special problems

During delayed embolectomy a cleavage plane between the embolus and the arterial wall may be difficult to identify. A ringstripper can then be used as a supplement to the balloon catheter, or a bypass graft is applied for revascularization.

Sometimes, the embolus may consist of atherosclerotic material from the proximal arterial tree. Removal of the source of embolus is indicated in most of these patients on an elective basis. If the limb ischaemia is caused by aortic dissection, revascularization of the extremity is performed, the anticoagulation therapy must be reversed and further investigation of the aortic dissection is carried out. When acute arterial thrombosis is found to be the cause of critical ischaemia during operation, the surgeon should be prepared to proceed with arterial reconstruction following angiographic investigation. Thrombosis of a popliteal aneurysm may also be the cause of ischaemia. The aneurysm is excluded from the circulation and arterial reconstruction is performed.

Complications

Complications following use of the balloon catheter include rupture of the balloon, intimal injury, arteriovenous fistula, fragmentation of the clot with distal embolization and inadequate removal of the material. Furthermore, dissection of arterosclerotic plaques may occur. Perforation is indicated by difficulties during withdrawal of the catheter. The balloon should be deflated immediately and the catheter removed.

Fasciotomy is performed in cases with preoperative severe ischaemia when repeated postoperative examinations indicate a closed compartment syndrome.

The post-perfusion syndrome can be suspected in the same group of patients. This syndrome is indicated by a urine specimen with Guajac positive pigments, but without red blood cells on microscopy. Prophylaxis by isolation of the femoral vein followed by withdrawal of 300–500 ml of blood during the first pass of arterial blood has been recommended and may be indicated in selected cases (Tawes *et al.*, 1985). If deep venous thrombosis is found following venotomy, a venous thrombectomy is undertaken.

Postoperative considerations

The patient should be observed in the intensive care unit during the first 24 h following the operation. In addition to general monitoring, the circulation of the first toe should be recorded continuously by a non-invasive technique. The patient can be mobilized on the first postoperative day. Heparin is given postoperatively by continuous infusion according to body weight, sex and age. Warfarin-sodium is started immediately following the operation. When a protrombine time of 5–10% of normal value is obtained heparin therapy is discontinued. In most patients, including those with cardiac disease, we find lifelong treatment with warfarin-sodium indicates prevention of recurrent emboli.

References

Abbott, W. M., McCabe, C., Maloney, R. D., Wirthlin, L. S. (1984). Embolism of the popliteal artery. *Surgery, Gynecology and Obstetrics* **159**, 533.

Bowles, C. R., Olcott, C., Pakter, R. L., Lombard, C., Mehigan,, J. T. and Walter, J. F. (1988). Diffuse arterial narrowing as a result of intimal proliferation: A delayed complication of embolectomy with the Fogarty balloon catheter. *Journal of Vascular Surgery* **7**, 487.

Busuttil, R. W., Keehn, G., Milliken, J. *et al.* (1983). Aortic saddle embolus. A twenty-year experience. *Annals of Surgery* **197**, 698.

Dale, W. A. (1984). Differential management of acute peripheral arterial ischemia. *Journal of Vascular Surgery* **1**, 269.

Dobrin, P. B. and Jorgenson, R. A. (1985). Balloon embolectomy catheters in small arteries: A technique to prevent excessive shear forces. *Journal of Vascular Surgery* **2**, 692.

Fogarty, T. J., Cranley, J. J., Krause, R. J., Strasser, E. S. and Hafner, C. D. (1963). A method for extraction of arterial emboli and thrombi. *Surgery, Gynecology and Obstetrics* **116**, 241.

Gwynn, B. R., Shearman, C. P. and Simms, M. H. (1987). The anatomical basis for the route taken by Fogarty catheters in the lower leg. *European Journal of Vascular Surgery* **1**, 129.

Schwarcz, T. H., Dobrin, P. B., Mrkvicka, R., Skowron, L. and Cole, M. B., Jr (1988). Early myointimal hyperplasia after balloon catheter embolectomy: Effect of shear forces and multiple withdrawals. *Journal of Vascular Surgery* **7**, 495.

Starck, E. E., McDermott, J. C., Crummy, A. B., Turnipseed, W. D., Acher, C. W. and Burgess, J. H. (1985). Percutaneous aspiration thromboembolectomy. *Radiology* **156**, 61.

Tawes, R. L., Harris, E. J., Brown, W. H. *et al.* (1985). Arterial thromboembolism. A 20-year experience. *Archives of Surgery* **120**, 595.

Initial lysis and catheter clot removal for occlusive disease in critical ischaemia

B. Nachbur
Department of Thoracic and Cardiovascular Surgery, University of Berne, Berne, Switzerland

F. Mahler
Medical Department of the University of Berne, Berne, Switzerland

Do-Dai-Do
Medical Department of the University of Berne, Berne, Switzerland

E. Schneider
Division of Angiology, Medical Department of the University of Zürich, Zürich, Switzerland

Introduction

Catheter clot lysis (CTL) is gaining increasing acceptance as it becomes evident that not all cases of critical ischaemia are best treated surgically. Our own experience in Berne comprises well over 150 cases with streptokinase, urokinase and tissue plasminogen activator (rt–PA) being used in that order. Although success rates, i.e. patency rates, have risen from 73 to 85%, the differences are statistically not significant, there being no proof that any one fibrinolytic agent is superior to the other as far as efficacy is concerned. If the results with streptokinase are somewhat less favourable it should be borne in mind that this is most likely attributable to a period during which experience with this new form of treatment had to be gained. In the light of this we look back upon our results with streptokinase with satisfaction and are actually using either this drug or urokinase again.

Although Hess and others (Hess, Mietaschk and Ingrisch, 1980; Hess et al., 1982; Schneider and Largiadèr, 1987) have advocated local clot lysis in the treatment of arterial occlusions with symptoms of complete ischaemia, we feel that it is best indicated for treatment of viable limbs presenting with acute thrombotic occlusion associated with localized or widespread atherosclerotic lesions.

It is agreed that acute thromboembolic occlusion of the iliofemoral segment is best treated by the Fogarty balloon extraction catheter; local thrombolysis is especially suitable for acute thrombotic lesions involving the femoral and/or popliteal arteries including the popliteal trifurcation. CTL is furthermore indicated in the treatment of early re-occlusions after percutaneous transluminal angioplasty (PTA) and recanalization of acute occlusions of femoropopliteal grafts.

As the clot is gradually being dissolved, underlying stenotic lesions are uncovered and thus become amenable to PTA, which on its own merit must be considered an integral part of catheter clot lysis therapy because it deals with the causative mechanism of thrombotic occlusion. The rate of local thrombolysis can be hastened by aspiration of extraction of loosened clots (CTE) whereby clearance of the vessel is more actively promoted.

General outline

1. Fluoroscopy.
2. Seldinger technique for introduction of a percutaneous catheter.
3. Percutaneous catheter introducer (PCI kit), for use with a 0.035–0.038 inch diameter guide-wire, manufactured by Argon, containing:
   - 6–9 (= 2.8 mm) French radiopaque sheath;
   - removable haemostasis valve with side-port extension for injection of heparin or dye and removable stopcock;
   - vessel dilator.
4. Introduction of a French 7 or 8 polyethylene catheter under fluoroscopy.
5. Gradual infusion of fibrinolytic agent.
6. Stepwise advancement of catheter tip.
7. Suction of fresh, loosened thrombi.
8. Percutaneous dilatation of atherosclerotic plaque.

1 & 2

For introduction of a percutaneous catheter the Seldinger technique is used with anterograde puncture of the common femoral artery. This can pose problems in obese patients because the puncture site should be below the inguinal ligament in order to avoid retroperitoneal haematoma.

Laboratory examinations during CTL include the analysis of prothrombin time, thrombin time, coagulation factors II, V, VII and X, reptilase time, an ethanol test and fibrinogen levels. During long-term lysis the thrombin time values were kept from exceeding twice the normal by adjusting the doses of heparin given.

We apply between 40 000 and 100 000 u of streptokinase in one 90-min session. When patency is achieved the procedure is terminated, and 5000 u of heparin are given.

If, after 90 min, the flow through the initially occluded segment is unsatisfactory, the procedure is continued on the ward as a long-term regional thrombolysis after insertion of a French-3 catheter via the introducer sheath. The dose of streptokinase is 4000 u/h for 8–72 h. Heparin is infused through the side branch of the introducer sheath to prevent pericatheter thrombolysis. Clinical assessment is confirmed by contrast injection through the indwelling catheter at inervals of at least 24 h.

Clinical success is defined by either a return of pedal pulses or a reduction in the arterial ankle pressure deficit of at least 50 mmHg.

Fibrinogen levels do drop somewhat in our hands, albeit not dramatically: from 2.1 ± 0.7 to 2.0 ± 0.5 g/l for streptokinase; from 2.6 ± 0.7 to 2.5 ± 1.2 g/l for urokinase; and from 2.7 ± 0.8 to 2.3 ± 1.0 g/l for rt–PA. Bleeding complications occurred in 8, 4 and 4% respectively for the fibrinolytic agents.

Radiopaque sheath

24 cm

① Vessel dilator

23 cm or more

Haemostasis valve (removable)

Vessel dilator of varying length

③ 6–8.9 radiopaque sheath (compressible)

② Side-port extension

⑤ Guide-wire

④ Removable stopcock

Contrast medium

Heparin

1

2

3

Illustration 3 shows a radiographic image of a long popliteal occlusion of thrombotic origin in a 74-year-old male patient. Radiologic signs of embolism are not present. Clinically, the patient presents in a state of critical ischaemia, the limb is viable but there is a certain degree of numbness in the toes. The percutaneous catheter shown in *Illustrations 1* and *2* is introduced via the common femoral artery into the superficial femoral artery. A vessel dilator, 40–60 cm in length, can be introduced directly into the superficial femoral artery or with the help of a bent guide-wire, which in PTA is advanced through the occluded segment down to the patent vessel lumen beyond the occlusion to ensure avoidance of subintimal catheterization. A guide-wire is used in this case for better orientation.

3

4

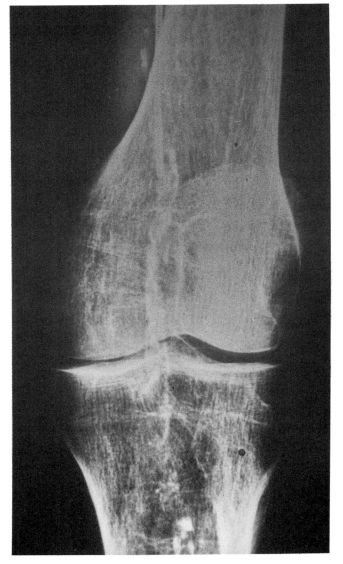

4

The guide-wire can be seen approximately 3 cm below the knee joint in the same patient as in *Illustration 3*. The tip of the catheter is recognizable at the level of the upper border of the knee cap. By comparison with *Illustration 3*, one can see that the catheter has been unmistakably advanced into the proximal part of the clot. This manoeuvre is performed very slowly and without undue force. Thrombolysis is induced by gradual infusion of streptokinase in doses of 2000–4000 u for each advancement of the catheter tip, allowing about 2–5 min per cm. If urokinase is used, the average dose necessary for each advancement is between 5000 and 10 000 u. For rt–PA, 1 mg is required. From time to time a little contrast medium is injected via the stopcock (see *Illustrations 1* and *2*) to ascertain the progress of clot lysis. It is possible to identify some contrast medium within the formerly totally occluded popliteal artery. The important aspects of this are shown in *Illustration 6*.

5 & 6

The same patient as shown in *Illustration 3*, 15 min after beginning clot lysis. The position of the intrathrombotic catheter and the guide-wire can be seen.

5

6

7

For the same patient as shown in *Illustrations 3–6* an angiogram shows that thrombolysis catheter treatment of acute and subacute thrombotic occlusions is possible and feasible. However, in some instances, CTL may keep the medical staff busy for several hours in the angiography laboratory, even though recanalization may be accelerated by catheter manipulation including suction, aspiration or even extraction of loosened clots. To decrease laboratory time, we have developed a two-stage programme for CTL. It consists of a short CTL for 90 min under fluoroscopy and, if patency is not achieved during this period, a subsequent CTL is performed in the ward up to 48 h later.

In the case presented here, complete thrombolysis was achieved within 24 h, at which time the angiograms shown in *Illustrations 7* and *8* were performed. The reader is urged to compare *Illustrations 3* and *7* carefully.

7

8

8

The completion angiogram for the same patient as in *Illustrations 3–7* shows the lower level of a formerly occluded popliteal artery 24 h after initiation of CTL. The popliteal trifurcation can now be seen clearly.

Note the well-defined circumscribed atheromatous plaque near the origin of the anterior tibial artery. This lesion might have been the reason for thrombotic occlusion. Once it is uncovered by thrombolysis, it can be dealt with by PTA, which is an integral part of the treatment modality.

9

CTL was started immediately after performing the initial angiogram on this 76-year-old female patient with sudden onset of arterial occlusion (*left*). Thrombolysis was accelerated by extracting considerable amounts of clot. In this case, an open distal run-off segment can be identified at the upper level of the femur condyles. As soon as complete thrombolysis is achieved, there is suddenly considerable reflux when the haemostasis valve is removed (see *Illustrations 1* and *2*). Loosened clots can then only be suctioned or extracted if the haemostasis valve is regularly removed and replaced afterwards for further manipulation. In the example presented here, there is residual subtotal occlusion of the proximal popliteal artery and a protruding plaque in the distal part of the superficial femoral artery. Both lesions underwent successful PTA. One year later, a control angiogram showed clear evidence of sustained patency of the femoropopliteal axis.

9

10a & b

Occlusions of femoropopliteal grafts are very suitable for CTL combined with CTE if discovered and diagnosed early (within days) after onset (*a*). CTL was performed in combination with clot extraction (CTE) in this patient for occlusion of a femoroinfragenicular Dardik biograft where surgical disobliteration was not deemed to be rewarding. The clot extraction was so abundant (see *Illustration 11*) that complete patency of the Dardik graft with both anastomoses to the anterior tibial artery and the tibiofibular trunk was achieved within a few hours.

10a

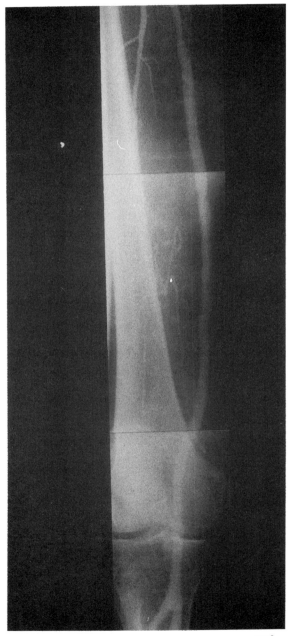

10b

11

Illustration 11 shows clot material retrieved by catheter extraction from the Dardik prosthesis after initial local lysis in the same patient as in *Illustration 10*. In this case, clot extraction was performed through a relatively large French 9 sheath.

11

12

The principle of clot extraction

The haemostasis valve with the side-port extension has been removed, and the radiopaque sheath French 8 or 9 is left in place to protect the vessel wall from injury due to catheter manipulation. Collaterals are likewise protected from being occluded by clots in dissolution. The catheter used for extraction is advanced into the loosened clots which are aspirated by some means of suction, e.g. with a syringe. The thicker the sheath, the larger the clots will be that can be extracted by a slightly smaller catheter. By using a large sheath, the danger of perforation increases.

12

Sheath

Catheter
Sheath 9 Fr

Haemostasis
valve with
side-port
extension
removed

Clot

Catheter for
lysis and/or
clot aspiration

Clot in
dissolution

Suction

Acknowledgement

B. Nachbur would like to acknowledge the help received from Ernst Schneider.

References

Do-Dai-Do, Mahler, F., Probst, P. and Nachbur, B. (1987). Combination of short and long-term-time catheter thrombolysis for peripheral arterial occlusion. *European Journal of Radiology* 7, 235.

Hess, H., Mietaschk, A. and Ingrisch, H. (1980). Niedrig dosierte thrombolytische Therapie tur Wiederherstellung der Strombahn bei arteriellen Verschlüssen. *Dtsch Med. Wschr* 105, 787.

Hess, H., Ingrisch, H., Mietaschk, A. and Rath, H. (1982). Local low-dose thrombolytic therapy of peripheral arterial occlusion. *New England Journal of Medicine* 307, 1627.

Schneider E. and Largiader, J. (1987). Therapiekonzept beim akuten Verschluss von Extremitätenarterien. *Therap. Umschau* 44, 653.

Reconstruction of, and to, the profunda femoris artery

Crawford Jamieson   MS, FRCS
Consultant Surgeon, St Thomas' Hospital, London, UK;
Honorary Consultant Surgeon, Hammersmith Hospital and Royal Postgraduate Medical School, London, UK

Introduction

The importance of restoration of flow to the deep femoral artery, as opposed to the superficial femoral artery, has long been recognized, but the first report of direct reconstruction of stenosis of the origin of this artery was made by Natali in Paris, and direct endarterectomy was popularized by Martin and Cotton. Martin published a large series of patients treated by 'profundaplasty' but 80% of them had a simultaneous proximal endarterectomy, or bypass of an iliac arterial stenosis or occlusion (Martin, Renwick and Stephenson, 1968). Cotton favoured an extended approach to the operation, patching the artery well down into the thigh, and claimed that the results were better the longer the reconstruction (Berguer, Cotton and Sabri, 1973). Martin, however, had preached the opposite, feeling that when disease extended beyond the first perforating artery, reconstruction tended to be unsuccessful owing to the prevalence of disease in distal branches. This dichotomy of opinion has never been resolved but, in the course of time, the operation of extended profundaplasty has fallen from favour and most surgeons now confine their attentions to stenoses localized to the proximal few centimetres of the artery.

This is an operation which is relatively safe and easy to perform, is capable of producing a new limited increase in the circulation of the limb but has excellent long-term patency (Hopkins *et al.*, 1983).

Indications

Profundaplasty is indicated only in the presence of a significant stenosis of the profunda femoris artery. This statement may appear obvious but it has been claimed that limb flow may be improved by widening a totally normal profunda femoris origin in the presence of a superficial femoral arterial occlusion (Berguer, Higgins and Cotton, 1975). The logic upon which this decision is made remains, however, rather dubious. It appears from the authors' interpretation of their haemodynamic model that a stenosis exists in the arterial tree which consists of the normal profunda femoris origin but, the branching arterial tree maintains, by an increase of area at each branch, a standard and even linear resistance. The decrease in resistance of the arterial tree from the heart to the foot achieved by a local profundaplasty of 2–3 cm is only an alteration in resistance, compared with the 1.3 m of artery from heart to foot, and cannot therefore be expected to be significant, and the operation of profundaplasty of an unstenosed vessel has generally been abandoned.

The operation is not indicated in patients with a patent superficial femoral artery, although theoretically they might suffer from intermittent claudication of the thigh with severe disease of the profunda femoris. This does not, however, seem to occur, and another cause must be sought for the aetiology of pain in the thigh if the superficial femoral artery is widely patent, even if disease exists in the profunda femoris. The operation is therefore indicated in patients with a stenosis of the origin of the profunda femoris artery and a co-existent superficial femoral arterial occlusion with or without proximal iliac or aortic disease. In the former circumstances, proximal reconstruction plus profundaplasty is indicated, whereas in the latter and less common situation, profundaplasty alone is indicated.

The most important and difficult decision lies in whether a patient with a profunda femoris stenosis and a superficial femoral arterial occlusion should be treated by profundaplasty, femoral popliteal bypass or a combination of both.

Successful femoral popliteal bypass restores flow in the foot to normal levels which profundaplasty in the presence of an untreated superficial femoral artery occlusion will never do (Jamieson, 1983). Bypass is therefore peferable to profundaplasty where circumstances are favourable and where a major increase in flow is necessary, either to relieve crippling intermittent claudication or to heal extensive ischaemic lesions of the foot. Profundaplasty is indicated in the relatively uncommon but well-defined alternative circumstances, particularly where there is critical ischaemia and where a rise of ankle blood pressure by 20 or 30 mmHg can be expected to relieve rest pain or allow healing of mild trophic lesions (Hill and Jamieson, 1977). Carefully selected profundaplasty in exactly this group of patients can produce excellent results and the general disenchantment with the procedure has, to a great extent, been due to unrealistic hopes for an increase in circulation by relief of such a local stenosis. Bernhard (1979) has pointed out that patients with a significant drop in pressure in the thigh, as opposed to across the knee on segmental thigh pressure, may be predicted to obtain a better result from profundaplasty than the latter group. Published results of the operation uncombined with a proximal reconstruction indicate that the mean increase in ankle pressure lies around 20% of the rise in the ankle brachial pressure index. The long-term patency of profundaplasty is excellent, late occlusion being rare within the life-span of the patient.

The major indication for a profundaplasty is as an adjunct to aortofemoral grafting or associated with reconstruction of a unilateral iliac arterial stenosis by direct endarterectomy or angioplasty. Profundaplasty may be vital to maintain an adequate flow and protect long-term patency of a proximal reconstruction, in addition to improving the results of the major proximal operation by increasing flow into the muscles of the thigh.

Simultaneous profundaplasty and femoral popliteal bypass

This is tempting when a superficial femoral block with a good run-off is associated with a severe stenosis of the origin of the profunda femoris artery, but is probably unnecessary, and may even be unwise, because theoretically it reduces the pressure gradient between the common femoral and the popliteal artery and, therefore, the flow rate through the femoral popliteal bypass. Although there is only shaky evidence that patency of femoral popliteal bypass is directly in proportion to the flow, there is no doubt that long-term patency is very poor when flow falls below the critical level of around 150 ml/min (Law and Roberts, 1983). It is probably better to perform the femoral popliteal bypass first, keeping profundaplasty in reserve in case of long-term failure of the bypass.

Preoperative preparation

In addition to the general assessment of the patient for fitness for surgery and the degree of ischaemia of his limb, it is important that angiograms be obtained in two planes, particularly an oblique view, as the profunda femoris origin may be obscured by dye in the origin of the superficial femoral artery in the conventional anteroposterior projection of an angiogram (Beales et al., 1971). Intravenous digital subtraction angiography (DSA) is frequently adequate in this preoperative assessment and direct arterial punture may be avoided, although DSA may not give adequate information on the popliteal run-off and patency of calf vessels when the choice lies between a long bypass and profundaplasty, in

which case an intravenous DSA to examine the iliac arterial system followed by a direct femoral puncture and conventional angiogram which gives the best view of the distal vessels of the leg is ideal. Bacteria swabs should be taken of necrotic lesions of the foot and appropriate treatment commenced prior to surgery.

The operation may be performed under local anaesthetic when a proximal reconstruction is not required and is, therefore, highly suitable for the frail patient.

Position of patient

The patient should be positioned supine upon the operating table with the leg slightly abducted. The whole limb should be prepared and exposed and the abdomen prepared to the costal, or even subclavian region, if there is any doubt over the quality of the inflow through the iliac artery. A patch of vein is required and it is inadvisable to remove this vein from the saphenous vein at the ankle, as the wound may not heal well. We prefer to prepare a segment of forearm to harvest a vein patch rather than sacrifice the saphenous vein itself in its more proximal course.

1

Incision

The incision follows a vertical route, slightly convex laterally, over the course of the iliac and femoral vessels to avoid lymphatic damage.

1

2

Exposure

The excision is deepened to the deep fascia and the common femoral artery exposed. The inguinal ligament is defined and the femoral pulse reassessed. If the femoral pulse is weak, it may be advisable to perform direct intrafemoral arterial pressure measurements with an intra-arterial injection of papaverine to assess the adequacy of iliac inflow. This test may be misleading when the superficial femoral artery is occluded and the profunda femoris artery is severely stenosed, because even following injection of papaverine peripheral resistance may be so high that a good femoral pulse may exist in the presence of a severe iliac stenosis. Inadequate flow may then only be detected when the artery is opened.

The superficial femoral artery is exposed and the common femoral artery and superficial femoral artery are snared and elevated. This exposes the origin of the profunda femoris artery which may be multiple and is crossed approximately 1 cm from its origin by a large vein, the circumflex femoral vein, draining into the termination of the profunda femoris vein. This vein may be up to 1 cm in diameter and must be carefully controlled and divided before the distal artery can be exposed. The exposed course of the vein is very short and it is safer to oversew both ends than ligate them. Distal to this vein, the artery tends to run more parallel to the superficial femoral artery, and as it plunges gradually into the muscles of the thigh, it is crossed by further veins at regular intervals which may require division. The branches of the artery, the circumflex femoral artery and the perforating arteries, tend to arise around the level of these veins and should be controlled individually by snares.

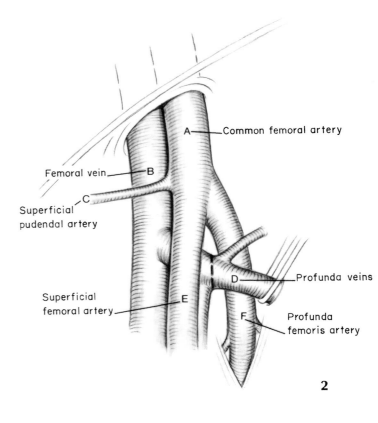

A — Common femoral artery

Femoral vein — B

C

Superficial pudendal artery

D — Profunda veins

Superficial femoral artery — E

F — Profunda femoris artery

2

3

3

Reconstruction

The arteries are clamped following intravenous administration of heparin 1.5 mg/kg. The direction and shape of the arteriotomy depends upon which method is selected, but it commences in the distal common femoral artery and is extended down the profunda femoris artery until an adequate lumen is reached. Local endarterectomy may then be performed if necessary, tailing off distally, making quite certain that there is no flap of intima to cause local occlusion. The loose intima should be anchored by a mattress suture inserted in through the endarterectomized segment and out through the unendarterectomized distal intima, to be tied on the exterior surface of the vessel. Avoidance of flaps is best achieved by avoiding endarterectomy where possible as Martin preferred. The adequacy of downflow and backflow are assessed – if downflow is inadequate, proximal reconstruction may be added at this stage, and the profundaplasty is then closed by Dacron end-to-side.

4

If backflow is inadequate, in spite of the gentle passage of Fogarty catheters, it may be necessary to reconsider the decision to perform a femoral distal bypass, but otherwise the arteriotomy is closed with a suitable vein patch. It can be an advantage to cut the vein square-ended as shown. The clamps are removed and anticoagulation is reversed. Operative angiography may be performed to assess the success of the reconstruction. The wound is closed over a suction drain.

5

A variety of permutations exist by which a stenosis of the profunda femoris origin can be relieved. These include use of the segment of endarterectomized occluded superficial femoral artery as a patch, dissected fully free as shown.

6

Alternatively, the endarterectomized superficial femoral artery is left attached and flapped over to widen the profunda origin as a square patch.

7

Widening of the profunda femoris origin can be achieved by suture of a patent or endarterectomized superficial femoral artery to a V-shaped arteriotomy between the superficial femoral artery and the profunda femoris.

6

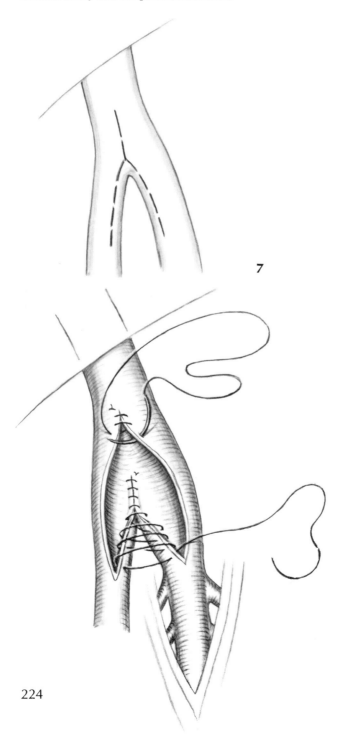

7

Postoperative management

There is little systemic disturbance from this operation and gastrointestinal function is normal. A urinary catheter is not required unless the iliac artery has been exposed, and the patient is allowed up after 24 h, provided there is no excessive lymph leak from the drain. If lymph drainage is considerable it is probably best that the patient be nursed supine until it decreases, as lymph flow is stimulated by exercise of the limb.

Ankle blood pressure is monitored daily for the first few days, though early failure of the reconstruction is most unusual. Antibiotic cover is not necessary as autogenous material alone has been used.

Complications

Apart from the general complications of any anaesthetic in a patient with a diffuse vascular disease and wound infection, the only significant complication is a lymphocoele, which is unusual, and almost always settles with time. It sometimes, however, develops after the suction drain has been removed and if it is large it is best treated by insertion of a further suction drain percutaneously by an oblique route which is left in until the drainage settles. Very rarely, this may take several days.

Profundaplasty combined with proximal reconstruction

The permutations of operation available in profundaplasty plus aortofemoral grafting are covered in elsewhere, but in spite of the popularity of bypass grafting there is still some place for local endarterectomy of iliac occlusions when the contralateral iliac artery is good. This operation may be performed by an extraperitoneal approach. It is safer, quicker and less traumatic than aortofemoral grafting (Martin, Renwick and Stephenson, 1968) and is associated with less systemic disturbance and ileus. Endarterectomy is technically more demanding than bypass, but it is a skill which should be available to every peripheral arterial surgeon and, although its detractors state that it only postpones the inevitable, similar operation on the contralateral side, this is not the case, as most patients treated by unilateral iliac endarterectomy do not survive to require an aortobifemoral graft within their limited life-span.

The preoperative preparation and positioning of the patient are identical to those of pure profundaplasty. The patient lies flat on the operating table.

8

Incision

A thin patient with external iliac occlusion is best treated by an incision carried vertically through the inguinal ligament and muscle layers of the abdominal wall just lateral to the origin of the common femoral artery, and extended proximally along the linear semilunaris. This incision, although apparently traumatic, gives excellent exposure of the external iliac artery and the distal common iliac artery, and is associated with a very low incidence of incisional hernia provided it is sutured carefully with continuous non-absorbable material of adequate strength. The incision is deepened through the external oblique aponeurosis and the conjoint muscles of internal oblique and transversus. A finger is inserted under the inguinal ligament and the peritoneum gently swept medially, taking great care to avoid damage to the deep circumflex iliac vein which crosses anterior to the distal part of the external iliac artery. The peritoneum becomes more adherent superiorly and medially to the posterior aspect of the rectus sheath and must be mobilized with great care to avoid opening the peritoneal cavity. It is, however, easily separated posteriorly from the anterior aspect of the vessels. The ureter is mobilized anteriorly with the peritoneum until the surgeon's fingers detect the normal pulse proximal to the iliac stenosis.

A Goligher retractor is inserted with a short blade against the iliac crest and a long blade protected by a large swab retracting the peritoneum and viscera. It is most important that this retractor should not exert pressure distally upon the femoral nerve which lies hidden under the fasica just lateral to the termination of the external iliac artery. The blades are opened giving excellent exposure of the external and internal iliac arteries and the common iliac artery. The inferior epigastric artery and deep circumflex iliac artery are controlled by snares as they originate from the distal part of the external iliac artery, and the deep circumflex iliac vein is divided.

Lymphatic tissue is cleared from the external iliac artery completely exposing the vessel. The internal iliac artery is snared taking great care to avoid damage to the internal iliac vein which lies deep to it. The distal part of the external common iliac artery is mobilized from the common iliac vein and similarly snared. Venous bleeding at this stage presents the only major hazard of the procedure and the common iliac artery may be so closely tethered to the common iliac vein by periarteritis that snaring is inadvisable, though it is difficult to control it adequately with a clamp unless it is mobilized.

8

Endarterectomy

The patient is anticoagulated with heparin 1.5mg/kg intravenously. The common iliac artery, internal iliac artery and branch of the common femoral artery are clamped and the distal common femoral artery is then opened in the same manner as for profundaplasty, but the arteriotomy is carried proximally to the distal extremity of the external iliac artery. Local endarterectomy is performed upwards from this point using loop or arc strippers to the patent common iliac artery. The arc stripper is extremely valuable for traversing a vessel or varying calibre but has the potential risk of catching in the arterial wall and must not be twisted during its upwards and downwards course in the plane of endarterectomy. It is best located by the surgeon's two fingers on each side of the points of its arc, as it is passed upwards. When the plaque has been loosened by one passage of the ring stripper or four passages of the arc stripper, an arterial clamp is gently closed on the unopened artery at the site of proximal mobilization of the plaque. The gentle closure combined with pressure from the fingers breaks the endarterectomized core, leaving the outer wall intact, and the core may be milked from the endarterectomized vessel.

The manoeuvre is not always successful and excessive force must not be used in attempting to break the plaque as it will result in damage to the external wall. If the plaque does not break open further, arteriotomy must be made at the proximal level of endarterectomy, the plaque divided under direct vision with scissors and the arteriotomy closed with continuous 4/0 polypropylene. Downflow is then assessed and if it is adequate the arteriotomy and the common femoral and profunda femoris arteries are closed with a vein patch as before.

Closure

The abdominal wall is closed with a continuous 2/0 nylon suture in two layers over a suction drain passed along the common femoral artery under the inguinal ligament to lie along the external iliac artery, and the groin wound is closed in layers.

Postoperative course

It is very similar to profundaplasty. Ileus is usually very slight unless the peritoneum has been inadvertently opened.

9

Combined common iliac endarterectomy and profundaplasty

9

The patient lies with a sandbag to raise the buttock if preferred. The incision described above does not give good exposure of the origin of the common iliac artery without such proximal extension that it risks weakening the muscles of the abdominal wall, and it gives less good exposure in the obese patient. Extensive unilateral iliac arterial occlusion is better treated by a combination of an incision over the common femoral artery and a separate oblique incision in the abdominal wall. The common femoral arterial exposure is extended proximally by division of the inguinal ligament for approximately 1 cm to allow control of the inferior epigastric and deep circumflex iliac arteries.

The abdominal incision is commenced at a point 3 cm above the pubic tubercle over the conjoint tendon and directed upwards and laterally towards the costal margin. It is deepened through the linear semilunaris in its lower part by a combination of splitting the external oblique and cutting the internal oblique and transversus muscles more proximally. The peritoneum is mobilized medially, as in the previous approach, and retracted by a Goligher rectractor as before. This exposure gives much better access to the common iliac artery and even the aortic bifurcation, and division of the inguinal ligament permits control of all the branches in the segment to be endarterectomized.

10

Common iliac endarterectomy requires a separate arteriotomy situated over the distal part of the common iliac artery. The external iliac endarterectomy is performed from a common femoral arteriotomy to the proximal arteriotomy, and common iliac endarterectomy is carried out using loop or preferably arc strippers. The atheromatous plaque in the common iliac artery is ruptured by gentle compression of the origin of the common iliac artery with an arterial clamp. It is obviously vital that this manoeuvre is performed with care, for rupture of the vessel at this point without adequate aortic control might be fatal. The atheroma in the proximal part of the common iliac artery is, however, in unilateral arterial occlusion, frequently soft and virtually non-existent. Frequently, the vessel occludes because of a development of atheroma in its distal part and, following a distal occlusion, thromboses back to the origin.

In rare circumstances, where external iliac endarterectomy proves to be impossible, it is convenient to insert a Dacron bypass from the common iliac arteriotomy to the common femoral arteriotomy as a unilateral iliofemoral bypass and, in the even rarer circumstance where flow cannot be restored to the common iliac artery, an aortofemoral graft must be used. This last alternative is used to rescue an incorrect clinical decision. These patients are better treated by an aorto-bifemoral graft if there is extensive distal disease.

The arteriotomy at the lower end of these procedures is always taken into the profunda origin if the superficial femoral artery is occluded and closure is by patch or Dacron graft as for a profundaplasty. Proximal reconstruction of one sort or another is always combined with profundaplasty if the aortoiliac disease significantly limits inflow to the profunda femoris artery.

10

References

Beales, J. S. M., Adcock, F. A., Frawley, J. S. *et al.* (1971). The radiological assessment of disease of the profunda femoris artery. *British Journal of Radiology* **44**, 854.

Berguer, R., Cotton, L. T. and Sabri, S. (1973). Extended deep femoral angioplasty. *British Medical Journal* **1**, 469.

Berguer, R., Higgins, R. F. and Cotton, L. T. (1975). Geometry blood flow and reconstruction of the deep femoral artery. *American Journal of Surgery* **130**, 68.

Bernhard, V. M. (1979). The role of profundaplasty in revascularisation of the lower extremities. *Surgical Clinics of North America* **59**, 681.

Hill, D. A. and Jamieson, C. W. (1977). The results of arterial reconstruction using the profunda femoris artery in rest pain and pre-gangrene. *British Journal of Surgery* **64**, 359.

Hopkins, N. F. G., Polyrakis, S., Jamieson, C. W. and Vaughan, G. M. M. (1983). Assessment of later patency of profundaplasty. *Surgery* **94**, 814.

Jamieson, C. W. (1983). Profundaplasty: An incomplete alternative to femoro-popliteal bypass. In *Controversies in Surgery* Vol. 2. Delaney, J. P., Varcos, R. L., eds. London and Philadelphia: W. B. Saunders.

Law, Y. F. and Roberts, V. C. (1983). Per-operative haemodynamic assessment of lower limb arterial surgery. *Journal of Biomedical Engineering* **5**, 194.

Martin, P., Renwick, S. and Stephenson, C. (1968). On the surgery of the profunda femoris artery. *British Journal of Surgery* **55**, 539.

Reversed saphenous vein for femoropopliteal bypass grafting

K. G. Burnand MS, FRCS
Assistant Director, Department of Surgery, St Thomas' Hospital, London, UK

N. L. Browse MD, FRCS
Professor of Surgery, Department of Surgery, St Thomas' Hospital, London, UK

Introduction

A good-calibre long saphenous vein remains the conduit of first choice for bypassing atherosclerotic obstruction of the femoropopliteal segment. Rest pain, pregangrene and frank gangrene of the digits or forefoot in the presence of a good femoral inflow and an adequate run-off via the popliteal artery constitute an absolute indication for the operation. The combination of severe ischaemia and an isolated femoro-popliteal occlusion rarely exists. There is almost always some concomitant aorto-iliac, profunda or distal vessel disease in limbs with severe ischaemia. Staged or simultantous aortic reconstruction may then be required and the distal end of the bypass may have to be taken below the popliteal trifurcation if there is a marked stenosis of the popliteal artery or occlusion of the crural vessels.

Intermittent claudication remains a relative indication for the operation: a good early symptomatic improvement must be weighed against the risks of operation and the uncertainty of long-term benefit. Younger, fit and fully employed patients with a unilateral block, a disease-free popliteal segment and a good-calibre saphenous vein are obvious candidates for surgery, although many would claim that such a combination of circumstances is unusual. Patients should ideally have given up smoking for a reasonable period of time and have stable or deteriorating symptoms of several months' duration, which are interfering with their occupation or hobbies to such an extent, that even after a full explanation of the risks and uncertain long-term benefits of procedure, they continue to request operation. Initial enthusiasm for operation in all patients with claudication has now waned in the UK, and more stringent selection criteria are applied to potential candidates for surgery.

Ischaemic leg ulceration, traumatic damage to the super-ficial femoral artery, cystic change in the popliteal artery, and popliteal aneurysms are alternative indications for vein bypass surgery.

There appears to be little difference in patency between *in situ* and reversed saphenous vein bypasses to the popliteal artery (Harris *et al.*, 1987) and the decision on which method to use appears therefore to be a matter of personal preference. Reversed grafts often lie better when made to the popliteal segment, whereas *in situ* grafts are almost always preferable below the trifurcation.

Assessment

Patients accepted for surgery on clinical grounds should have the basic screening tests outlined in the chapter on 'Operation planning', carried out before proceeding to aortography or digital subtraction angiography. If this shows a satisfactory aorto-iliac segment with an isolated femoro-popliteal occlusion and satisfactory run-off, we obtain bilateral saphenograms (Senapati, Lea Thomas and Burnand, 1983) to assess the morphology and diameter of both long saphenous veins before surgery is considered. Duplex Doppler scanning is an alternative method of assessing the calibre and branches of the long saphenous vein. Confirmation of a single lumen saphenous vein of adequate length and diameter in either leg makes recommendation of vein bypass surgery much easier in patients with moderate claudication, whereas a multichannelled or narrow vein may argue against surgery in all but the severely handicapped. In patients with rest pain, demonstration of a poor saphenous vein on saphenography may prevent an extensive dissection through poorly vascularized tissue. A prosthetic graft of human umbilical vein, Dacron or polytetrafluoroethylene can then be selected as an alternative bypass.

Preoperative preparation

The affected limb should be fully shaved together with the genitalia and iliac fossa of the same side. Naseptin drops are administered twice a day to the nasal passages for 48 h before operation and the patients have chlorhexidine added to their bath water for the same period. Flucloxacillin 250 mg four times a day is started 24 h before operation and 2 u of blood are cross-matched.

Anaesthesia

The operation is carried out under normotensive general anaestheisa. Good peripheral intravenous access for fluid and blood replacement is essential and an ECG recording and central venous pressure monitoring may be indicated if severe cardiac disease coexists. A Swan-Ganz catheter, an arterial line and continuous bladder drainage are not routinely required.

228

The operation

1 & 2

Position of patient

The patient lies supine on the operating table with the end flap of the table lowered to remove the opposite leg from the operating field and provide better access to the popliteal space. The affected leg is supported by a rubber-padded steel strip which is held in place between the metal base of the operating table and the weight of the patient on the antistatic rubber cushion. A large sandbag is placed under the thigh to produce slight knee flexion which aids access to the popliteal space, but excessive knee flexion is avoided because this makes tailoring of graft length difficult. Dissection of the popliteal fossa can then be carried out from the opposite side of the table with the surgeon seated on an adjustable stool. The affected side is painted with chlorhexidine or iodine from ankle to mid-abdomen. The unprepared foot is wrapped in a sterile plastic bag, which allows its colour to be inspected and the pulses to be palpated when the reconstruction is completed. The prepared skin is covered with one or two large plastic drapes.

1

2

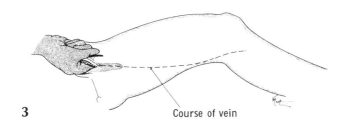

3   Course of vein

3

Exposure of the vein

Confirmation of an adequate saphenous vein and avoidance of vein damage are the first two steps of the operation. Our preference is to find the upper end of the vein by a vertical incision placed over the saphenofemoral junction which is then extended up across the front of the inguinal ligament. This incision also allows adequate access to the common femoral artery. Using a combination of blunt and sharp dissection, the vein should be found in the subcutaneous fat as it dips down through the cribriform fascia. The junction of the saphenous with the common femoral vein must be confirmed. If this step is omitted it is possible to trace a large anteromedial or posterolateral thigh vein instead of the main saphenous trunk. Once the vein has been found and exposed to its termination, the initial short incision may be extended along the course of the vein by sliding a finger along the perisaphenous space superficial to the vein and carefully incising the skin overlying the surface of the finger with a scalpel. The subcutaneous fat can then be divided with scissors. The finger prevents inadvertent damage to the vein and identifies the direction of its course, so preventing an inaccurate incision and undercutting of the wound edges which predisposes to skin necrosis.

4 & 5

Dissection of the vein

The skin and subcutaneous tissue over the vein are divided, exposing the appropriate length required for the bypass, using the sliding finger technique already described. It is advisable to over-estimate the length of a vein which is required since unused vein may be easily discarded while insufficient length may prejudice successful surgery. The vein becomes more superficial just above the knee and the finger dissection technique may have to be abandoned in favour of blunt tunnelling with scissors under direct vision with scissor division of the overlying skin. Blind tunnelling may perforate and damage the vein. Dabs of patent blue violet are applied to the superficial surface of the vein before it is lifted from its bed. This enables the vein to be carefully aligned without twists when it is later positioned in the tunnel. When the required length of vein is completely exposed two operators working from opposite ends free the vein from the surrounding fat and stringy periadventitia by a combination of sharp and blunt dissection, ligating each small branch of the long saphenous vein with 3/0 silk ties on the vein side and 2/0 chromic catgut at the tissue end. The ligatures must not be tied so close to the main vein that it is constricted.

When there is still some doubt over the length of vein that will be required for the bypass, it is better to leave the vein *in situ* (*see Illustration 5*) and to explore the popliteal artery to determine its suitability (*see Illustration 8*) before proceeding to harvest the vein (*see Illustration 6*).

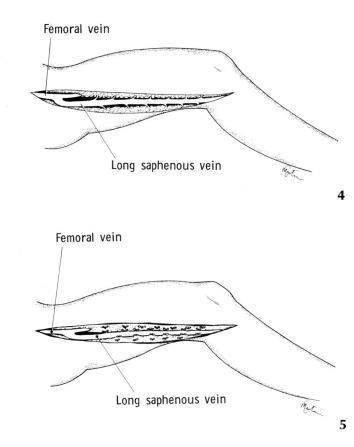

Femoral vein

Long saphenous vein

4

Femoral vein

Long saphenous vein

5

6

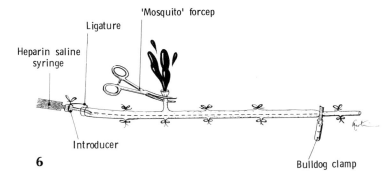

'Mosquito' forcep

Ligature

Heparin saline syringe

Introducer

6

Bulldog clamp

Vein distension

When the vein has been lifted from its bed, both attached ends are tied off with 2/0 silk ligatures, before the vein is divided and removed. A cannula is tied into the distal end of the vein. Then, 20 ml of 1:400 000 heparin saline solution or heparinized blood are drawn up into a syringe which is attached to the cannula. A bulldog clamp is then placed across the vein and a segment is gently distended by depressing the plunger of the syringe. Side branches that were not ligated when the vein was dissected out are revealed when they emit small jets of perfusate. The stumps of unligated side branches can usually be picked up with accurately placed mosquito forceps and ligated. A small 6/0 polypropylene stitch is used to close any sideholes in the vein where branches have torn off flush with the main channel. Great care must be taken to avoid narrowing the lumen of the graft when picking up small branches or placing a stitch in the side of the vein wall.

When the entire vein has been distended and rendered watertight, adventitial bands are divided with small curved scissors and the outer layers of adventitia are divided longitudinally to allow maximal venous dilatation. Overdistension of the vein must be avoided, since this has been shown to separate and damage endothelial cells, exposing the underlying collagen, which is known to promote platelet adhesion and thrombosis. Devices to prevent overdistension are now marketed, but we do not use them at present, relying instead on careful technique to prevent damage.

7

Femoral artery exposure

The common femoral pulse is palpated through the upper end of the incision which was used to expose the vein. Self-retaining Travers' retractors are inserted to hold the wound edges apart and the subcutaneous fat and deep fascia over the pulse is then divided in the long axis of the limb by sharp dissection until the vasa vasorum on the anterior surface of the artery are clearly seen. The common femoral artery is displayed from the inguinal ligament to its division into the superficial femoral and profunda branches. The three main vessels are dissected free and taped with polythene snares; small branches are ligated and divided or controlled by looped silk sutures.

8

Low popliteal artery exposure

The segment of popliteal artery between the knee joint and the trifurcation is usually the least diseased and this is the segment of vessel usually chosen for the lower anastomosis. The posteromedial border of the tibia is identified by palpation through the lower end of the incision used to expose the saphenous vein. The deep fascia of the calf is then incised vertically about 1 cm behind this bony attachment. This incision is extended upwards, until the tendons of sartorius, gracilis, semimembranosus and semitendinosus are encountered at about the level of the knee joint, and downwards as far as is required. A finger pushed in front of the medial head of gastrocnemius which lies beneath the deep fascia separates loose areolar tissue between this muscle and the posterior border of the tibia. This space is enlarged by inserting the twin Browse retractors which open up the lower part of the popliteal fossa. These retractors are 'rake-type' paired self-retaining retractors similar to Travers' but with a long and short blade. The short blades sit against the tibia while the long blades 'hold back' the calf muscles. The popliteal vessels lie anteriorly on the posterior surface of the bone with the vein lying on the medial side of the artery and the nerve lying behind. The vein is gently dissected off the artery which is freed at one point and taped with a plastic snare. A reasonable length of artery is then dissected free and a second snare is placed around the artery. Small branches between the snares should be ligated. A Lahey forceps is then passed behind the artery and the vessel is gently palpated against the rigid forceps. This confirms the presence of a satisfactory lumen and allows the distribution of the atheroma to be gauged. The optimum site for the lower anastomosis can then be selected. Control of blood flow from the segment of artery to be used for the anastomosis can usually be obtained by gently pulling up the snares and holding them taut over the central pinion of the self-retaining retractor. This avoids cluttering the wound with bulldog clamps. Access to the upper part of the artery may be improved by dividing the medial head of gastrocnemius and the tendons attached to the upper end of the tibia. If exposure of the tibial vessel is required, the origin of soleus and anterior tibial veins can be divided.

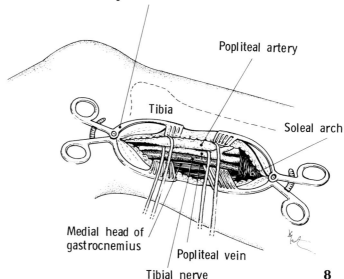

High popliteal exposure

Some surgeons have claimed better results from a short bypass ending above the knee provided the upper popliteal artery is found to have a lumen and is relatively disease-free. The anterior border or sartorius is found and freed above the knee through the incision used to expose the saphenous vein. This muscle is then retracted posteriorly and the upper part of the popliteal fat is exposed. The fat is separated by blunt dissection and the vessels are found lying deeply within the popliteal space. They lie close to the back of the bone and after insertion of the self-retaining retractors are dissected and prepared in an identical manner.

9

The tunnel

A Wilson's or Taylor's tunneller is pushed upward between the heads of gastrocnemius through the apex of the popliteal space, into the thigh medial to the tendon of adductor magnus. The tunneller passes along Hunter's canal deep to sartorius and in front of the superficial femoral artery to emerge in the femoral triangle. The upper end of the saphenous vein is attached to the tunneller or its introducer by a silk suture and pulled back down from the groin to the popliteal space taking great care not to twist the vessel during its passage. This is checked by watching the dye marks previously applied to the surface of the vein, and making sure that they point in the same direction. The proximal end of the vein should lie over the common femoral artery and the distal end should lie over the prepared segment of popliteal artery without tension. The vein should be trimmed at the top end since this is usually its narrowest portion.

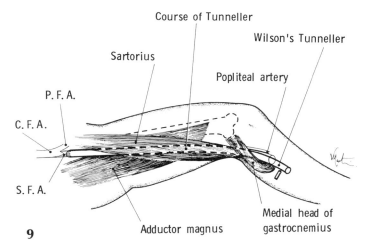

Course of Tunneller

Wilson's Tunneller

Sartorius

Popliteal artery

P. F. A.

C. F. A.

S. F. A.

Medial head of
gastrocnemius

Adductor magnus

9

The popliteal anastomosis

The upper and lower anastomoses are carried out in an identical manner and may be performed simultaneously if two experienced surgeons are available with adequate assistance. This has the benefit of saving time and reducing the period of distal ischaemia. Heparin 5000 u is given by the anaesthetist and allowed to circulate. This dose is sufficient to prevent thrombosis during 1 h of arterial occlusion in normal-sized individuals, but it may be increased if the patient is very fat. Further increments of 2000 u are given if the anastomosis takes longer than 1 h.

The surgeon who is seated on a stool on the opposite side of the patient occludes the popliteal artery by tensing the snares over the central pinion of each self-retaining retractor. A small arteriotomy is then made in the centre of the prepared segment of popliteal artery using a No. 15 blade on a long-handled scalpel. A small quantity of blood escapes when the lumen of the vessel is entered. Bulldog clamps are applied if bleeding persists, which may occur in a heavily diseased or calcified vessel. The initial arteriotomy is then enlarged using Potts' scissors, angled on the vertical, until the length of the arteriotomy exceeds the width of the vein (usually 1 cm or more). The arteriotomy should finish well short of both snares. They are then released to assess the volume of back- and downbleeding before heparin saline is instilled into the distal and proximal segments via a catheter of appropriate size. The end of the saphenous vein is then tailored to the length of the arteriotomy by cutting it obliquely while ensuring that there is adequate vein to reach the distal point of the arteriotomy. The cut end of the vein should be matched for size against the arteriotomy.

10

A double-ended 6/0 polypropylene suture is used for the anastomosis, inserting both needles into the 'heel' of the vein as shown. The needles are then passed out through the proximal end of the arteriotomy on either side of its apex and a knot is tied on the superficial side of the vessel. One needle is then passed back between the attached vein and artery to the far side of the vessel in order to carry out the 'deep side' of the anastomosis.

10

11

A standard continuous suture is then begun, entering the vein from out to in and the artery from in to out. Three or four sutures are placed on either side of the 'heel' under direct vision before the backhand side is sutured towards the apex of the graft.

11

12

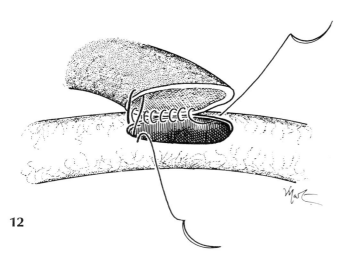

12

13

When the 'toe' has been passed, the over-and-over suture is completed on the near side, tying off both ends in the middle of the forehand side.

A bulldog clamp is then placed on the graft just proximal to the suture line and both snares are relaxed to allow the anastomosis to be checked for leaks and to allow the blood to perfuse the distal vessels again.

Carefully placed smaller bites are taken at the apex or 'toe' to ensure that the distal vessel is not narrowed or occluded. This part of the anastomosis must be carefully made to avoid picking up the far side of the vessel and to prevent narrowing.

Alternatively, a number of loops may be inserted under direct vision and pulled tight when the apex has been completed, or the continuous suture may be tied off and a series of carefully placed interrupted sutures put in around the apex.

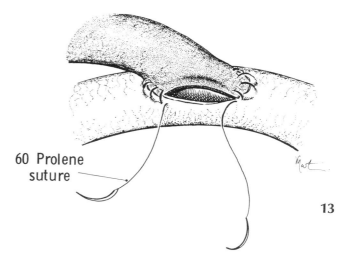

60 Prolene suture

13

14

Alternative anastomosis technique

A parachute technique may be used on both the heel and the apex of the anastomosis in seeking a number of 'loose' loops on both sides without tying down a knot. After six sutures have been inserted, the vein may be slid down to the artery while gentle traction is applied to the sutures. The central part of the anastomosis can then be completed in the usual manner.

14

15

Upper anastomosis

A small, angled Fogarty clamp is placed across the common femoral artery as close to the inguinal ligament as possible. Bulldog clamps are used to occlude the profunda and superficial femoral vessels. An arteriotomy is made in the common femoral artery which may be extended into the profunda femoris artery in the presence of a localized stenosis near its origin. The inflow is checked by releasing the proximal clamp and the backflow from both superficial and profunda vessels is examined by releasing the bulldog clamps. A few millilitres of heparin saline are instilled into both distal vessels which are then reclamped. The anastomosis is made in an identical manner to that described for the popliteal vessels. When the anastomosis nears completion, the upper clamp is released to expel any thrombus which may have developed on the iliac artery above the clamp, and the final sutures are inserted. The ends are tied together as before. The bulldog clamp is removed from the lower end of the saphenous vein and the clamps on the superficial and profunda vessels are released. The Fogarty clamp is then released and the anastomoses at either end are examined for bleeding. Leaks are occluded by accurately placed single 6/0 polypropylene sutures inserted, if necessary, after the brief reapplication of the upper Fogarty clamp. A reversing dose of protamine 25–50 mg is given by the anaesthetist when it is certain that the vessel will not need to be reclamped again.

Confirmation of patency – operative arteriography

When the anastomoses are dry, the popliteal artery distal to the graft is carefully palpated to confirm the presence of pulsatile flow. The foot pulses are also examined through the sterile plastic bag. A green butterfly needle is inserted into the common femoral artery and an X-ray plate wrapped in a sterile Mayo table cover is placed behind the knee. The common femoral artery is briefly occluded and 20 ml of contrast (Conray or Hexobrix) are injected slowly through the butterfly to outline the graft. A spot film is taken of the popliteal anastomosis and run-off to detect any technical errors which might lead to early occlusion of the graft.

Closure

If the films are satisfactory, the wound is closed. Suction drains are inserted near both anastomoses to prevent haematoma formation. The deep fascia and subcutaneous fat are closed with interrupted 2/0 chromic catgut. The skin is closed with 2/0 or 3/0 interrupted nylon mattress sutures or by disposable metal clips if preferred. The wound is covered with sterile adhesive dressings or a thin layer of gauze held in place by zinc oxide tape. Care is taken not to occlude the graft or its outflow by tight circumferential bandaging of the limb.

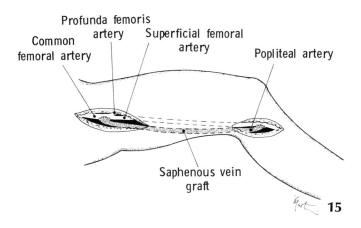

15

Postoperative care

The knee is flexed to 10° or 15° by supporting the lower leg on a soft pillow. The ankle is kept free of the bed clothes by a cradle placed over the feet, and the patient is kept in the recovery ward overnight in order that the pulses can be carefully monitored by well-trained staff. Doppler ankle pressures are used if severe distal disease makes the foot pulses impalpable. Some surgeons prefer to use a continuous pulse volume monitor.

The patient returns to the ward the following day provided that the pulses remain palpable and the Doppler pressures are satisfactory. Any disappearance of a previously palpable pulse or a marked deterioration in Doppler pressure is investigated by urgent digital subtraction angiography, conventional arteriography, or re-exploration and operative angiography. Confirmation of graft occlusion is an indication for urgent reoperation unless the run-off is deemed too poor to allow satisfactory graft function to be maintained. The suction drains are removed after 24 or 48 h if the postoperative course is uncomplicated. The patients should begin to walk on the third or fourth day after operation. Our patients normally remain in hospital until the sutures are removed on the tenth day.

Complications

The main complications are early graft closure, haemorrhage, infection, skin necrosis and leg swelling. A careful technique reduces these problems to a minimum.

References

Harris, P. L., How, T. V. and Jones, D. P. (1987). Prospective randomised clinical trial to complete *in situ* and reversed saphenous vein grafts for femoropopliteal bypass. *British Journal of Surgery* **74**, 252.

Mosley, J.G., Manhine, A. R., Raphael, M. and Marston, J. A. P. (1983). An assessment of long saphenous venography to evaluate the saphenous vein for femoropopliteal bypass. *British Journal of Surgery* **70**, 673.

Senapati, A., Lea Thomas, M. and Burnand, K. G. (1983). A trial of saphenous phlebography compared with surgical dissection as a method of assessing suitability of long saphenous veins for use as a bypass graft. *British Journal of Surgery* **70**, 688.

The use of cephalic vein as a conduit

George Andros MD
Robert W. Harris MD
Leopoldo B. Dulawa MD
Robert W. Oblath MD
Sergio X. Salles-Cunha PhD
Vascular Laboratory, Saint Joseph Medical Center, Burbank, California, USA

Introduction

The choice of cephalic (arm) vein as an arterial conduit requires the surgeon to consider the relative merits and shortcomings of all currently employed grafts for leg revascularization.

The long saphenous vein remains the gold standard of small-diameter arterial bypass grafts. Its advantages include the greatest short- and long-term patency and limb salvage rates, freedom from additional cost for a synthetic prosthesis, relative ease of implantation and low complication rate. It fulfils the surgeon's natural desire to use an autologous material. In the original venous position, the saphenous vein remains patent at low flow rates and retains this quality when transposed to the pulsatile arterial system. Nevertheless, many prosthetic materials, both biological and non-biologcial, are more easily procured and prepared, add only slightly to the overall cost of the procedure, are in some cases more easily implanted and, in others, more easily thrombectomized.

In 1969 cephalic veins were first successfully employed as bypass grafts (Kakkar) and were shown to have adequate length and bursting strength. They were presumed to share other virtues of their autologous saphenous vein counterparts.

Since that time, we have employed these grafts as our second choice after ipsilateral or contralateral saphenous vein for leg revascularization. Our recent as yet unpublished, 10-year follow-up of 70 cephalic vein bypass grafts, 55% of which extended to the tibial level, demonstrated a long-term patency rate closely approximating that obtained with saphenous veins. This experience forms the basis of this report on the technique of their use.

Decision to use cephalic vein

Cephalic veins are indicated in all clinical situations calling for saphenous veins. These include bypass of lower limb lesions extending as far as the foot, upper limb and visceral lesions, and coronary artery occlusive disease. They are useful for patch angioplasty.

Intraoperative discovery of an inadequate long saphenous vein, either because of past phlebitis, varicose veins or a small vein with single or multiple trunks, occurs in 10–25% of cases. This necessitates a bold decision to explore the arms for a cephalic vein. Preoperative knowledge of previous saphenous vein stripping or previous excision permits planned preparation of the patient and direct cephalic vein harvesting. However, upon exploration, cephalic veins are found to be inadequate in 20–30% of cases. Past cutdown or phlebitis, usually from intravenous fluid therapy, accounts for the majority of non-usable veins. Satisfactory veins can be harvested on the side of permanent pacemaker implantation or previous subclavian catheter insertion.

Occlusion of the brachial artery following cardiac catheterization creates a special indication for the use of arm vein. In this case, a short segment of antecubital vein can be harvested under local anaesthesia through the lengthened antecubital incision; it may be applied as an interposition graft or as a patch graft.

Preoperative

1

Preserving a potential graft

The characteristics of size, length and superficial position, which make the cephalic vein a desirable arterial conduit, also predispose it to potentially damaging venipuncture. Education and protection are needed to prevent vein injury. The patients are shown their own cephalic and basilic veins and given a diagram of the anatomy of the area (*see Illustration 2*). They are instructed to prohibit cephalic vein puncture for any reason. Venipuncture is limited to the dorsum of the hand. Teaching programmes for phlebotomy nurses emphasize techniques which spare these veins. Precautionary signs are placed on the patient's room door, hospital bed, hospital chart and nursing records. The arm is wrapped with gauze held in place with non-allergenic tape upon which is written: NO IV'S or VENIPUNCTURES.

1

2

2

Arm vein assessment

Arm veins are evaluated preoperatively and intraoperatively. The cephalic and basilic veins are assessed, preferably in a warm room, by inspection and palpation, employing tourniquets, exercise and dependency. Special attention is directed to the antecubital fossa as variations in venous anatomy are sometimes encountered. Inexact preoperative assessment may result from hair, obesity or tattoos. The latter, however, do not produce vein damage. Arm phlebograms and preparatory cephaloradial arteriovenous fistulae are not employed, although their use has been described.

3

Cephalic vein anatomy

The cephalic vein originates distal to the anatomical snuff box on the radial aspect of the wrist. Coursing medially to the antecubital fossa, it joins the median antecubial vein and then continues proximally (centrally), first on the lateral aspect of the biceps brachii and then in the deltopectoral groove, terminating in the axillary vein.

The median antecubital vein receives a deep muscular branch and the forearm branch of the basilic vein; thereafter it continues as the basilic vein to the axilla. In the forearm the basilic vein diameter is smaller and more variable than the forearm portion of the cephalic vein. Moreover, it lies posteriorly and its excision is awkward; it is not a useful saphenous vein substitute. Males and females appear to have equally usable cephalic veins. Cephalic vein diameter, generally 5–6 mm distally and 6–8 mm proximally, tends to be more uniform than that of the saphenous vein. If the basilic vein is used proximally (centrally), its diameter is 8–10 mm. At their proximal ends, both veins tend to be gossamer-thin. Surprisingly, the true cephalic vein from wrist to clavicle is only 15% shorter than the long saphenous. If the proximal cephalic vein is not usable, then use can be made of forearm cephalic → median antecubital → upper arm basilic, but the length is reduced an additional 15%. The latter is sufficient to extend from the common femoral artery to the infrageniculate popliteal artery; the former will extend to tibial vessels in the mid-calf.

Some reports of arm veins as arterial conduits have differentiated between basilic and cephalic veins. Although both extend from the wrist to the shoulder, only the upper portion of the basilic vein is satisfactory as a bypass graft. Long grafts suitable for femoropopliteal bypass and beyond must necessarily include at least the forearm segment of the cephalic vein and in sequence the remainder of the cephalic or basilic vein of the upper arm. For practical purposes, all arm veins used as lower limb arterial conduits are in part cephalic veins; all venous grafts harvested from the upper limbs are therefore termed 'cephalic vein' grafts.

4

Preoperative preparation of the arm

Leg bypasses are generally performed under regional anaesthetic. The intravenous line is placed in the dorsum of the hand with the less desirable cephalic vein. When the decision is made to employ the cephalic vein, a general anaesthetic is administered. If both arms must be explored for veins, a jugular intravenous line is inserted. If the patient lacks a saphenous vein, and cephalic vein graft is contemplated preoperatively, the general anaesthetic is administered with a jugular intravenous catheter in place. The arm is shaved from the wrist to the clavicle, including axilla, and placed on a moveable arm board. The hand is draped out with a towel. A sterile tourniquet is useful to review venous anatomy after the arm has been prepared.

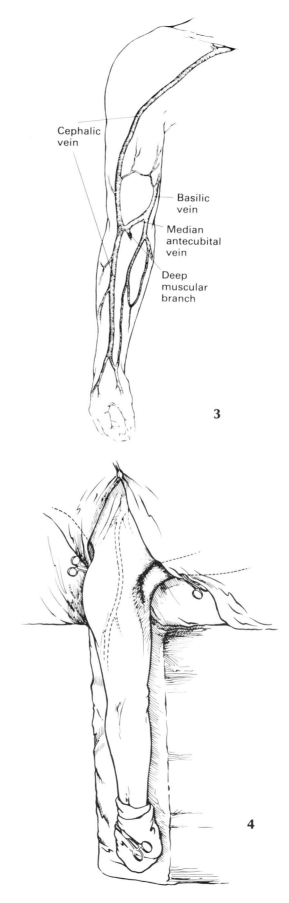

Cephalic vein

Basilic vein

Median antecubital vein

Deep muscular branch

3

4

The operation

5a–d

Unroofing

Before any excision is undertaken, the entire vein is completely unroofed, beginning at the wrist and incising the skin directly over the vein. A No. 15 scalpel is used to start each incision for 2–3 cm. Incisions are extended using scissors. Two manoeuvres help to prevent harm to the vein: (1) spreading the scissors between the skin and the vein creates a space (shown as a stippled area) for the scissors' blade when the skin is cut (b); (2) only the body of the blade, and not the tips, are used to cut the skin (c).

Very few branches arise anteriorly and are easily seen as the vein is unroofed. One 2–3 cm skin bridge is generally placed in the forearm and one in the upper arm. The antecubital incision is always transverse. The proximal (central) cephalic vein is mobilized in the deltopectoral groove to its junction with the axillary vein (d). The skin is undermined for 5 cm or more to decrease the length of the incision.

5a

5b

5c

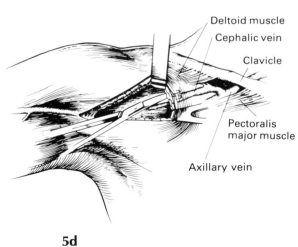

Deltoid muscle
Cephalic vein
Clavicle
Pectoralis major muscle
Axillary vein

5d

6

The antecubital decision

As the cephalic vein is unroofed proximally along the lateral biceps brachii for 5–8 cm, it may be found to be scarred or small. If these conditions are seen, the vein is usually inadequate all the way to the clavicle. The course of unroofing is then redirected. The transverse antecubital incision is extended medially along the median antecubital vein. The basilic vein is unroofed through one long incision to the axillary vein, terminating the skin incision at the hairline. This graft of cephalic and basilic veins in sequence is employed in about 20% of cases.

6

7

In situ distension

In situ distension with heparinized saline at 20°C introduced through a No. 14 or No. 16, 5-cm plastic catheter placed in a side branch is helpful in deciding whether to use the cephalic or the basilic vein. Finger pressure or soft bulldog clamps are applied at various sites to permit distension of the segments in question. Indeed, much of the vein may be unusable and the decision to use the other arm or alternate graft material can be reached without excising the entire vein or even completely unroofing it.

Saline-soaked gauze sponge

7

8a–d

Excision

Excision of the unroofed vein is begun at the wrist. The vein is tied with plain catgut as distally as possible under the skin to obtain maximum length. It is divided, gently mobilized and rolled on to a wet gauze sponge; the unexcised portion is covered with wet sponges frequently irrigated with saline.

The vein and its branches are circumferentially dissected. It is important to tie branches 1–2 mm from the cephalic vein to prevent adventitial gathering; 4/0 silk ligatures are used. The vein is divided so that a 2–3 mm stump extends beyond the tie. Branches are tied or haemoclipped distally. The vein is freed under the skin bridges and passed to the successive next incision. The vein is doubly tied with 2/0 silk at the axillary vein and divided. Venous scarring produced by antecubital venipuncture makes dissection more difficult and risks damage to both the cephalic and basilic veins. If the veins in the forearm and upper arm are usable, the median antecubital vein is not employed. If a short segment of vein is diseased it is excised and a long spatulated venovenous anastomosis is constructed using 7/0 Prolene or Tevdek.

8a

8b

8c

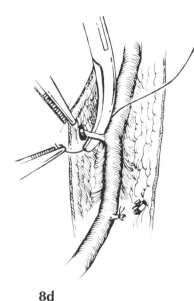

8d

Distension

Reversed venous conduits are minimally distended. By inserting a No. 14, 5-cm plastic catheter (Angio-Cath) a short distance into the distal end of the vein, it can be generously irrigated with heparinized saline to assess ease of irrigation and to remove all blood. With a bulldog clamp on the central end, the vein is gently distended only enough to determine the length of vein necessary to construct the bypass. At this stage, large and easily identified branches are ligated with 4/0 silk.

9

Implantation

With the vein reversed, the proximal anastomosis is performed using 6/0 Prolene or Tevdek (*see* chapter on 'Techniques of anastomosis'. If a soft area in the artery is not available, a vein patch is considered for the anastomotic site. Whenever possible, prosthetic grafts and endarterectomized vessels are avoided for the proximal anastomosis. Grafts maintain long-term patency when originating from the common, superficial or deep femoral arteries and from the popliteal artery as well.

With the proximal anastomosis completed and inspected, the vein graft is allowed to distend with heparinized blood. Constricting adventitial bands are carefully divided. Since damage to the vein can occur with this manoeuvre bands are best managed by prevention. Removing the original silk ligature with a No. 11 scalpel and religating the branch is sometimes desirable. Divided branches lacking a discrete neck are ligated or sutured after the proximal anastomosis is completed and opened. Finally, the blood flow from the end of the graft is observed. The end of the graft is led down to the distal anastomotic site in a previously formed deep tunnel adjacent to the native artery. By passing the graft when it is distended with blood, the risk of twisting an inappropriate graft length is minimized. The distal anastomosis and leg closure are described in the chapter on 'Techniques of anastomosis'.

Completion and postoperative angiograms are not routinely employed. Attempts to use cephalic veins as leg bypass grafts may be aborted at all stages from the time of inspection of the arms before incisions are made, up to when the vein is completely implanted. Vein fragility, haemorrhage, or inadequate graft or distal pulse have prompted graft removal and insertion of another saphenous vein substitute.

Postoperative anticoagulants are not employed. Active leg exercises are begun on the first postoperative day and ambulation on the second.

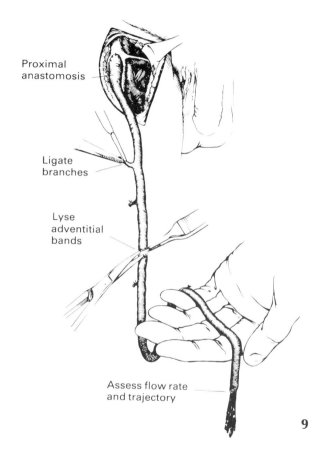

Proximal anastomosis

Ligate branches

Lyse adventitial bands

Assess flow rate and trajectory

9

10 & 11

Wound closure

A one-layer closure of running vertical mattress sutures of 3/0 nylon is preferred. Incisions are covered with povidone-iodine ointment, dry dressings, a gauze wrap and padding over bony prominences. The entire area is finally wrapped with a 10-cm elastic bandage from the base of the fingers to the axilla. Dressings are removed on the second or third day and sutures removed on the eighth or ninth day.

No morbidity has been observed in arms from which cephalic veins have been harvested. Surprisingly little postoperative pain or swelling is experienced. The cosmetic appearance is well accepted by men and women.

Povidone-iodine ointment

Gauze dressing

Gauze wrap

Elastic wrap

10　　　　**11**

Complications

Six weeks after implantation, arm veins have become thickened, resembling saphenous veins on gross *in vivo* inspection, yet retain their compliance. Cephalic veins are susceptible to all of the early and later complications encountered with saphenous veins. Haemorrhage and infection are very infrequent and are treated as with saphenous vein. Thrombectomy within the first day of operation is difficult and should not be performed *in situ*. The entire vein is removed, gently stripped of clot, irrigated with heparinized saline and reimplanted. Alternatively, the proximal anastomosis may be retained, the distal anastomosis taken down, and the thrombectomy performed on the surface of the leg with the vein removed from the tunnel. Balloon embolectomy catheters can be hazardous and are best avoided. Late complications of inflow occlusion, proximal neointimal fibrodysplasia, vein valve hypertrophy, aneurysmal dilatation with secondary embolization and progression of outflow occlusive disease have all been observed and are treated as with saphenous veins. Early and late complications are similar in kind and frequency to those observed with long saphenous vein.

Acknowledgement

We are grateful to Mrs Sheila Pastor for her contribution to this chapter.

Reference

Kakkar, V. V. (1969). The cephalic vein as a peripheral vascular graft. *Surgery, Gynecology and Obstetrics* **128**, 551.

Popliteal aneurysm and entrapment

Norman M. Rich MD, FACS

Professor and Chairman, Department of Surgery, and Chief, Division of Vascular Surgery, F. Edward Hebert School of Medicine, Uniformed Services University of the Health Sciences, Bethesda, Maryland, USA;
Co-Director, Vascular Fellowship Program, Walter Reed Army Medical Center.

Introduction

The popliteal artery is approximately 20 cm in length extending from the adductor hiatus to the lower border of the popliteus muscle. Identification of the many structures in the popliteal area is considerably different from the medial and posterior approaches. The anatomy can be confusing and those with limited experience are frequently at a higher location on the popliteal artery than recognized. An anatomic surface landmark is the head of the fibula, which is usually at the level of the origin of the anterior tibial artery with the continuation of the tibial-peroneal trunk continuing for approximately an additional 3 cm before dividing into the posterior tibial artery and the peroneal artery. Anatomic classification can be confusing because there is frequent description of a popliteal trifurcation which exists in only a very small percentage of patients. There are numerous anatomic variants which should be recognized appropriately. Aneurysms may be difficult to palpate, particularly in the upper third. Aneurysms contain laminated thrombus which can detach an emboli with movement and muscular action. This is an unfortunate complication. Elongation and kinking can accompany dilatation of the popliteal artery and occlusion may occur.

Popliteal aneurysmectomy has been generally abandoned in place of popliteal aneurysmorrhaphy because of the frequent trauma to the popliteal vein which is closely adherent to the wall of the aneurysm. Thrombosis of the popliteal vein with subsequent lower extremity swelling was a frequent complication when aneurysmectomy was performed. A bypass can be used successfully in the majority of cases; however, decompression of a large popliteal aneurysm may be valuable with an incision into the wall of the aneurysm opposite the vein with extraction of the thrombus. Occasionally, there might still be consideration for proximal Hunterian ligation in the very elderly who are at increased risk, especially when the aneurysm is ruptured.

The medial approach for popliteal aneurysmorrhapy

While general anaesthesia can be used and the patient is monitored as described in the chapter on 'Operation planning', regional anaesthesia may be utilized, particularly in the elderly who are at high risk. The leg is semi-flexed at the knee with support in that position and the foot can be held by a cushion or a heel-ring. The surgeon has the advantage by facing the medial side of the leg.

1

Incision

The incision is usually continuous. It can be placed conveniently over the greater saphenous vein which can be harvested easily. Efforts should be made to prevent undermining skin flaps which may lead to poor healing of the incision. The vein may be obtained at this level or from the groin area and prepared as described in the chapter on 'Reversed saphenous vein for femoropopliteal bypass'.

1

Facia over the adductor canal

Site of Hunterian ligation

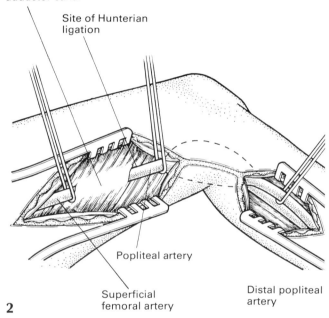

Popliteal artery

Superficial femoral artery

Distal popliteal artery

2

2

Approach to the artery

Initially, the popliteal artery is identified as it emerges below the adductor hiatus by separating the sartorius and vastus medialis muscles. Proximal arterial control is obtained by use of a vascular loop (it is also the site of Hunterian ligation which might be considered for a ruptured popliteal aneurysm in the compromised elderly patient). The superficial femoral artery above the adductor hiatus may also be encircled with a vascular tape if this is the intended site of the upper anastomosis.

The popliteal artery distally is approached as described in the chapter on 'Reversed saphenous vein for femoropopliteal bypass'. The sartorius, gracilis, semimembranosus and semitendinosus muscles are encountered and usually do not require division. It is usually not necessary to divide the soleus tunnel. The popliteal artery is separated from the popliteal vein and tibial nerve and a vascular loop is placed for distal control. The anterior tibial artery origin is usually easily identified.

3

Anastomosis for the graft

With the patient's blood heparinized, atraumatic vascular clamps can be applied both proximally and distally. At this stage a ligature of strong suture is used to ligate the popliteal artery just proximal to the aneurysm and the distal popliteal artery is ligated as high as possible. An end-to-side proximal anastomosis of the reversed greater saphenous vein bypass is usually accomplished most easily in the distal superficial femoral artery. The distal anastomosis can either be end-to-side or end-to-end using 5/0 vascular suture.

After completion of the proximal anastomosis and near completion of the distal anastomosis, the arterial clamps are removed to fill the vein and to eliminate any air, followed by completion of the anastomosis.

3

4

Tunnelling and the upper anastomosis

There may be variation in the best route for the vein bypass. This may require incision into the aneurysm to evacuate thrombis to prevent tension against the vein. Care must be taken to prevent entrapment of the bypass by the long medial tendons. A subcutaneous route may be elected and satisfactory. The proximal anastomosis may be end-to-end as well as end-to-side. Precise suture techniques are described in the chapter on 'Techniques of anastomosis'.

The incision is closed in layers. The use of suction drains for 12 h is a matter of choice.

4

Popliteal entrapment and the posterior approach to the popliteal artery

Since the anomalous course of the popliteal artery was first identified in 1879 by a medical student in Edinburgh, a variety of forms of entrapment of the popliteal artery, and vein, have been identified and one classification includes five separate varieties. Most commonly, however, there is an abnormal lateral insertion of the medial head of the gastrocnemius muscle which can entrap and displace the popliteal artery medially (Rich et al., 1979; Bouhoutsos and Daskalakis, 1981). There can also be accessory slips of the medial head of the gastrocnemius muscle, fibrous bands and an assortment of more unusual anatomic variations.

The posterior approach is preferred to identify the anatomic variants easily, which might be missed when utilizing the medial incision to the popliteal neurovascular bundle. Yet, there might be an associated aneurysm with the entrapment, and the medial approach and bypass might also be selected. For the posterior approach, the patient is prone and the ankle is slightly raised to flex the knee.

5

Incision

The incision is 'S' shaped, being reasonably vertical and midline to follow the course of the artery. At the popliteal fossa the skin crease is included in the incision in an attempt to avoid later skin contracture.

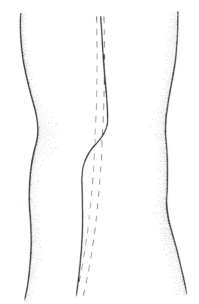

5

6

The incision is extended through the fascia into the popliteal fossa approaching the neurovascular bundle, and then the artery is separated carefully from the vein and the tibial nerve. Vascular loops are placed proximally and distally on the popliteal artery. Usually, it is necessary to divide the small branch of the nerve to the medial head of the gastrocnemius muscle to aid in exposure. Incision through the fibrous portion of the abnormal lateral attachment of the medial head of the gastrocnemius muscle may be all that is required, or similar incision through fibrous bands or accessory muscles may release the popliteal artery, and possibly the vein from the entrapment. If there is poststenotic dilatation which has progressed to aneurysm formation, bypass or replacement with a reversed segment of autogenous greater saphenous vein may be required. If thrombosis of the artery has occurred, an onlay saphenous vein patch graft with thromboendarterectomy may be successful.

The wound is closed in layers. Drainage is not usually required.

6

Complications

Thrombosis of any arterial reconstruction may be due to technical fault. Re-exploration and removal of the thrombus with a Fogarty catheter is recommended. These problems can be minimized by confirming patency and suture line integrity using on-table angiography at the completion of the reconstruction.

With a popliteal aneurysm care must be taken to see that there is no unnecessary manipulation so as to prevent distal embolization of thrombus from the aneurysm.

Thrombosis of the popliteal vein can occur and this is a reason to avoid unnecessary dissection around the popliteal vein. Elevation of the limb, early inactive calf movements, physiotherapy and compression hose are all adjunctive measures that can be utilized to prevent this complication. If thrombosis occurs, heparin and warfarin therapy should be utilized.

References

Bouhoutsos, J. and Daskalakis, E. (1981). Muscular abnormalities affecting the popliteal vessels. *British Journal of Surgery* **68**, 501.

Rich,. N. M., Collins, G. J., McDonald, P. T., Kozloff, L., Clagett, G. P. and Collins, J. T. (1979). Popliteal vascular entrapment. *Archives of Surgery* **114**, 1377.

Sites and approaches for tibial anastomoses

Charles N. McCollum   MD, FRCS
Reader in Surgery, Charing Cross and Westminster Medical School, London, UK
Consultant Surgeon, Charing Cross Hospital, London, UK

Introduction

A feature in the development of vascular surgery in recent years has been the increasing willingness to extend arterial bypass to smaller distal arteries in an attempt to avoid amputation. The posterior tibial artery was first used as the 'run-off' vessel approximately 30 years ago (Palma, 1960; Dale, 1963), but these techniques were not widely accepted until recently. Where an adequate vein is available, and with careful case selection, graft patency rates of 50–70% at 1 year have produced worthwhile limb salvage in these cases (Noon et al., 1969; Davies, Davies and Mannick, 1975). However, where the vein is not adequate and a prosthetic substitute has to be used, the results are considerably less encouraging, with graft thrombosis sometimes exceeding 50% within 6 months (Klimach and Charlesworth, 1983). In the absence of a dramatically new material or approach to the bypass of small arterial disease, we can only expect improvement by attention to three main areas. First, the use of saphenous vein could be extended to a greater proportion of patients by one of the techniques for *in situ* vein bypass (Hall and Rostad, 1978; Leather, Powers and Karmody, 1979). Secondly, it may be possible to improve patency by increasing the blood flow within the graft using a distal arteriovenous fistula as suggested by Ibrahim et al. (1980) and further discussed in the chapter on 'Adjuvant arteriovenous fistula at the distal anastomosis of a femorotibial bypass graft'. Thirdly, patency may be improved in vascular reconstructions by prescribing platelet inhibitory drugs, although good evidence of their benefit in peripheral reconstruction is only available in patients receiving prosthetic bypasses (Green, Roedershecmer and De Weese, 1982; Goldman et al., 1983).

The quality of popliteal 'run-off' is important in femoropopliteal bypass with the best results obtained when two to three tibial arteries are patent. It therefore seems logical in bypasses below this level to consider implanting the distal anastomosis to more than one calf artery. This approach has recently been described using both inverted Y vein grafts and sequential anastomoses at and below the knee (Edwards et al., 1976; Piccone et al., 1978). The combination of *in situ* saphenous vein bypass with the use of either a natural or a sutured bifurcation might extend the use of vein, improve total graft flow and increase perfusion to the distal calf and foot. By these means it may be possible to prevent the few frustrating amputations that have to be performed in the presence of a patent femorotibial bypass.

Indications and preoperative assessment

The almost exclusive indication for tibial bypass is ischaemic rest pain or frank tissue necrosis or ulceration of the foot. Occasionally, patients with severely ischaemic feet and lower legs may suffer a minor injury which ulcerates and fails to heal. In these cases reconstruction may have to be considered in the absence of typical rest pain. Reconstruction to the proximal posterior tibial artery may, very rarely, be indicated for severe claudication alone, but the author doubts that reconstruction to the other calf arteries, particularly at the distal sites of anastomosis, should ever be performed for this indication. The peripheral distribution of arterial disease in these patients is such that calf claudication is rarely an important feature in the history. Many of the patients undergoing these procedures will be diabetic and some will have thrombangitis obliterans. These conditions are not contraindications but it is unlikely that a successful outcome will result when none of the calf arteries cross the ankle and communicate with the foot. This does not of course prohibit the use of the peroneal artery where one of the other two arteries is reconstituted at or just below the ankle and may then be filled by collaterals.

Most patients requiring arterial bypass to the distal calf are elderly and usually unfit. The preoperative assessment must obviously include careful evaluation of all the factors already described in the chapter on 'Operation planning'. Angiography is almost always required, not only to assist in the selection of distal anastomotic sites, but to confirm the adequacy of the proximal arterial system. Often with a distal distribution of disease typical in these patients it is possible to site the proximal anastomosis at the superficial femoral artery just above the adductor canal, thereby shortening the length of bypass. The quality of image obtained in the distal calf is often poor, and selective angiography to each limb is essential. It is now well recognized that despite the most carefully performed angiography, patent distal arteries may not opacify. Patency can be detected with greater sensitivity using a standard Doppler flow probe to insonate the three arteries at ankle level which also allows assessment of the pedal arch (Simms, 1988). Angiography detects only a mean of 1.3 patent arteries per leg in patients requiring femorotibial bypass, whereas Doppler insonation will detect a mean of 2.2 arteries per leg. It must of course be recognized that those arteries detected by arteriogram may be more suitable for distal anastomosis and that a higher rate of failure may be associated with Doppler detection alone.

Preoperative preparation

Many patients requiring tibial bypass will already have had either an operative or a chemical lumbar sympathectomy. On the basis that a few patients do improve with sympathectomy alone we usually perform a chemical sympathectomy during the period of evaluation. Although sympathectomy may only increase the flow of blood in arteriovenous shunts in the distal limb this may augment the total graft flow following implantation and theoretically improves the chances of subsequent patency (Terry, Allan and Taylor, 1972). Once it has been determined that a femorotibial bypass is possible, the patient is started 2 days preoperatively on the platelet inhibitory combination of aspirin and dipyridamole given orally. At this stage a plan is made as to which arteries should be explored and in what order. Obviously, where two patent calf arteries are known to cross the ankle the selection of distal anastomoses is easy. Finally, on the day before surgery the saphenous vein and, where possible, its natural branches, are marked on the skin to aid the subsequent dissection.

Operative technique

1

Medial incisions and long saphenous vein exposure

The medial incisions are placed over the long saphenous vein to minimize dissection in the subcutaneous fat. The author's preference is for separate incisions with the upper one extending 12 cm below the saphenofemoral junction in order that the first two valves and the upper branches can be seen. Further incisions are made centred 12–15 cm above the knee and 8–10 cm below the knee as these are regions where sizeable branches are usually found. Where there are many branches from the long saphenous vein or where the valve stripper does not pass easily, the incision may be converted to full length without hesitation.

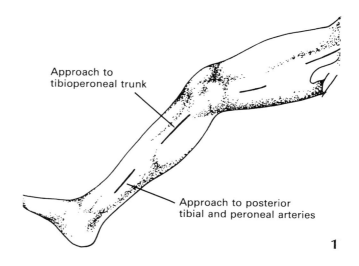

1

2

Exposure of tibioperoneal trunk

The incision used to expose the saphenous vein just below the knee is deepened. The deep fascia is incised 1–2 cm posterior to the upper tibia as shown. The gastrocnemius muscle is retracted posteriorly and in the upper part of the incision the tendons of semitendinosis and gracilis are exposed. Where the distal popliteal artery above the bifurcation of the anterior tibial artery is of adequate quality to receive the graft, these tendons may need to be divided to gain adequate access. The tibioperoneal trunk is found deep to the arch of the soleus which is most easily divided 1 cm posterior to its origin on the tibia. A mass of soleal veins usually obscures the anterior tibial artery which must be exposed by gentle dissection with ligation of the venae comitantes that lie superficial to the artery. It is interesting that with severe ischaemia of the distal limb the soleal veins are often found to be thrombosed. Distal anastomosis of a single stem bypass may be placed anywhere along the tibioperoneal trunk, providing its bifurcation into the posterior tibial and peroneal artery is not severely diseased. It may also be placed directly over the peroneal artery to widen the origin, but with disease of the proximal peroneal and posterior tibial artery, bypass to the distalf calf seems preferable.

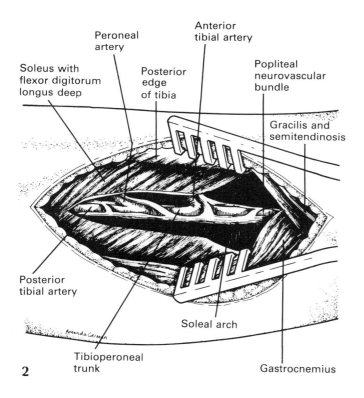

2

249

3

Exposure of posterior tibial and peroneal arteries distally

The exposure of the posterior tibial and peroneal artery of the lower calf can best be achieved by placing the incision well distally in the medial calf (*see Illustration 1*). The lateral approach to the peroneal artery should ideally be avoided and only be used when a bifurcated graft to both the anterior tibial and peroneal arteries is planned. The incision is centred approximately 10 cm above the medial malleolus even if the calf arteries are patent above this level. The deep fascia is incised 0.5–1 cm posterior to the medial border of the tibia and the incision is deepened posterior to flexor digitorum longus (*a*). The soleus muscle is retracted posteriorly using a self-retaining retractor which engages the posterior tibia. The arteries are still surrounded by the venae comitantes but these are more easily dissected free farther distally. Approximately 5 cm of the healthiest length of artery is mobilized and gently retracted posteriorly. The peroneal artery is exposed by deepening the plane of dissection and incising flexor hallucis longus longitudinally (*b*). This may be done by finding the peroneal vascular bundle in the upper wound and then dividing the overlying muscle over the jaws of a curved clamp passed in the plane just superficial to the vessels. Dissecting the peroneal artery from its venae comitantes is tedious and demands both good light and magnification.

3a

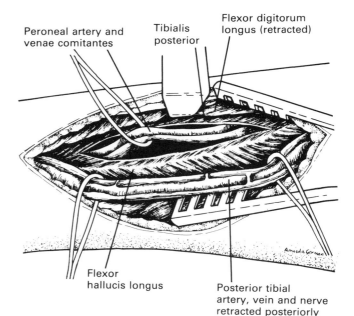

3b

4a, b & c

Anterior and lateral leg incisions

Exposure of the anterior tibial artery

The anterior tibial artery may be easily exposed throughout its length in the anterior tibial compartment (*a*). The incision is placed just lateral to the centre of the anterior tibial compartment and is deepened between tibialis anterior and the two extensor muscles (digitorum longus and hallucis longus) (*b*). In practice, the plane between these muscle groups is not always immediately apparent but it is easy to split the muscles of tibialis anterior. If it is planned to route the graft to the anterior tibial artery from the medial aspect of the leg, a sufficient length should be mobilized and a cruciate incision in the interosseous membrane made 2 cm above the proposed anastomosis (*c*).

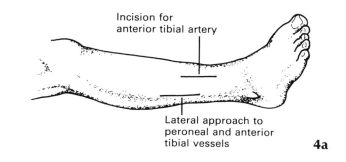

Incision for anterior tibial artery

Lateral approach to peroneal and anterior tibial vessels

4a

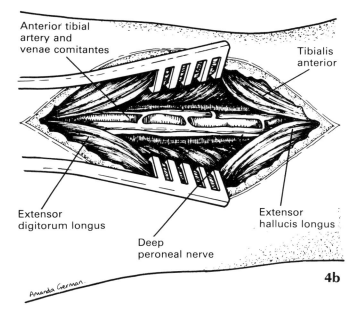

Anterior tibial artery and venae comitantes

Tibialis anterior

Extensor digitorum longus

Deep peroneal nerve

Extensor hallucis longus

Amanda German

4b

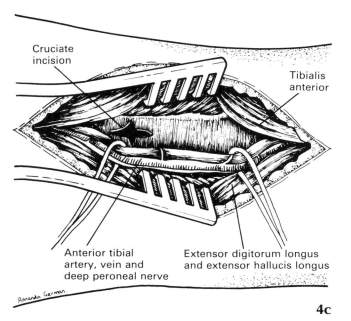

Cruciate incision

Tibialis anterior

Anterior tibial artery, vein and deep peroneal nerve

Extensor digitorum longus and extensor hallucis longus

Amanda German

4c

251

5a & b

Lateral approach to both anterior tibial and peroneal arteries

As previously stated, this approach is rarely required. However, where preoperative Doppler evaluation or angiography indicates that the anterior tibial and the peroneal artery are patent, with an occluded posterior tibial artery, then the lateral approach with a view to a bifurcated bypass to these two vessels may be appropriate. The incision is placed directly over the fibula (*see Illustration 4a*) and deepened between the soleus and the peroneal muscles. The periosteum over the fibula is elevated and a 10–12 cm segment is excised using rib shears (*a*). Incision of the periosteum posterior to the interosseous membrane leads to the peroneal vessels and incision anterior leads to the anterior tibial neurovascular bundle. *Illustration 5b* depicts a suitable layout for a sequential bypass routed from the medial calf with a side-to-side anastomosis to the peroneal artery and an end-to-side anastomosis to the anterior tibial artery.

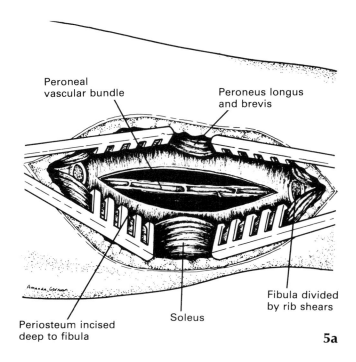

Peroneal vascular bundle

Peroneus longus and brevis

Periosteum incised deep to fibula

Soleus

Fibula divided by rib shears

5a

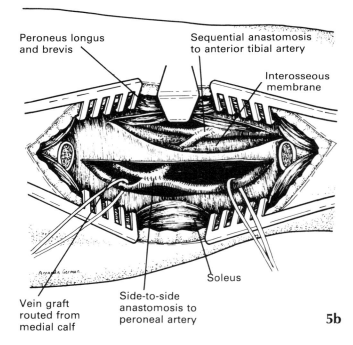

Peroneus longus and brevis

Sequential anastomosis to anterior tibial artery

Interosseous membrane

Vein graft routed from medial calf

Side-to-side anastomosis to peroneal artery

Soleus

5b

252

6

Routes for bypass

When performing *in situ* saphenous vein bypasses it is undesirable to mobilize the long saphenous vein from its bed. Clearly, the distal and proximal ends have to be dissected free in order to route them to the proposed site of anastomosis, but this dissection should be restricted to the shortest length possible. In effect, this means that the graft should be routed from the medial calf in nearly every case. In bypassing to the upper tibioperoneal trunk or distal popliteal artery it may be necessary to route the distal part of the vein through the popliteal fossa to avoid excessive angulation. However, this is not necessary when bypassing to the distal tibioperoneal trunk or to the posterior tibial artery throughout its length. Routing the vessel to the peroneal artery when exposed through the medial incision is quite simple in that the graft merely lies in the plane of dissection already developed between soleus and flexor digitorum longus. In the vast majority of cases, we prefer to take the same route for anastomosis to the anterior tibial artery, tunnelling between flexor digitorum longus and flexor hallucis longus and through the interosseous membrane. It is important that the cruciate incision in the interosseous membrane is made at least 2–3 cm above the proposed site of anastomosis, so that the vein can curve laterally around the anterior tibial artery, allowing the anastomosis to be performed on the anterolateral aspect.

Where saphenous vein is being mobilized from its bed, either in a reversed or '*in situ*' orientation, some surgeons prefer to route grafts to the anterior tibial or peroneal artery subcutaneously across the front of the thigh, and then lateral to the knee, passing just anteriorly to the head of the fibula. This route can also be used when a prosthetic graft or human umbilical vein is employed. It is doubtful that it confers any real advantages. However, where the distal anastomosis is to the dorsalis pedis or anterior tibial artery at or just above the ankle, the graft may have to pass from medial to lateral anterior to the tibia. This is far from ideal as necrosis may develop in the overlying skin.

Planning bifurcated grafts

In considering approaches to bifurcated bypass to distal calf arteries it is usually possible to select preoperatively which vessels are most likely to be adequate. In practice there are three possible combinations: posterior tibial and peroneal; posterior tibial and anterior tibial; or peroneal and anterior tibial. Wherever possible the bypass will be routed to anterior or posterior tibial arteries as these cross the ankle but the peroneal artery is available more often as it is relatively spared by atherosclerosis.

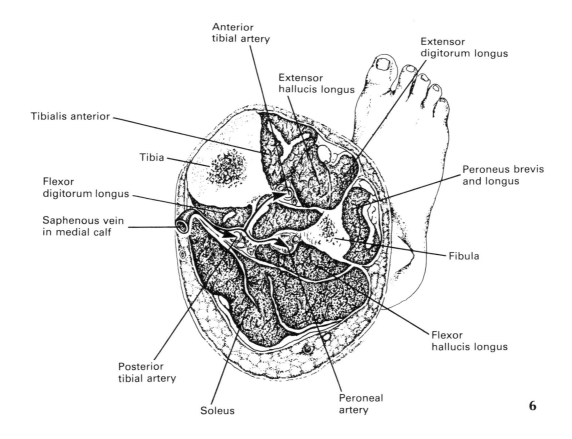

Anterior tibial artery

Extensor digitorum longus

Extensor hallucis longus

Tibialis anterior

Tibia

Flexor digitorum longus

Peroneus brevis and longus

Saphenous vein in medial calf

Fibula

Posterior tibial artery

Flexor hallucis longus

Soleus

Peroneal artery

6

Postoperative complications

Patients undergoing femorotibial bypass are usually old, in poor health and may have diabetes. As the major body compartments are not opened, the perioperative mortality should be low, but over the following months and years a substantial number of these patients will die from myocardial or cerebral ischaemia. In contrast, postoperative morbidity often leads to prolonged hospital stay.

Pressure sores are avoided by carefully padding the patient on the operating table and immediately turning the patient and massaging the pressure areas on completion of the procedure. Wound edge necrosis which predominantly affects the distal wounds is related to ischaemia but can be minimized by keeping wound edges moist with saline swabs and releasing the pressure from self-retaining retractors whenever possible. Occasionally, vein grafts may become exposed with the risk of secondary haemorrhage.

Lower leg swelling and oedema occurs in nearly all patients and can be treated symptomatically with leg elevation and gentle elastic compression. Persistent arteriovenous fistulae and anastomotic problems will be reduced to a minimum if intraoperative assessments, including on-table angiography, are used.

References

Dale, A. W. (1963). Grafting small arteries. *Archives of Surgery* **86**, 22.

Davies, R. C., Davies, W. T. and Mannick, J. A. (1975). Bypass vein grafts in patients with distal popliteal artery occlusion. *American Journal of Surgery* **129**, 421.

Edwards, W. S., Gerety, E., Larkin, J. *et al.* (1976). Multiple sequential femoral tibial grafting for severe ischaemia. *Surgery* **80**, 722.

Goldman, M., Hall, C., Dykes, J. *et al.* (1983). Does indium-platelet deposition predict patency in prosthetic arterial grafts? *British Journal of Surgery* **70**, 635.

Green, R. M., Roederschecmer, R. L. and De Weese, J. A. (1982). Effects of aspirin and dipyridamole on polytetrafluorethylene graft patency. *Surgery* **92**, 1016.

Hall, K. V. and Rostad, H. (1978). *In situ* vein bypass in the treatment of femoro-popliteal atherosclerotic disease: a ten year study. *American Journal of Surgery* **136**, 158.

Ibrahim, I. M., Sussman, B., Dardik, L. *et al.* (1980). Adjunctive arteriovenous fistula with tibial and peroneal reconstruction for limb salvage. *American Journal of Surgery* **140**, 246.

Klimach, O. and Charlesworth, D. (1983). Femoro-tibial bypass for limb salvage using human umbilical vein. *British Journal of Surgery* **70**, 1.

Leather, R. P., Powers, S. R. and Karmody, A. M. (1979). A reappraisal of *in situ* saphenous arterial bypass: its use in limb salvage. *Surgery* **86**, 453.

Noon, G. P., Diethrich, E. B., Richardson, W. P. *et al.* (1969). Distal tibial artery bypass – analysis of 91 cases. *Archives of Surgery* **99**, 770.

Palma, E. C. (1960). Treatment of arteritis of the lower limbs by autogenous vein grafts. *Minerva Cardioangiologica* **1**, 36.

Piccone, V. A., Moon, W., Harry, H. *et al.* (1978). Limb salvage by inverted Y vein grafts to below-knee arteries. *Archives of Surgery* **113**, 951.

Simms, M. H. (1988). Is pedal arch patency a pre-requisite for successful reconstruction? In *Limb Salvage and Amputation for Vascular Disease.* Greenhalgh, R. M., Jamieson, C. W. and Nicolaides, A. N., eds. London and San Diego: W. B. Saunders.

Terry, H. J., Allan, J. S. and Taylor, G. W. (1972). The relationship between blood flow and failure of femoro-popliteal reconstructive arterial surgery. *British Journal of Surgery* **59**, 549.

The *in situ* saphenous vein arterial bypass by valve incision

Robert P. Leather   MD, FACS
Professor of Surgery, Albany Medical College, Albany, New York, USA

Dhiraj M. Shah   MD, FACS
Associate Professor of Surgery, Albany Medical College and Veterans Administration Medical Center, Albany, New York, USA

Benjamin B. Chang   MD, FACS
Associate Professor of Surgery, Albany Medical College, Albany, New York, USA

Jeffrey L. Kaufman   MD, FACS
Associate Professor of Surgery, Albany Medical College and Veterans Administration Medical Center, Albany, New York, USA

Introduction

The provision of a normal functioning endothelium which will retain a non-thrombogenic surface even in low flow situations is the theoretical ideal in vascular surgical conduits. Smooth tapering and matching of the sizes of the conduit at both ends of the arterial bypass has definite and obvious haemodynamic flow advantages. The unique qualities of the saphenous vein when used *in situ* for infrainguinal bypass, first described by Hall (1964), have extended our ability to perform a successful bypass with consistent operative success and long-term patency in most situations (95%), including those with severely limited outflow tracts such as isolated or discontinuous tibial or peroneal arteries, the dorsalis pedis and plantar arch arteries. In addition, in over 1200 such cases performed exclusively for chronic limb-threatening ischaemia, we have achieved a 93% vein utilization rate. Since the flow-limiting constraints applied to other bypass conduits

do not appear to affect the performance of this bypass, the evolution of the procedure has concomitantly increased the three crucial parameters, i.e. patency, operability and vein utilization, which has lead to a marked improvement in limb salvage (Karmody *et al.*, 1984). Although the potential arteriovenous fistulae of the saphenous vein when used *in situ* must be controlled, the most important aspect of this procedure is the efficient removal of the valvular obstructions to distal arterial flow. This has been achieved by our method of valve incision (Leather and Karmody, 1979). The technique which has been used and improved throughout this experience to obtain these results is now described. The preparation of the saphenous vein *in situ* as a bypass conduit will receive the greatest concentration in this chapter because the techniques of anastomosis are similar to those described earlier in the book.

The operation

1

Accurate preoperative knowledge of the course of the patient's saphenous vein and its specific anatomy will forestall many potential intraoperative technical problems. With the patient standing, the path of the vein is marked out by digital percussion and/or Doppler ultrasound if the vein is too deeply placed. In most cases, Duplex ultrasonographic mapping or an ascending phlebogram is also obtained preoperatively. The injection is made into a dorsal vein of the foot which, with heparin flushing, ameliorates any chemical damage to the saphenous vein. The phlebogram accurately portrays the frequent (30%) anatomical variations of the vein, e.g. presence of double systems, large perforators, other major branches and valves. The size of the vein on phlebography sometimes correlates poorly with the true vein size so that an attempt at an *in situ* procedure should not be precluded on the basis of this information alone (Veith *et al.*, 1979). The diagram shows these details together with two possible double systems, i.e. the communicating branch of the medial accessory vein and the posterior accessory vein in the calf.

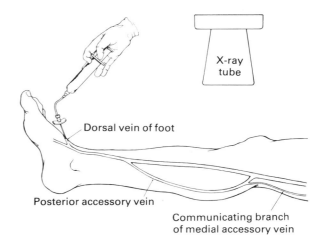

1

2

An incision is made in the groin crease and is extended downwards over the saphenous vein. By sharp dissection, 10 cm of the upper end of the vein is identified. Its tributaries are ligated with silk and divided, and the vein is dissected from its bed. The saphenofemoral junction lies at a level which always corresponds to the bifurcation of the common femoral artery into the superficial and profunda artery. Hence, detachment of the entire saphenous bulb with, if necessary, a small portion of the anterior wall of the common femoral vein will ensure that the upper end of the bypass reaches the common femoral artery.

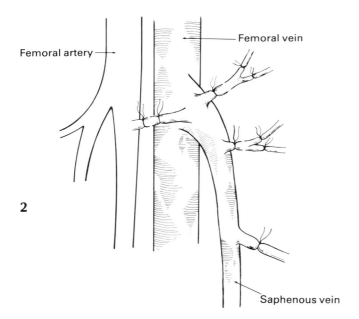

3

A curved vascular clamp (e.g. Paediatric Satinsky) is placed across the saphenofemoral junction on the common femoral vein in such a way that this extension (femoral patch) is achieved. The saphenous bulb is detached from the femoral vein and the resulting common femoral venotomy within the clamp is closed with a continuous suture of 6/0 polypropylene. Postoperative phlebography has demonstrated that this manoeuvre, when carefully done, does not result in narrowing of the femoral vein. A lightly sprung vascular clamp (e.g. Heifetz) is placed on the mobilized and detached end of the saphenous vein to control bleeding through its proximal end.

3

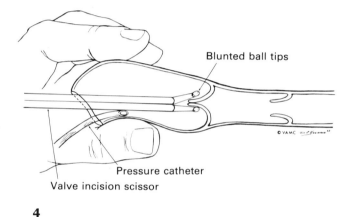

4

4

The most proximal valve, the saphenofemoral, is now easily seen at the saphenofemoral junction. This valve is excised by lifting each cusp with a fine forceps and excising it through the base of the leaflet with a microscissor. All other valves down to the point of the distal transection of the vein are thereafter removed by the specifically developed valve incision instruments. For the three proximal valves, a valve scissor is used. The scissor has a slide action and blades with blunted ball tips. It engages the valve most efficiently when it is in the closed position. The valve can be kept closed by a pressurized column of fluid introduced through a 6 Fr catheter. Fresh heparinized autogenous blood is best for these purposes but Dextran 70 containing heparin 2500 i.u. and papaverine 125 mg has also been used without adverse effects. The venous distension created by this mechanism is maintained by the fingers around the scissor so that the valves are closed and therefore efficiently engaged by the scissor blades.

5

After the most proximal valves have been incised, the venous anatomy determines the subsequent techniques for valve incision. When the saphenous vein is greater than 4 mm with a single trunk in its thigh portion, a detachable intraluminal valve cutter is used which divides the cusps up to the level of the knee without the necessity of surgical exposure of the vein (Leather, Corson and Karmody, 1984). A small incision is made posterior to the previously marked vein below the level of the knee joint. The vein is examined for suitability at this point because it is, in general, at its narrowest here. A branch of suitable size is located and divided. Through this, a 3 Fr traction catheter is passed into the saphenous vein and advanced through the detached proximal end. Any redundant length of the traction catheter is cut obliquely and the cutter is prepared as shown in *Illustration 6*.

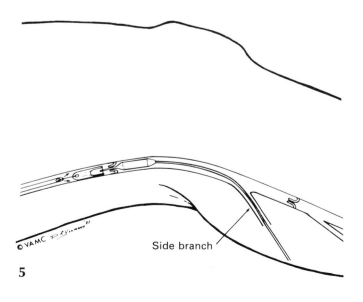

5

6a & b

Illustration 6(a) shows the construction of the cutter, which is made of moulded polystyrene in two sizes – 2.5 and 3.0 mm. An 8 Fr catheter through which pressurized fluid is delivered into the vein is attached to the upper end of the cutter ('follower') with a 6/0 monofilament suture. The two blades of the cutter are on either side of a thin stalk which connects the 'follower' to the 'leader'. The oblique end of a traction catheter is screwed firmly into a self-tapping screw in the leader before the pressure catheter is attached. *Illustration 6(b)* shows the orientation of the cutter within the saphenous vein. The fluid pressure distends the vein, closes the valves so that they will be efficiently engaged by the cutter blades, and provides a fluid interface on which the cutter 'floats' away from the vein wall. The 'leader' centres the device in the saphenous vein and prevents it from engaging any side branches.

6a

6b

7

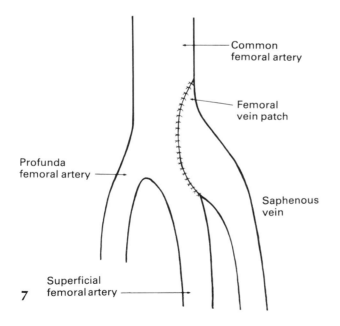

The valves are serially cut and defunctioned to the level of the knee joint by two or three passes of the valve cutter. The cutter is then withdrawn with the traction catheter through the proximal end of the vein and dismounted. The upper end of the saphenous vein is anastomosed to the common femoral artery just across its bifurcation. If an inflow procedure, e.g. endarterectomy, has to be carried out in the common femoral artery, the arteriotomy for this is incorporated into the upper anastomosis. As shown, the femoral vein patch greatly facilitates placement of the upper anastomosis directly on to the common femoral artery. If the superficial and profunda arteries are competent, these can also be used as inflow sources. The latter is particularly useful if the common femoral artery is competent but heavily calcified or has been the site of previous surgery.

8a & b

Once arterial pressure has been established at the knee level, the valvulotome is used for all subsequent valve incisions. Below the knee use of the valve cutter is riskier because the vein is smaller. In addition, since in this area, the vein is usually exposed concomitantly with the incisions for arterial exposure, efficient use of the valvulotome is readily possible. It should be noted that the valvulotome can also be used for valve incision in the region of the thigh, particularly if the vein is too small for safe passage of the cutter. When possible, the saphenous vein should be arterialized before its distal end is mobilized, since electron microscopic study has shown that this is most protective of endothelial stability.

The valvulotome consists of a 20 cm long, 1 mm flexible shaft, a blade at right angles to the shaft and a ball-tip which protects the vein wall. The instrument is passed either through a side branch (*a*) or through the open end of the vein after it has been distally detached (*b*). Note that at each point of valve incision, the vein should be distended by arterial pressure to close the valve. Before the instrument is passed through the detached end of the vein, the unarterialized segment of vein should be gently dilated with irrigant solution so that the valvulotome does not rub along the vein wall. Valve incision with the valvulotome should always be performed under direct vision because the valvulotome may become lodged in the small venous branches which are in close proximity to the valve sinus, thus causing damage to the vein wall when it is drawn downward.

8a

8b

9

The mechanism of progressive arterialization of the vein by means of serial valve incisions with the valvulotome is shown down to the point at which the vein is transected before mobilization for distal anastomosis.

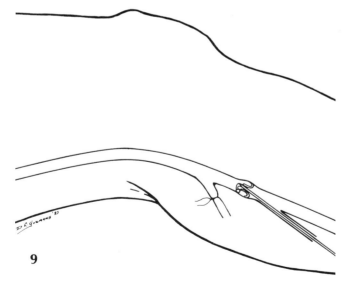

9

10a & b

Illustration 10(a) shows the distal end of the vein which has been mobilized before arterialization. Two branches are securely tied and the lower branch which has been used for passage of the valvulotome is secured with a temporary clip. Note that the valve remnants are barely discernible on the vein wall. However, once the vein is arterialized, the mobilized end readily undergoes torsion while under pressure (*b*). This problem must be recognized and the vein returned to its anatomical position by alignment of the branches before distal anastomosis is begun. Sufficient length of vein should be mobilized so that the clamp end can subsequently be discarded.

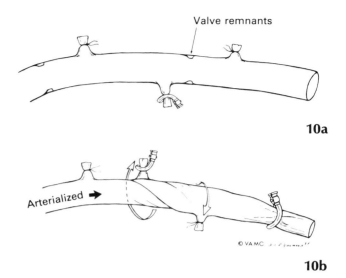

Valve remnants

10a

Arterialized ➤

© VAMC

10b

11a

© VAMC

11b

11a & b

The details of distal tibial arterial anastomosis are shown here. An arteriotomy and corresponding venotomy is made which is 1.5–2 times the diameter of the distal vein. The proximal end (heel of the anastomosis) is usually sutured with a loop or parachute technique to ensure maximum accuracy of suture placement. Use of a monofilament suture (7/0 or 8/0 polypropylene) ensures smooth subsequent approximation of vein to artery and easy completion of the anastomosis. In the tibial arteries, 4.5–6 × magnification is routinely used. In the completed anastomosis (*b*) attention is drawn to the close matching of the size of the vein and artery together with the use of small, softly sprung (40 g pressure) and unobtrusive vascular clamps which do not crowd the operative area. These are preferred to elastic loop control which requires greater arterial dissection and may also cause plaque separation (Leather, Shah and Karmody, 1981).

12

Elimination of arteriovenous fistulae is not a difficult part of the procedure. The position of most of the branches which will become fistulae will be already identified either from the preoperative venogram or during venous exposure for valve incision as discussed previously. Residual arteriovenous fistulae (usually no more than two) are initially determined by the use of intraoperative Doppler probe as shown here. Sequentially the probe placed in the proximal position provides a flow signal when a fistula is present and an obstructive signal when the vein is compressed proximal to this point. After this, an intraoperative arteriogram (considered to be mandatory) is carried out.

12

13

On the completion arteriogram, remaining fistulae can be readily identified and the technical accuracy of the distal anastomosis can be seen. A 22-gauge plastic sheath is inserted into the proximal part of the vein and contrast is injected. A needle grid shown numerically allows rapid location of the fistulae. The perforating vein which connects directly with the femoral vein is shown at the third needle position. Note that the valve in the vein is directed towards the deep system. A subcutaneous vein which forms a fistula beyond the fifth needle is not of haemodynamic value and can safely be left if desired. Most such fistulae subsequently become occluded because of the formation of true phlebitis within the vein wall.

The distal anastomosis must also be examined on the arteriogram. Its adequacy should be confirmed in this way as well as by Doppler ultrasound of the flow at this point.

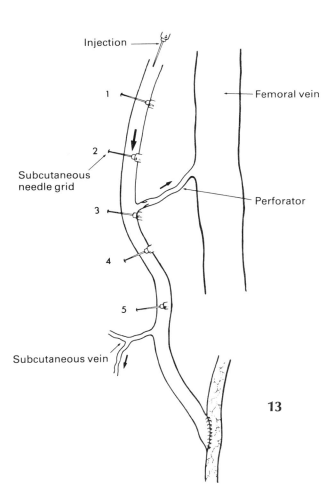

13

Complications

Occasionally, pathological difficulties within the saphenous vein may occur during the operative procedure. These consist of platelet deposition at the site of injured endothelium, unyielding valves because of previous fibrosis, a missed valve cusp, or laceration of the vein wall. Vein wall lacerations are easily identified because of leakage of blood and haematoma formation of the vein wall. A missed valve will cause intermit- tent or even total cessation of flow within the vein. When deposition occurs within the vein, this will be seen on the operative angiogram as a foamy filling defect and the Doppler ultrasound will reflect a diminished flow signal. These difficulties, though rare, must be diagnosed and managed intraoperatively if early failure of the bypass is to be avoided.

14, 15 & 16

When such problems occur, they can usually be treated by the technique of vein branch angioplasty. The vein is opened in order to visualize its endothelial surface. Platelets can be removed through the venotomy and/or missed valves dealt with. The venotomy is subsequently closed by patch angioplasty using a venous branch opened in continuity with the diagnostic venotomy.

This technique is in keeping with and preserves the complete *in situ* nature of the entire procedure (Corson *et al.*, 1984). It is stressed that at the termination of the procedure, the predicted physiological criteria resulting from the bypass should be confirmed in the distal limb by non-invasive methods, e.g. Doppler ultrasound, systolic pressures and waveform analysis. In this respect, the intraoperative arteriogram should also be helpful. The patient should not leave the operating suite until the surgeon is satisfied that these criteria have been met.

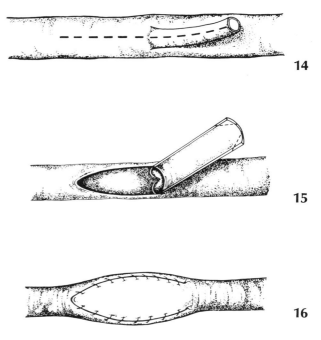

14

15

16

References

Corson, J. D., Leather, R. P., Shah, D. M. and Karmody, A. M. (1984). *In situ* vein branch angioplasty. *Surgery, Gynecology and Obstetrics* **159**, 283.

Hall, K. V. (1964). The great saphenous vein used *in situ* as an arterial shunt after vein valve extirpation. *Acta Chirurgica Scandanavica* **128**, 365.

Leather, R. P. and Karmody, A. M. (1979). A reappraisal of the *in situ* bypass, its use in limb salvage. *Surgery* **86**, 453.

Leather, R. P., Shah, D. M. and Karmody, A. M. (1981). Infrapopliteal arterial bypass for limb salvage: increased patency and utilization of the saphenous vein used *in situ*. *Surgery* **90**(6), 100.

Leather, R. P., Corson, J.D. and Karmody, A. M. (1984). Instrumental evolution of the valve incision method of *in situ* saphenous vein bypass. *Journal of Vascular Surgery* **1**, 113.

Leather, R. P. and Shah, D. M. (1988). Experience with *in situ* lower extremity saphenous vein bypass procedures. In *Surgery Annual*. New York: Appleton and Lange.

Leather, R. P., Shah, D. M., Chang, B. B. and Kaufman, J. L. (1988). Resurrection of the *in situ* vein bypass: 1000 cases later. *Annals of Surgery* **208**, 435.

Veith, F. J., Moss, C. H., Sprayregen, S. and Montefusco, C. (1979). Preoperative saphenous venogrpahy in arterial reconstructive surgery of the lower extremity. *Surgery* **85**, 253.

Vein and PTFE bypasses to infrapopliteal arteries

Frank J. Veith MD

Professor of Surgery and Chief of Vascular Surgical Services, Albert Einstein College of Medicine and Montefiore Medical Center-Albert Einstein College of Medicine, New York, New York, USA.

Introduction

Arterial reconstructions distal to the popliteal artery can be performed in the upper, middle or lower third of the leg as well as in the ankle region or foot. The approaches to each of these levels will be described separately. However, there are several generalizations applicable to any bypass that is inserted into the posterior tibial, anterior tibial, dorsalis pedis or peroneal arteries.

These are technically demanding, time-consuming procedures that should only be performed by vascular surgeons with skill, patience and a commitment to conduct the operation with great care and attention to detail. Even if these small vessel bypasses are performed with technical perfection, 5–10% of them will fail within several days. If this occurs, the circulatory status of the involved limb may be worsened. Therefore, these operations should never be performed for intermittent claudication alone but only to salvage limbs that have gangrene, a non-healing ulcer or severe true rest pain.

Complete preoperative angiography to identify patent arterial segments and distal obstructions is an absolute prerequisite to these operations. Occasionally, this will have to be supplemented by intraoperative angiography. This may be required after an acute occlusion in which no contrast media reaches the distal vasculature. Rarely, it may be required to visualize adequately patent arteries in the distal leg and foot with occlusive disease.

The patient's ipsilateral long saphenous vein, if available, is presently the vascular graft of choice for small vessel bypasses. It may be difficult to obtain sufficient length of this graft, particularly if the bypass is to an artery in the distal third of the leg or beyond. For this reason, we perform the proximal anastomosis to the superficial femoral artery or, occasionally, the popliteal artery, if it is of good quality and has a normal or only minimally narrowed lumen on preoperative angiography. Similarly, to minimize the length of saphenous vein required, we perform the distal anastomosis to the most proximal portion of any leg artery that has a direct course into the foot. Small vessel bypasses to leg arteries that are obstructed distally usually do not remain patent and should be avoided if possible. On the other hand, we would perform a bypass to an isolated popliteal segment in preference to a more distal small vessel bypass in patients without extensive gangrene or infection in the foot. Good results have been achieved with such operations (Veith, Gupta and Daly, 1981a; Veith *et al.*, 1986).

If an ipsilateral segment of long saphenous vein is not available, or if its smallest diameter is less than 3 mm, we attempt to find other segments of autologous vein elsewhere in the same or another extremity. Duplex ultrasonography or contrast venography can be helpful in the search. In our experience, upper extremity veins have often been found abused by previous intravenous therapy and scarred segments are common, so that other lower extremity veins are more useful in this setting. The short saphenous, an accessory long saphenous or the opposite long saphenous vein are our usual grafts if the ipsilateral long saphenous is inadequate. If absolutely no adequate autologous vein is available as a graft after a diligent search, a PTFE graft may be employed and is a better option than using a poor vein or performing a primary amputation. Some of these grafts have functioned for several years or more; and even if such grafts fail after 1–2 years, the foot lesion is healed and remains so in a substantial proportion of patients. Thus even though late patency rates for infrapopliteal PTFE bypasses are poor, they can contribute to important periods of limb salvage in patients who have a threatened leg and no suitable autologous vein graft (Veith *et al.*, 1986).

Vein utilization can be increased if arteries distal to the common femoral are used to provide bypass inflow for a short vein graft. Obviously, this strategy can only be used if there is no important stenosis proximal to the site used to provide bypass inflow. In our experience, we have found that an important proportion of our patients who require bypasses to the lower leg or foot can have their grafts originate from the superficial femoral, the deep femoral, the popliteal or even tibial arteries (Veith *et al.*, 1985). Vein utilization is thereby enhanced.

Although *in situ* vein graft techniques have become very popular and although this technique offers some theoretic advantages over the reversed vein graft techniques to be presented, we remain unconvinced that the *in situ* method is best for all lower extremity bypasses. No adequate or conclusive comparative study has demonstrated such superiority, and many patients are not suitable for an *in situ* bypass but are candidates for ectopic reversed vein graft. Accordingly, any surgeon performing lower extremity bypasses to distal arteries must be capable of performing careful reversed vein grafts irrespective of their beliefs about the superiority of *in situ* grafts.

We prefer a single, long vein-harvesting incision, although multiple small ones can be used effectively. Most of this incision is stapled closed temporarily during performance of the bypass to avoid drying and necrosis of the subcutaneous fat. After the bypass is completed and the heparin neutralized, the vein harvest incision is reopened, all blood is removed, meticulous haemostasis is obtained, and the wound is carefully reclosed with sutures or clips.

The long saphenous vein is mobilized by ligating all branches close to the main vessel without catching any adventitia in the ligatures. If the adventitia of the main vein is so caught, stenosis can result after it is distended. For speed, the peripheral end of branches may be clipped, but clips on the main vein should be avoided since they may be caught during tunnelling and produce distortion or injury to the graft.

1

1

After the vein graft is removed, it is immersed in and distended gently with chilled (4°C) Hank's solution or chilled heparinized autologous blood. This is best accomplished using a long (12.5 cm) plastic cannula attached to a 20-ml plastic syringe. In this way the vein can be distended and tested for leaks in segments.

If unligated branches are present, they are discovered during distension and ligated. Avulsed branches leave holes in the main vein, and these must be carefully sutured with 6/0 silk to avoid any constriction of the main vein. After preparation and measurement, the vein is placed in the chilled Hank's solution until it is used. Drying and warming are avoided as much as possible even while the vein is being sutured into place.

Small vessel bypass in the upper and middle thirds of the leg

2

This may be performed to the tibioperoneal trunk, the posterior tibial artery, or the peroneal artery, using a medial approach below the knee joint to gain access to these vessels. The anterior tibial artery requires an additional anterior incision.

The positions of the incisions required to perform bypasses from the femoral artery to the tibioperoneal trunk or the posterior tibial and peroneal arteries in the upper third of the leg are shown in heavy lines. The upper incision provides access to the common or superficial femoral artery. The above-knee incision allows tunnelling under the sartorius muscle and along the course of the popliteal vessels behind the knee. The dashed extension to the lower incision provides access to the posterior tibial and peroneal arteries in the middle third of the leg. If the saphenous vein is to be used, all incisions should be placed over the vein and access to deeper structures obtained when needed by raising thick flaps.

2

3

The below-knee incision is made through the skin, subcutaneous fat and deep fascia of the popliteal space. The gastrocnemius muscle is retracted posteriorly. The more superficial popliteal vein is encircled with a Silastic loop to facilitate dissection of the underlying popliteal artery which can be seen disappearing deep to the fibres of the soleus muscle.

3

4

A finger or right-angled clamp is placed deep to this muscle prior to cutting it at its origin from the fibrous band that is attached to the back of the tibia and fibula. This exposes the origin of the anterior tibial artery and its accompanying vein or veins.

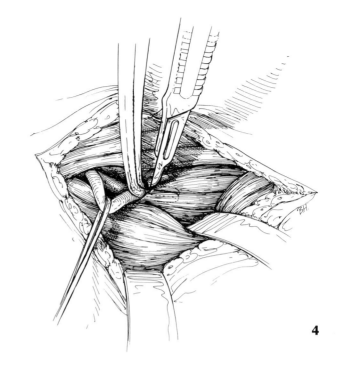

4

5

Division of these veins allows further retraction of overlying veins and exposure of the tibioperoneal trunk and its terminal branches.

5

6

Tunnels are fashioned by blunt finger dissection (as shown here), use of a plastic tube, passage of a larger gentle curved clamp (*see Illustration 23*), or a combination of two or more methods. When this is completed, the patient is given systemic heparin (1.5 mg/kg).

6

7

The artery for distal anastomosis is elevated by gentle traction of Silastic vessel loops which may be held taut by clamping them to the appropriate drapes or self-retaining retractors. Frequently, such gentle traction is adequate to provide haemostasis during arteriotomy and anastomosis. If not, microvascular clips, small atraumatic vascular clamps, double looping of the vessel loops, or passage and inflation of a No. 3 balloon catheter may be used. Although it is essential to have a bloodless field so that perfect visualization can be obtained, it is important to note that any of the above haemostatic methods may damage the delicate small vessel, which may also be calcified or thick-walled. We, therefore, prefer to use whatever method requires the least force and produces the least vessel distortion, and we take as much time as necessary to perform this phase of the operation with the least trauma to the artery. Side branches, although always dissected free, are only encircled with ligatures or Silastic loops when necessary, and this is not usually the case.

All arteriotomies and anastomoses must be performed with extreme care and magnification with excellent illumination is essential for these technically demanding procedures (*see* chapter on 'Techniques of anastomosis'. Arteriotomies are usually performed with a new-bladed (No. 15 blade) scalpel (as shown), so that all layers of the arterial wall are cut evenly. This is particularly important if the artery is diseased.

7

8a & b

After the initial incision in the artery, placement of a fine mosquito clamp within the vessel can facilitate the rest of the arteriotomy (*a*) and prevent injury to the opposite wall. Fine scissors are only used if the artery is small and thin-walled (*b*). In general, the length of the arteriotomy and the

anastomosis is 2–3 times the diameter of the graft, which in turn is 1.5–3 times the diameter of the recipient distal artery, although this relationship may vary if a saphenous vein graft is employed.

8a

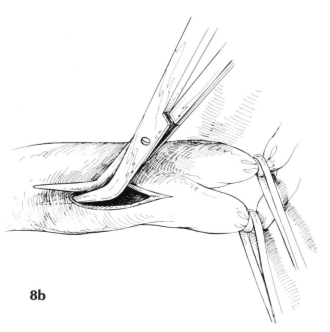

8b

9

All anastomoses are constructed with fine monofilament polypropylene or PTFE continuous sutures (6/0). Every stitch must be perfectly placed under direct vision using Castroviejo needle-holders and fine atraumatic forceps, so that small even bites of intima and other layers of the arterial wall are included in every stitch. We prefer to start the distal anastomosis with a double-armed toe suture and then run each side of the suture halfway down the anastomosis. Thereafter, the double-armed heel stitch is placed and tied. Each half is run to the mid-portion of the anastomosis and tied to the appropriate end of the toe stitch. Interrupted stitches at the toe of the anastomosis, which have been advocated by some, are almost never necessary if the described method is employed.

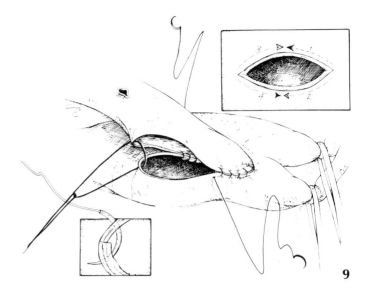

9

10

The completed distal anastomosis with the graft in place is shown. If more distal exposure of the posterior tibial or peroneal arteries is required, further separation of the soleus muscle from the posterior surface of the tibia and its overlying muscles provides access to the neurovascular bundles. Careful dissection of the veins with ligation of crossing branches provides access to the more deeply placed arteries. These can be dissected free, taking great care to preserve all branches, so that the appropriate segment of artery can be elevated and controlled to perform the distal anastomosis.

After completion of the distal anastomosis, all haemostatic elements are removed, and the graft and recipient artery are flushed gently with heparinized normal saline. Large leaks are visualized and carefully fixed, usually by adventitial sutures; small or moderate leaks are ignored and stop spontaneously.

The saline-filled graft is then drawn through the previously fashioned tunnels by using a large clamp or by placing a plastic tube (Argyle Thoracic Catheter Container) through the tunnel, cutting off the end, and then drawing the graft through the tube using a bronchoscopy grasping forceps. Care is taken to prevent rotation of the graft within the tunnel and to avoid redundancy, excessive tension or sharp angulation.

The segment of artery to be used for the proximal anastomosis is then isolated between gently applied vascular clamps, again using the minimum amount of force and distortion consistent with a bloodless operative field so as to minimize clamp injury. Proximal anastomoses are generally begun by placement of a double-armed distal heel stitch. Each arm of this is run proximally to the midpoint of the anastomosis. The proximal apical suture is then placed and tied, and each arm of this is run to the midpoint of the anastomosis and tied. Since the vein component in this anastomosis may be small, care is taken to make the suture bites in the vein small, catching equal portions of all layers.

After completion of both anastomoses and removal of all occluding clamps, heparin is neutralized by protamine, and meticulous haemostasis is obtained from the anastomoses and all other wounds. Usually, this requires considerable patience, particularly for anastomoses in which PTFE grafts are employed. Intraoperative angiography is performed if indicated, and all wounds are closed using meticulous plastic techniques. Dressings are applied, and any necrotic or infected tissue in the foot is widely debrided. This may require removal of one or more toes or a partial or total transmetatarsal amputation. Generally, these debridements are best left open. Although we continue our patients on aspirin (0.6 g/day) and dipyridamole (50 mg/day) postoperatively, there is no firm evidence in humans that this is helpful. No other anticoagulants are used postoperatively.

Excellent anaesthesia is required to keep the 30-day operative mortality rate between 3 and 5% (Reichle and Tyson, 1972; Veith et al., 1978, 1981b).

10

Bypass to the anterior tibial artery in the upper and middle thirds of the leg

11

An anterloateral incision is made in the leg midway between the tibia and fibula over the appropriate segment of patent artery. Additional small medial incisions are also required for tunnelling.

11

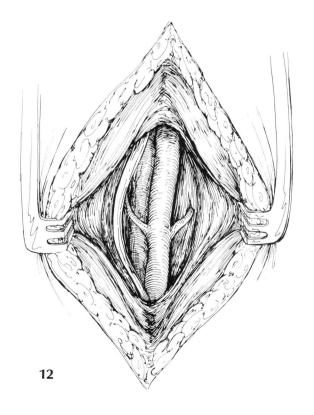

12

12

The anterior incision is carried through the deep fascia, and the fibres of the anterior tibial muscle and the long extensors of the toes are separated to reveal the neurovascular bundle. Mobilization of accompanying veins with division of branches allows visualization of the anterior tibial artery which can then be carefully mobilized as already described.

13

After the artery is freed, it is elevated and retracted along with the accompanying veins using Silastic loops. This permits further posterior dissection, which allows the interosseous membrane to be visualized and incised in a cruciate fashion.

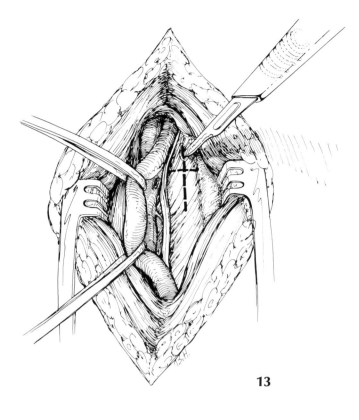

13

14

Careful blunt finger dissection from this anterior approach and from the popliteal fossa via the medial incision facilitates creation of a tunnel without injuring the numerous veins in the area.

14

15

By elevating the anterior tibial artery, a meticulous distal anastomosis can be constructed. This is shown in progress with a PTFE graft.

Other operative anastomotic details are similar to those already described.

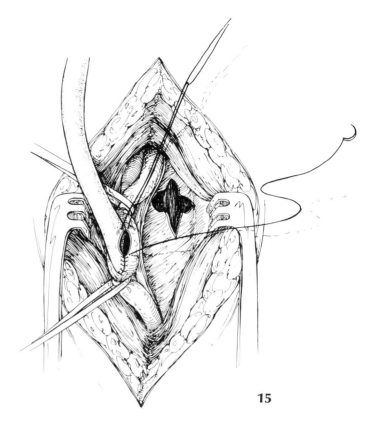

15

16

16

The resulting graft in place.

The anterior tibial artery can also be approached by a lateral incision with fibulectomy, but the author believes this approach to be bloodier and more time-consuming than the one described. However, it may be useful in patients who require a reoperation and who have extensive scarring or infection.

Bypasses to the distal third of the leg and the foot

17

Bypasses to the anterior tibial, posterior tibial, or peroneal arteries in the distal leg can be performed by techniques similar to those already described, with the exception of the following features.

Anterior tibial artery

Peroneal artery

Posterior tibial artery

17

18

18

The distal posterior tibial artery can be approached by an incision along the posterior edge of the tibia. By deepening this incision along the tibialis posterior muscle and the posterior surface of the tibia, the distal peroneal artery can also be located and isolated just medial to the medial edge of the fibula. By dividing restraining fascia and fibres of the flexor hallucis longus muscle, it is possible to free this artery and elevate it into the wound so that a careful anastomosis can be constructed.

19

However, in most patients, particularly those with a stout calf and ankle, this vessel is best approached by a lateral incision with excision of the fibula.

Lateral approach to peroneal artery

Anterior approach to anterior tibial artery

19

20

A long segment of fibula is freed from its muscle attachments using a combination of blunt and sharp dissection. Particular care should be taken in the dissection along the medial edge of the bone, since the peroneal vessels are just deep to this edge and are easily injured by instruments. Once a finger has been passed around the fibula, this free edge of bone can be further developed by pushing a right-angled clamp forcefully inferiorly and superiorly.

20

21

21

A right-handed retractor is then passed behind the bone and a hole drilled in it.

22

The fibula is easily and cleanly divided with rib shears.

The peroneal artery is then dissected free from surrounding veins so that it can be used for construction of a distal anastomosis. Gentle blunt finger dissection is required to develop a tunnel from this lateral wound to the lower popliteal fossa. Great care is taken to avoid injury to the numerous veins in the area. From there, the tunnelling to the femoral artery wound is performed in the previously described fashion. Because it is the least accessible of the three leg arteries and normally has the poorest connections with the arteries of the foot, the author recommends use of the peroneal artery as a distal implantation site only when the anterior and posterior tibial arteries are not suitable for use.

22

23

23

The tunnel from the distal posterior tibial artery to the popliteal fossa is made just deep to the deep fascia. This is best accomplished with a long, gently curved clamp.

24

The distal anterior tibial artery is approached by an anterior incision midway between the tibia and fibula (*see also Illustration 19*). For bypasses to this vessel, a tunnel is made from the distal popliteal fossa, deep to the deep fascia, to a point 5–7 cm above the medial malleolus. This is best accomplished with a large, gently curved clamp.

From this point, the tunnel is made subcutaneously in a gentle curve across the tibia and adjacent tendons to reach the anterior tibial wound. The underlying tendons are those of the anterior tibial muscle and the long extensors of the toes. The tunnels are marked with umbilical tapes for subsequent identification.

After completion of the distal anastomosis and drawing the graft through these tunnels, any tendons that distort or compress the graft in its course around the tibia are divided. This is usually required in the very low anterior tibial bypasses.

24

25 & 26

When no more proximal procedure is possible, bypasses to the ankle region or foot can be used to salvage limbs (Veith *et al.*, 1978a, 1981b). The dorsalis pedis artery can be easily approached via an incision on the dorsum of the foot. We place this incision laterally, curve it and raise a flap so that the incision will not be directly over the anastomosis. If this artery must be approached at the ankle, it is necessary to divide the extensor retinaculum. Otherwise, the operation is performed as already described for the distal anterior tibial bypass. The posterior tibial artery can be approached down to a point several centimetres below the medial malleolus. Below this level the artery divides into a medial and lateral plantar branch, either of which can be used for successful distal bypasses (Ascer, Veith and Gupta, in press).

All other details in this procedure are similar to those already described for posterior tibial bypasses in the lower leg.

25

26

References

Ascer, E., Veith, F. J. and Gupta, S. K. (in press). Bypasses to plantar arteries and other tibial branches: An extended approach to limb salvage. *Journal of Vascular Surgery*.

Reichle, F.A. and Tyson, R. R. (1972). Bypasses to tibial or popliteal arteries in severely ischemic lower extremities: Comparison of long-term results in 233 patients. *Annals of Surgery* **176**, 315.

Veith, F. J., Moss, C. M., Fell, S. C., Daly, V. and Haimovici, H. (1978). New approaches to limb salvage by extended extra-anatomic bypasses and prosthetic reconstructions to foot arteries. *Surgery* **84**, 764.

Veith, F. J., Gupta, S. K. and Daly, V. D. (1981a). Femoropopliteal bypass to the isolated popliteal segment: Is polytetrafluoroethylene graft acceptable? *Surgery* **89**, 296.

Veith, F. J., Gupta, S. K., Samson, R. H. *et al.* (1981b) Progress in limb salvage by reconstructive arterial surgery combined with new or improved adjunctive procedures. *Annals of Surgery* **194**, 366.

Veith, F. J., Ascer, E., Gupta, S. K., *et al.* (1985). Tibiotibial vein bypass grafts: A new operation for limb salvage. *Journal of Vascular Surgery* **2**, 552.

Veith, F. J., Gupta, S. K., Ascer, E., *et al.* (1986). Six-year prospective randomized comparison of autologous saphenous vein and expanded polytetrafluoroethylene grafts in infrainguinal arterial reconstructions. *Journal of Vascular Surgery* **3**, 104.

The use of the vein cuff and PTFE

Justin H. Miller   MBBS, FRCS, FRACS, FACS
Royal Adelaide Hospital and Repatriation General Hospital, Adelaide, South Australia, Australia

Introduction

The cuff (or 'sleeve' as it is often, but less correctly called) is a cylinder of vein interposed between a PTFE tube and small artery. It was introduced in 1981 (Miller *et al.*, 1984) to facilitate the anastomosis of large (6 mm diameter) stiff PTFE grafts to small (often < 2 mm diameter) tibial arteries.

Its application has now become very widespread, gradually replacing all direct PTFE anastomoses, such as those to the popliteal and profunda femoris arteries. In selected cases, it is also used at the proximal common femoral inflow anastomosis.

Likewise, a recent innovation has been to facilitate the side-to-side anastomosis between the PTFE and an artery, such as sequential ilio-profunda-popliteal reconstructions, or sequential composite PTFE-vein femoro-popliteal-tibial grafts.

While the main advantage of the cuff over direct anastomosis remains its technical facility, evidence is accruing that it leads to improved long-term patency. Another major advantage is that the presence of the cuff facilitates later thrombectomy. The cuff mimics vein in as much as neointimal hyperplasia at the cuff/artery anastomosis is minimal, leading to preservation of the original outflow artery. Moreover, the cuff has less fibrotic reaction than PTFE directly in contact with artery, thereby minimizing the amount of dissection required to control the vessel.

Indications

Femorodistal bypass

It is emphasized that autogenous saphenous vein is still the preferred conduit in all forms of femorodistal grafting. However, PTFE remains a satisfactory alternative when vein (for numerous reasons, not the least of which are multiple previous operations in the same limb) is not available.

The cuff is indicated in all situations where PTFE is to be anastomosed to tibial arteries and is strongly recommended when the anastomosis is to the below-knee popliteal artery, a situation hitherto considered to be a contraindication to the use of any prosthesis. The use of the cuff for the above-knee popliteal artery is not essential but is useful in situations where extensive atheroma makes direct suturing difficult. In the sequential bypass (femoro-popliteal-tibial), the cuff facilitates the side-to-side anastomosis of PTFE (or composite PTFE-vein).

Aortofemoral or cross-over bypass surgery

Aortofemoral surgery often requires the distal end of the graft to be anastomosed to the profunda femoris vessel. Mismatch of the graft vessel diameters requires the use of a long tapering graft down the profunda femoris. The cuff is ideal in this situation, reducing the extent of the dissection required and actually reducing the operating time for the anastomosis. The cuff is equally applicable when a cross-over femoro-profunda graft is required. When an inflow operation is combined with a distal bypass (aorto- or ilio-profunda-popliteal graft), a cuff applied to the profunda greatly facilitates the side-to-side anastomosis between that vessel and the PTFE graft.

Special considerations for infrainguinal PTFE grafts with cuff

The total experience in femorodistal bypass grafting has been with 6-mm PTFE, initially with the standard graft, but exclusively with thin-walled grafts since 1984. With the profunda femoris as outflow vessel, 8-mm tubing has been used.

Infection

Contrary to accepted belief, the risk of infection (from foot necrosis, nearby wound breakdown after failed surgery or removal of infected graft) has not been a problem. This is provided that the new PTFE graft lies in a new non-devitalized tract, that the suture line of PTFE to cuff is properly buried in living tissue and that the graft remains patent (and this aided by the cuff). Apart from this, prosthetic grafts are at higher risk of infection than vein and the use of preoperative intravenous antibiotics is essential. The agent selected should have good activity against *Staphylococcus aureus* as well as any local cultured organisms, and should be continued for 48 h postoperatively.

Dissection

Anastomosis with prosthesis needs a good blood supply. Local tissue ischaemia should be avoided by minimal and gentle dissection at anastomotic sites. Approaches to arteries should not transect lymph channels and should avoid collaterals. This is especially so in the groin. A less extensive exposure is required for the cuff than a direct anastomosis with PTFE. Often in the presence of difficult atheroma at the inflow common femoral artery anastomosis, deliberate use of the cuff will simplify the operation compared with direct anastomosis.

Graft length

PTFE is more unforgiving than vein and in judging the length of the graft it is better to err on the side of making the graft too slack rather than too tight. A rule of thumb is to extend the leg fully, distend to arterial pressure and cut the graft to the exact length plus 1 cm.

Clotting

PTFE is intolerant to either stasis of blood within the graft or slow flow, and this must be carefully avoided as follows:

1. Adequate peroperative systemic heparinization is essential. There is little evidence regarding the exact dose to be used but our experience has been to use a bolus of 5000 u of heparin, supplemented by 1000 u/h if the clamp time exceeds 1 h. The advantage of this regime is that it almost never requires reversal with protamine.
2. Heparinized saline (5000 u/500 mls) is used liberally to irrigate the graft and the artery. Once the proximal anastomosis is completed, heparinized saline is forcibly refluxed upstream into the proximal artery of supply prior to clamping of the graft (*see Illustration 4(a)*). Although there is little evidence of its value in an effort to reduce platelet adherence, the author uses heparinized rheomacrodex as well as saline.
3. Postoperative systemic heparinization is not used routinely, but it is recommended for at least 48 h or until maximum perfusion is manifest by pulses and reactionary warmth in the foot in redo situations, or when there is poor distal run-off.

Operating time

The execution of the sleeve takes about the same length of time as a conventional hood of a vein graft. The extra time needed for this technique is for the suturing of the PTFE to the sleeve, but this amounts to less than 15 min in most cases.

Preparation of the patient: choice of vein for the cuff

The whole limb (or both, if veins are scarce) is prepared in the usual way, and the outflow artery is exposed to establish operability. The vein is chosen from the following sites:

1. Long saphenous vein on the shelf of the medial malleolus, unless as in very critical limb ischaemia the site is unlikely to heal. This can be a problem if there is no boost to the local blood supply by the operation.
2. The lateral saphenous vein in the groin incision. (The main trunk makes an excellent and even better cuff but would be more appropriate in some other capacity, e.g. as a sequential composite graft.) Saphenous vein seems to have the right muscular strength; others such as arm veins can be used but are generally too fragile.
3. The beginning of the short saphenous vein behind the lateral malleolus.
4. In the lower edge of a below-knee approach to the popliteal artery. This segment of long saphenous vein is often spared after coronary artery surgery or previous femoropopliteal bypass. Sometimes an *in situ* vein graft is abandoned at an early stage beause the vein is too small at this site; however, it is still adequate for a cuff.

Procedure

The usual order is to suture the cuff on the outflow vessel, then to make the proximal inflow anastomosis, place the graft, cut to length and then join the PTFE to the cuff as the final procedure. Completing the distal anastomosis before the proximal, as is often done with reversed vein graft, is not recommended. PTFE is not as tolerant of stagnant blood as is vein. To shorten operating time it is usually possible for a second operator to execute the proximal anastomosis, while the cuff is being made.

Cuff and inflow anastomosis

Most consider that a cuff is not necessary at the upper inflow anastomosis, and this is certainly true if it is beyond the take-off of the profunda femoris. However, a direct anastomosis to the common femoral vessel does constitute a risk to the integrity of the flow of the profunda artery, especially if there is a chance of early graft occlusion and need for removal, e.g. desperate attempts at limb salvage by femorotibial grafting. To minimize this risk the following steps can be taken:

1. Bring a direct anastomosis wholly on to the superficial femoral vessel by enlarging the outlet of the common femoral artery with a vein patch, so that no PTFE intrudes into the main vessel.
2. Sometimes in very complex atheromatous situations it is more expeditious (in the interests of minimal dissection and avoidance of lymph nodes) to simply let in a cuff in any soft spot free from plaque. The cuff helps avoid what experience has shown to be a bad combination (especially in the groin) – endarterectomy and direct suturing of PTFE.

Concomitant profunda disease at the inflow anastomoses

The decision as to whether to combine a profundaplasty with a distal bypass is always difficult. There are times however when the need cannot be ignored. With vein, the two procedures combine well by using the hood of the proximal anastomosis as the vein patch for the profundaplasty (Greenhalgh, 1980). The combination of cuff and PTFE can be utilized in a similar and simple manner:

1. Simple orifice stenosis is easily handled by siting the cuff partly on the soft profunda and partly on the common femoral artery without endarterectomy. It is often possible to incorporate the lateral circumflex artery orifice as well.
2. When extensive endarterectomy is necessary (e.g. common femoral orifice coralline atheroma), the combined patch and cuff is useful (see Illustration 5 (f)). Here the cuff can be sited over the junction of endarterectomized profunda and normal intima, so that any tendency to lift will be in the mid-portion of the cuff.

1a–d

Technique of creating the cuff

This is the standard technique for any anastomosis, and despite the many modifications which have been suggested, it remains essentially unchanged since it was first developed in 1981.

A total of 3–4 cm of saphenous vein with a diameter of 2–4 mm is opened up longitudinally (a). A larger diameter makes an even better cuff, but this is an extravagant use of vein. An arteriotomy (b), 1–1.5 cm in length, or approximately twice the diameter of the graft, is made in any soft portion free of plaque. The sleeve is then sutured with continuous prolene sutures (6/0 for popliteal, 7/0 for tibial) to the inferior edge of the arteriotomy (c). Some surgeons prefer the traditional method of commencing at the distal apex (or 'toe') using the parachute technique to view the lumen first (d). In either case, it is essential to stitch the artery from within out, so that the vein fixes the intima against the medial coat.

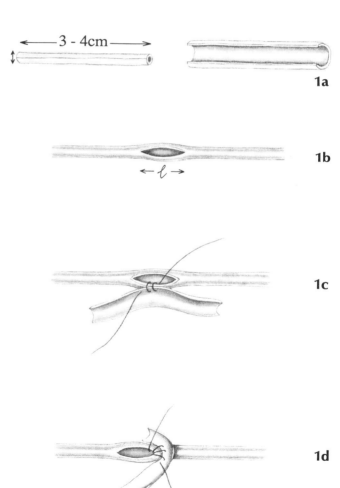

1a

1b

1c

1d

2a–d

Suturing the apices

In the middle portion of the arteriotomy, the bite of artery should be larger than that of vein, so as to take the vein well down into the artery to fix the intima (a). As the apex is approached, this bite should be reduced so as to prevent the vein intruding into the lumen. The interval between sutures should be small and they should be left loose to be tightened later (with a nerve hook if necessary) (b). The heel is treated in the same way as the apex. As each suture is placed at both ends, the lumen of the vessel beyond should be clearly visible.

This is to preserve outflow in both directions, so that in the event of graft occlusion, artery patency is preserved (c). This is vital at the level of the tibial artery. Suturing is continued on the upper edge until the two separate sutures meet (d), when they are tied together. A sealing corner suture is made by passing one needle out–in through the vein and then in–out through the other edge of the vein, where it is tied to the free length of suture.

2a

2b

2c

2d

3a–d

The vein ends are squared off, leaving a little extra for suturing. One thread is cut or used as a stay. The remaining suture is used to approximate the square ends of the vein carefully with frequent bites until the corners meet, where the suture is tied to itself, clipped and used as a stay suture for the next part of the procedure (*a*). The upper anastomosis is then made and the graft is placed in its appropriate tract. Heparinized saline is forcibly refluxed upstream (see *Illustration 4a*) and the graft is clamped distally.

The PTFE is cut at the appropriate angle with a blade (conveniently along a clamp). The angle at which it is cut will determine its circumference, which should equal the circumference of the cuff. This in turn should be twice the length of the arteriotomy ($c = 2l$). If half the circumference ($c/2 = \pi d/2$) of a 6-mm tube cut at right angles = 9.4 mm, then $c/2$ cut at an angle of 60° = 10.8 mm (9.4/sin 60), $c/2$ cut at 45° = 13.3 mm, and an 8-mm tube cut at 60° = 14.5 mm (*c*).

The circumference of the cut PTFE should now approximate to that of the sleeve. If there is to be a disparity in length, it is better that the cuff diameter exceed that of the PTFE, so that 'tenting' takes place in the vein rather than the PTFE (this makes extra suturing easier). By squaring off the tip of the PTFE with a blade, its circumference can be shortened (*d*). It is a simple matter to join the PTFE and cuff end-to-end (*d*). A parachute technique using 7/0 Goretex is appropriate.

Prior to the completion of the anastomosis, backbleeding from both directions is checked to flush out any thrombus. After a final irrigation both proximally and distally, the suture line is completed and the clamps released. A peroperative arteriogram is performed through a 21-gauge butterfly needle inserted into the PTFE near the distal anastomosis and facing upstream. This allows the minimum amount of contrast to be used to display the distal anastomosis. This is important with tibial artery outflow, where excessive contrast can be harmful.

3a

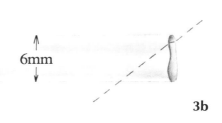

6mm

3b

$\theta = 60°$

$\dfrac{C}{2}$ d = 6mm $\dfrac{C}{2} = l = 10.8\text{mm}$

45°

d = 6mm $l = 13.3\text{mm}$

60°

d = 8mm $l = 12.5\text{mm}$

3d

4a–d

Care of the graft and prevention of clotting

Considerable care is taken to ensure that the graft is of the correct length and that at no stage is there any stationary blood, either in the graft or the well of the cuff and artery, where blood is inclined to accumulate during the execution of the proximal anastomosis. After the proximal anastomosis is made, the graft is placed in its selected tract by a tunneller or sponge-holding forceps. Heparinized saline is then forcibly refluxed upstream through the graft and inflow artery with a 20-ml syringe and malleable cannula (e.g Oschner), and the graft is clamped distally (*a*). This has the effect of ironing out any kinks or malrotation and of ascertaining the optimal length under arterial pressure at the moment the graft is cut(*b*). It also makes absolutely sure that there is no stagnant blood in the graft.

Just prior to completion of the anastomosis, the downflow is checked. A cannula is gently inserted between the loose continuous suture and the cavity of the cuff, and then the graft is flushed with heparinized saline with the arterial clamps removed (*c*). The suture is tightened and the graft clamp is released. This variation in the technique is important with tibial arteries, where backbleeding is often negligible. The perfect tibial clamp is yet to be designed, and therefore clamping and unclamping should be kept to a minimum.

Most suture line bleeding stops within 5 min with gentle swab pressure. 'Tents' from excess vein to PTFE cause 'spurters', which may require individual suturing with the graft reclamped. At no stage should there ever be stationary blood in the PTFE graft. If clamping longer than 1 min is required for any reason, heparinized saline solution should be refluxed back up the graft (clamped distally) to the proximal anastomosis via the scalp vein needle used for the arteriogram (*d*).

4a

4b

4c

4d

5a–f

Pitfalls

When the vein is too short, stretching it under tension (*a, b*) predisposes to necrosis and bleeding at a later date. It is better to cut another piece of vein and suture this in place, tedious though this might be (*c*). If the arteriotomy is too long, the resultant sleeve becomes aneurysmal (*d*). To compensate, part of the vein is sutured in as a patch leaving sufficient for the cuff to accommodate the cut PTFE. It is usual to place the sleeve component at the downstream end so as to provide for the vital distal outflow lumen (*e*). The use of this procedure is sometimes made in concomitant profundaplasty. The patch component widens the proximal profunda, and the cuff accommodating the PTFE is placed distally over uninvolved vessel (*f*).

5a

5b

Rx

5c

5d

Rx

5e   Popliteal →

Profunda →   5f

6a–c

Sequential composite femoro-popliteal-tibial graft

The accepted method for composing a femoro-popliteal-tibial graft by making use of a short segment of vein is to make a direct anastomosis of the PTFE to the popliteal artery and run a jump graft from the PTFE to the tibial vessel (Finn *et al.*, 1980), or to join the PTFE distal outflow anastomosis and the vein inflow anastomosis sequentially to the popliteal artery. There are two problems, however. Technically, the proximal portion of the vein is narrow (at the best 4 mm, otherwise it would have been used in its entirety as a complete vein graft) and therefore likely to be narrow immediately at the heel. Secondly, in the long term, neointimal hyperplasia may develop as a consequence of the compliance mismatch.

By applying a cuff to the intermediate popliteal anastomotic site first (*a*), the PTFE and the vein can be joined using the sleeve as an intermediary (avoiding the direct vein – PTFE join or the vein to thick-walled artery). The critical heel of the small-diameter vein is first parachuted on to the mid-distal point of the sleeve, and then the wider heel of the PTFE on to the proximal or cephalic side of the sleeve. The apical opened-out part of the vein becomes a long patch on the PTFE (*b*). Alternatively, a single tube of PTFE can be anastomosed side-to-side to the popliteal artery via the cuff (*c*). A direct side-to-side anastomosis between the PTFE and the artery is very difficult.

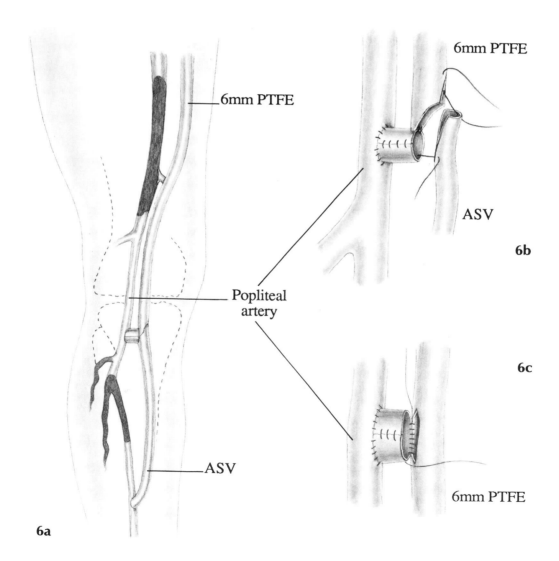

6mm PTFE

Popliteal artery

ASV

6a

6mm PTFE

ASV

6b

6c

6mm PTFE

7a & b

Late thrombectomy of occluded PTFE graft and cuff

When a PTFE graft occludes (often years later), the presence of a cuff facilitates the thrombectomy. Usually, the original outflow artery remains open and shows up on the arteriogram. If not, it can sometimes be cleaned out by local infusion of streptokinase via the graft. Failing this, the main body of the graft can be thrombectomized and extended with a fresh piece of PTFE to a new site lower down via a cuff. It is unlikely that simply clearing the graft at its midpoint with a Fogarty catheter will have any lasting outcome. Both ends must be exposed and cleaned under direct vision.

7a

Clearing the distal anastomosis

The junction of the PTFE and cuff is exposed by sharp dissection, as are both the upstream and downstream arteries, sufficient to control backbleeding using straight clamps and without formal taping. It is best not to bare the original vein-to-artery stitching. An arteriotomy is made across the PTFE and cuff (*a*).

Thrombus is then lifted from within the vein–artery cavity. This results mostly in backbleeding from either end. It is not usually necessary to pass a Fogarty catheter, but this can be decided upon using the arteriogram. Very occasionally, a vessel full of clot can be cleared from here, but it is more likely that the artery lining will be damaged. On rare occasions, neointima may line the junction of the PTFE and vein cuff, possibly extending to the arterial lumen. This will endarterectomize cleanly (it is quite distinct from atheroma), leaving natural endothelium. No attempt should be made to clear out above with a Fogarty catheter at this stage.

Inguinal ligament

7b

Clearing the upper anastomosis

The upper graft is exposed by sharp dissection and followed up to the anastomosis. It is preferable to avoid laying bare the previous sutures. The common femoral artery is then similarly dissected just under the inguinal ligament, separating the femoral vein to the lateral side and the femoral nerve laterally. This should be virgin territory. Taping, which risks damaging the back wall, is not necessary; a Bainbridge DeBakey clamp directed backwards will suffice. Profunda backbleeding is controlled using a similar clamp across the superficial femoral and profunda artery complex (*b*). Again it is preferable that the profunda femoris is not taped.

The hood of the PTFE is opened and the cavity is cleared of fibrin. This is facilitated if there has been a previous cuff. The downflow is then checked and, if found to be inadequate, a Fogarty catheter or sound may be gently passed to ascertain the need for a patch above the anastomosis. It may be necessary to have profunda backbleeding during the final stages of cleaning. This is obtained using a blunt paediatric sucker and irrigation. A common mistake is to shift to a new anastomosis more proximally. Ultimately, this only prejudices the profunda circulation, lengthens the graft and leads to a lower patency rate. It is possible to use the original anastomosis over and over again.

8a—e

The graft is then cleared through both openings. A No. 4 Fogarty catheter is passed from below upward to extract the main thrombus (*a,b*). Often there is surprisingly little. This procedure should be carried out with care unless a thin layer of fibrin is disturbed. The passage of the catheter from above downward is to make sure there are no kinks. Finally, a large malleable cannula (e.g. Oschner) is introduced from above and the graft is vigorously flushed downwards with heparinized saline (*c*).

The upper opening is then closed (after checking downflow). Sometimes, a protruding mound ('cervix') presents from the original heel of the PTFE graft. If so, it is preferable to add a patch of PTFE or vein (*d*). It is best not to clamp

just beyond this suturing, in case clot accumulates. Instead, heparinized saline (or rheomacrodex) should be refluxed against the bloodstream as described (*see Illustration 4a*), and a clamp attached just above the distal opening. This allows any debris to separate and prevents it from going down the outflow vessel. A brisk outflow when the clamp is released ensures the flow is not impeded.

Finally, the bottom opening is closed. Usually, a patch is required (preferably vein), especially if there is a protuberance of the original PTFE heel. The apex of the patch parachutes nicely into the previous cuff (*e*). After thrombectomy, it is recommended that immediate full heparinization and long-term anticoagulation be instituted.

8a

8b

8c

8d

Heel

8e

Heel

References

Finn, W. R., Flanigan, D. P., Verta, M. J., Bergan, J. J. and Yao, Y. S. T. (1980). Sequential femoro-tibial bypass for severe limb ischaemia. *Surgery* **88**, 357.

Greenhalgh, R. M. (1980). Profunda femoris reconstruction with and without distal bypass. In *Operative Techniques in Vascular Surgery*, 1st ed. Bergan, J. J., Yao, J. S. T., eds. London and Orlando: Grune and Stratton.

King, T. A., Rhodes, R. S. and De Palma, R. G. (1980). Use of the profunda femoris artery for secondary revascularization. In *Operative Techniques in Vascular Surgery*, 1st ed. Bergan, J. J., Yao, J. S. T., eds. London and Orlando: Grune and Stratton.

Miller, J. H., Foreman, R. K., Ferguson, L. and Faris, I. (1984). Interposition vein cuff for anastomosis of prosthesis to small artery. *Australian and New Zealand Journal of Surgery* **54**, 283.

Repair of the failing femorodistal graft

John H. N. Wolfe MS, FRCS
Consultant Vascular Surgeon and Honorary Senior Lecturer, St Mary's Hospital Medical School, London, UK;
Consultant Vascular Surgeon and Honorary Senior Lecturer, Royal Postgraduate Medical School, Hammersmith Hospital, London, UK

Peter R. Taylor MA, FRCS
Senior Clinical Vascular Fellow, St Mary's Hospital, London, UK

Introduction

In recent years the number of bypass grafts performed to the more distal arteries in the lower limb has increased considerably. Despite experience and improved operative techniques, the failure of these arterial grafts continues to be a problem of considerable magnitude. Reported failure rates of femoropopliteal and femorocrural grafts range between 20 and 50% at 5 years. Brewster and colleagues (1983a) showed that 65% of graft failures occurred within the first postoperative year, and that 79% of grafts occluded within 2 years of operation.

Graft failures can be divided into three groups, based on the postoperative time interval:

1. *Immediate failures.* These occur within 1 month and are almost invariably attributable to errors of surgical technique or judgement. Such failures can be minimized by careful objective intraoperative assessment with Doppler probes and arteriography (Whittemore *et al.*, 1980).
2. *Early failures.* This group accounts for the majority of graft failures and spans the time period from 1 month to 1 year following operation. This group may benefit particularly from graft surveillance techniques. (Wolfe and McPherson, 1987).
3. *Late failures.* These occur after 1 year and are usually secondary to progression of the original atherosclerotic disease process. Although graft surveillance may be useful, the failure rate at this stage is only 2.5% per annum for vein grafts and 7% per annum for prosthetic grafts (Berkowitz *et al.*, 1981).

Techniques of graft surveillance

1. *Serial ankle Doppler pressure measurements.* Initial reports using this technique were encouraging (Taylor and Fox, 1977). However, more recent studies show that if this method is used alone, many graft stenoses are missed (Wolfe *et al.*, 1987; McShane *et al.*, 1987).
2. *Serial intravenous digital subtraction angiography.* This is a reliable method for detecting graft stenoses, providing that the patient has a good cardiac output. However, patient compliance remains a drawback despite the introduction of non-ionic contrast medium.
3. *Serial duplex Doppler assessment.* This non-invasive method can detect graft stenoses before they become haemodynamically significant. Graft flow measurements are inaccurate (Grigg *et al.*, 1988), but changes in peak systolic velocity of 50% or more within a 2-cm length of graft suggest the presence of a stenosis (Grigg, Nicolaides and Wolfe, 1988).

If patients are monitored regularly for the first year, approximately 20% of grafts will develop stenoses (Wolfe *et al.*, 1987; Cohen *et al.*, 1986). However, not all stenoses will be haemodynamically significant. Our current policy is to monitor their progression. When the change in velocity suggests a 50% reduction in diameter (equivalent to a 75% reduction in cross-sectional area), we intervene, since we believe that the graft is at risk of occlusion from a haemodynamically significant stenosis. Whittemore *et al.* (1980) have shown that the results of thrombectomy are much worse compared with those of graft repair before occlusion. Not all stenoses progress to become significant, and in approximately half no progression is seen so that intervention is not indicated. Difficulties in imaging may be encountered when the graft is very deep to the skin, such as the area immediately adjacent to a popliteal anastomosis. Distal grafts to the crural vessels are more superficial and reliable recordings can be obtained. Colour flow Doppler imaging may be useful in this regard since the deeper grafts are more easily identified. This policy of graft surveillance leads to a number of re-operations on arterial bypass grafts. These secondary procedures can be classified into the following three categories: (1) inflow problems, (2) graft problems, and (3) outflow problems.

Secondary procedures

Inflow problems

1a & b

In the presence of ipsilateral iliac artery occlusion, vein grafts may remain patent even though clinically they do not pulsate (*a*). In these patients an appropriate procedure is performed to improve the inflow of the graft. This may include a femorofemoral cross-over graft, iliofemoral cross-over graft (*b*), unilateral iliofemoral graft or an aortobifemoral graft.

The upper end of the graft is anastomosed, end-to-side, to the new graft using the usual anastomotic technique. There seems little purpose interposing parent artery between the two grafts. Clamp injury may damage the common femoral artery, but in our experience this is rare (Grigg, Nicolaides and Wolfe, 1988).

1a

1b

2a & b

A more common problem is aggressive myointimal hyperplasia occurring at the site of femoral endarterectomy performed to facilitate the proximal anastomosis (*a*). This can be repaired with a vein patch (*b*) across the stenosed segment.

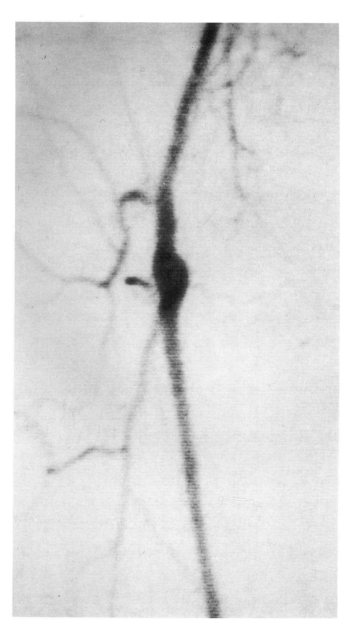

2a

2b

Graft problems

3 & 4

Short fibrotic stenoses occurring in vein grafts are frequently related to valve cusps. These can be treated by either vein patch (taken from either the arm or the short saphenous vein) or percutaneous balloon angioplasty. However, balloon angioplasty is not as successful as surgery (Whittemore *et al.*,

1980; Cohen *et al.*, 1986; Brewster *et al.*, 1983b; Veith *et al.*, 1984), but is probably useful in selected patients. The use of a 2.5-mm cardiac balloon may improve results since it is more difficult to disrupt vein grafts with these small, softer balloons.

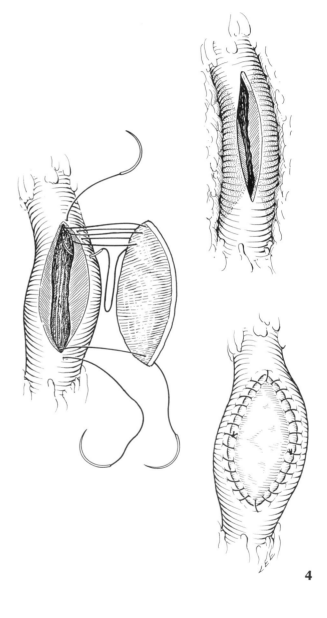

3

4

5a, b & 6

Longer stenoses should be treated operatively by using either a vein patch or 'jump' graft to bypass the stenosed segment. End-to-end venovenous anastomoses give better flow characteristics and the use of a long oblique anastomosis using 7/0 Prolene protects against stenosis. When long or multiple segments of graft are affected by a stenotic process, surgery is of little value.

5a

5b

6

Outflow problems

7a, b & 8

We have had some success with balloon angioplasty in treating stenoses close to the distal anastomosis, but others are more sceptical (Thompson *et al.*, in press). The alternative is to perform a bypass 'jump' graft from the graft to a crural vessel distal to the stenosis using arm vein or short saphenous vein. The graft is tunnelled subcutaneously. The dissection of the distal vessel is relatively straightforward providing the previous operating field can be avoided.

7a

7b

8

9

Except under rare circumstances, no attempt should be made to dissect out the previous anastomosis. The dense scar tissue resulting from the previous operation makes this a procedure fraught with hazard. When it is necessary to dissect a graft

from this scar tissue, it can be extremely difficult to visualize or palpate, and a hand-held Doppler probe placed within a sterile operating glove may be invaluable in localizing the graft.

9

References

Berkowitz, H. D., Hobbs, C. L., Roberts, B., Freiman, D., Oleaga, J. and Ring, E. (1981). Value of routine vascular laboratory studies to identify vein graft stenoses. *Surgery* **90**, 971.

Brewster, D. L., La Salle, A. J., Robison, J. C., Stranghorn, E. C. and Darling, R. C. (1983a). Factors affecting patency of femoro-popliteal grafts. *Surgery, Gynecology and Obstetrics* **157**, 437.

Brewster, D. C., La Salle, A. J., Robison, J. G. *et al.* (1983b). Femoro-popliteal graft failures: Clinical consequences and success of secondary reconstructions. *Archives of Surgery* **118**, 1043.

Cohen, J. R., Mannick, J. A., Couch, N. P. and Whittemore, A. D. (1986). Recognition and management of impending vein graft failure. *Archives of Surgery* **121**, 758.

Grigg, M. J., Nicolaides, A. N. and Wolfe, J. H. N. (1988). Femoro-distal bypass graft stenoses. *British Journal of Surgery* **75**, 737.

Grigg, M. J., Wolfe, J. H. N., Tovan, A. and Nicolaides, A. N. (1988). The reliability of duplex haemodynamic measurements in the assessment of femoro-distal grafts. *European Journal of Vascular Surgery* **2**, 171.

McShane, M. D., Gazzard, W.H., Clifford, P. C., Hacking, C. N., Fairhurst, J. J., Humphries, K. N., Birch, S. J., Webster, J. H. H. and Chant, A. (1987). Duplex ultrasound assessment and femoro-

distal grafts – correlation with angioplasty. *European Journal of Vascular Surgery* **1**, 409.

Taylor, R. S. and Fox, N. D. (1977). Ultrasonic prediction of graft failure. *Journal of Cardiovascular Surgery* **18**, 309.

Thompson, J., McShane, M., Gazzard, V., Webster, J. and Chant, A. (in press). Intervention for graft stenoses: Experience following 206 femoral-distal reconstructions. *British Journal of Surgery*.

Veith, F. J., Weiser, R. K., Gupta, S. K., Ascer, E., Scher, L. A., Samson, R. H., White Flores, S. A. and Sprayregen, S. (1984). Diagnosis and management of failing lower extremity arterial reconstructions prior to graft occlusion. *Journal of Cardiovascular Surgery* **25**, 381.

Whittemore, A. D., Clowes, A. W., Couch, N. P. and Mannick, J. A. (1980). Secondary femoro-popliteal reconstruction. *Annals of Surgery* **193**, 35.

Wolfe, J. H. N. and McPherson, G. A. D. (1987). The failing femoro-distal graft. *European Journal of Vascular Surgery* **1**, 295.

Wolfe, J. H. N., Thomas, M. L., Jamieson, C. W., Browse, N. L., Burnard, K. G., and Rutt, D. L. (1987). The early diagnosis of femoro-popliteal graft stenoses, a prospective one year follow up. *British Journal of Surgery* **74**, 268.

The use of glutaraldehyde-stabilized umbilical vein for lower extremity reconstruction

Herbert Dardik   MD, FACS

Chief, General and Vascular Surgery, Englewood Hospital, Englewood, New Jersey, USA;
Clinical Associate Professor of Surgery, New Jersey Medical School, Newark, New Jersey, USA

Introduction

Significant developments in the technology for performing lower limb revascularization procedures have eclipsed the historical importance and continued current value of synthetic materials for lower extremity bypass. Autologous venous tissue is the bypass material of choice and should be employed wherever possible. My personal experience supports this view, with availability and utilization of autologous tissue for arterial conduits in the vast majority of cases exceeding 90%. Is there any role for synthetics in lower limb bypass procedures, particularly those terminating at infrapopliteal levels? The answer, in my opinion, is decidedly yes.

Based on our experience with more than 1000 glutaraldehyde-stabilized umbilical vein graft implantations in the lower extremity, we have recognized the special technical requirements essential for the successful implantation of this graft material. The results of vascular surgical reconstruction depend on many factors including precise selection of cases, classification and staging of the disease process, and judicious application of appropriate therapeutic modalities. We previously discussed some of these factors with regard to selecting patients for vascular reconstruction of the lower extremities (Dardik *et al.*, 1975, 1979). However, once the appropriate patient and a particular procedure have been selected, the technical expertise and the intraoperative judgement exercised by the surgeon are essential to achieving long lasting success.

Graft selection

The glutaraldehyde-stabilized umbilical vein graft (Biograft™, Meadox Medicals, Oakland, New Jersey) is an appropriate choice of graft material in the absence of a suitable autologous saphenous vein or if circumstances militate against its use, such as limited life expectancy of the patient. Our experience over the past 14 years with glutaraldehyde-stabilized umbilical veins has convinced us of its excellent qualities and applicability for lower extremity bypass reconstructions, yet being aware of its deficiencies, notably the increasing likelihood for biodegradation after implantation for 5 or more years (Dardik *et al.*, 1988).

The most important factor governing graft selection is the required length. This is determined by intraoperative measurement of the distance between the proximal and distal anastomoses with the extremity in full extension. It is obviously prudent to add an additional few centimetres to compensate for any error in measurement and to allow for better trimming of the graft at the anastomotic areas. In the absence of a single long graft long enough to reach from the proximal to the distal site, composite grafts are perfectly acceptable, whether they are constructed at the time of surgery or presutured by the manufacturer.

Graft preparation

Irrigation

All umbilical vein grafts must be thoroughly washed with a heparinized solution prior to implantation.

1 & 2

The graft is first removed from its container in an area away from the irrigation basin and is gently compressed manually from above downwards in order to milk out excess fluids.

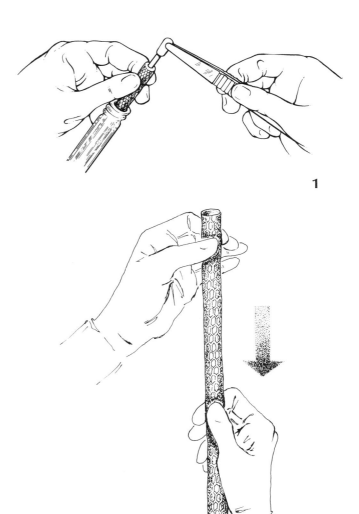

1

2

3

Soaking the graft in a basin containing 1 litre of heparinized saline solution is the method employed to dilute and wash out residual alcohol and glutaraldehyde. It is important to avoid airlocks in the graft by manual irrigations at intervals during the 15-min soak. This is done most conveniently by the scrub nurse with several 50-ml aliquots of dilute heparin solution injected directly into the graft via a soft rubber catheter as the graft is immersed in the soaking basin.

3

4

4

After the actual irrigation or soaking is completed, several millilitres of undiluted concentrated heparin are instilled directly into the graft. This is then simply flushed from its lumen with an additional 30–40 ml of dilute heparin solution. It has been suggested that concentrated heparin bonds to the flow surface and increases thromboresistance (Hufnagel, 1979). The residual high concentration of heparin is flushed out because any spillage into the patient's tissues during the anastomotic procedure might result in an excessive degree of anticoagulation.

The operation

Anaesthesia

The anaesthetic management of patients requiring lower limb revascularization should be performed by physicians skilled in caring for the diverse medical problems that are indigenous to this patient population. Although general anaesthesia is frequently employed and is even desired by many patients, our preference is for epidural anaesthesia. This method is very effective, is acceptable to patients after an explanation of the procedure, and it avoids many of the potential debilities associated with inhalation anaesthesia. Postoperative injections of analgesics into the epidural space provide prolonged pain-free periods, thereby avoiding many of the undesirable effects of systemic analgesics.

Instrumentation, sutures and anastomoses

5a–e

Standard metallic vascular instruments are not used to clamp the graft. The umbilical vein graft is fragile and subject to intimal fracture and splitting if excessive pressure, whether manual or instrumental, is applied. We have devised a special clamp ('D' clamp) and to date it appears to function very well in securing vascular occlusion with minimal, if any, trauma. Although special clamps or intraluminal balloon tamponade can be employed, we still prefer either reclamping of the host arterial system or simple digital compression of the graft for vascular control.

Intraluminal   **5a**

5b   Reclamp host artery

"D" Clamp   **5c**

5d   Digital control

Berlin (Silastic) Clamp   **5e**

6a–d

Proper trimming of the graft is important and should be done with sharp scissors. The distal end of the graft should have a squared-off taper to avoid sutures tearing through at this point. All arteriotomies should be long, ranging from 20 to 25 mm.

Monofilament polypropylene has been our choice for suture material, but any of the standard types can be used. Number 6/0 is generally employed, but in the distal areas and particularly for the peroneal artery and construction of adjunctive arteriovenous fistulae, 7/0 is recommended to avoid or minimize bleeding through needle holes.

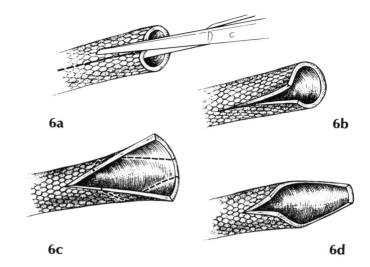

6a

6b

6c

6d

7

Over the past 5 years, it has become our preference to perform the distal anastomosis first. We have encountered no problem from the graft or the presutured composite anastomosis. Nevertheless, it is perfectly feasible to do the proximal anastomosis first if this is the surgeon's preference. Although we have employed diameters of 4–6 mm, we prefer the 5-mm diameter graft for all reconstructions in the lower extremity.

Umbilical vein grafts are now prepared so that the wall thickness varies from less than 1 mm to slightly more than 1 mm. Thus the surgeon will need some experience to become accustomed to the management and suturing of this wall. It is interesting that no matter how thick the wall may be at the time of implantation, it becomes thinner within a short time thereafter because of resorption of extracellular fluid and compression from intraluminal forces.

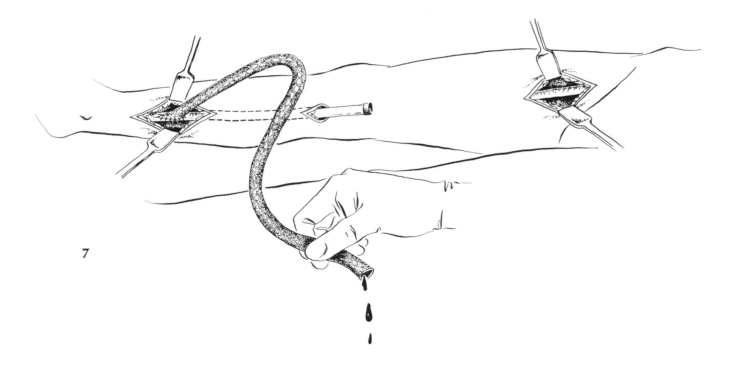

7

8–11

Interrupted suture technique is advocated at both the proximal heel and distal toe of the distal anastomosis. This avoids shearing of the tissue as well as purse-stringing of the anastomosis. This may help to minimize compliance mismatch. Just prior to completion of the final suture line, calibrated coronary artery dilators are passed beyond the anastomosis to overcome any clamp compression effects.

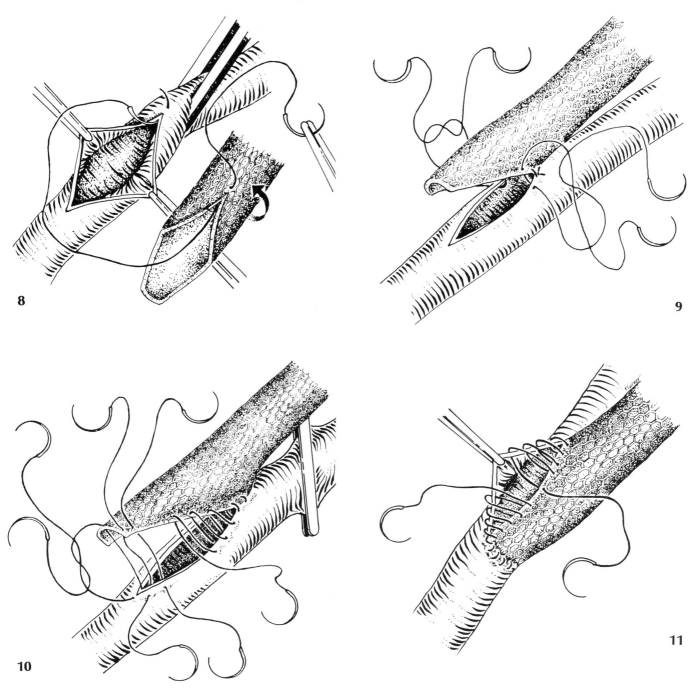

8

9

10

11

12–15

The proximal anastomosis is performed with a continuous technique. The 'parachute' method is particularly helpful at the heel and toe areas.

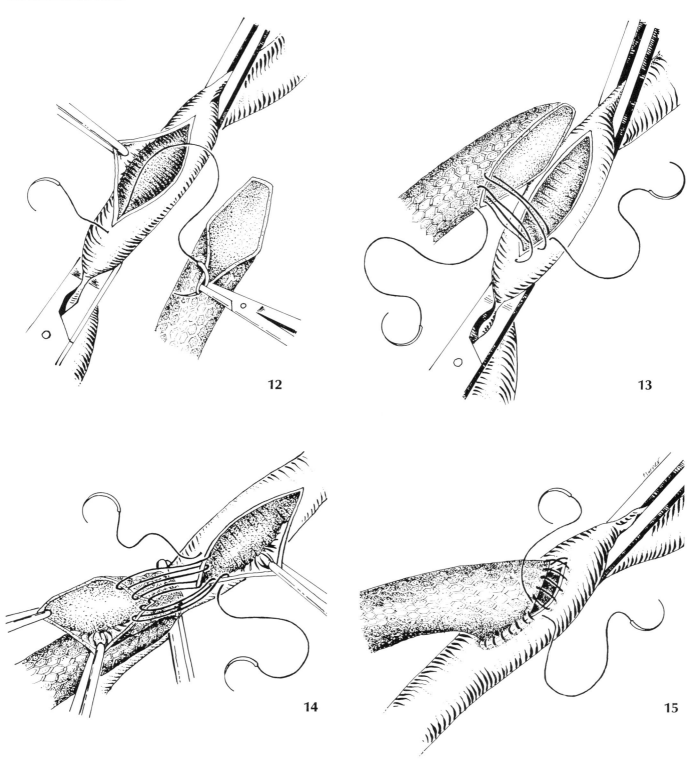

12

13

14

15

16

The mesh is incorporated with each suture, but it is not particularly critical if one or more areas are missed. What is important, however, is that each needle bite should penetrate the actual intimal component of the graft, which can be recognized as a slightly deeper beige-coloured tissue compared to the major outer component of the graft. Anastomotic aneurysms and intramural dissection can be prevented by precise suturing technique. For the same reasons, it is also essential to avoid needle penetration of the intima of the opposite wall when taking an outside-in bite, particularly at the beginning of the suture line at or adjacent to the acute angle. Both inside-out and outside-in needle passage are acceptable provided the above cited precautions are taken. The only exception for overlooking 'missed intima' would be on one or two needle passages of a continuous suture line of a distal anastomosis where the downstream flow direction precludes intimal lifting and mural dissection. It is not critical if the mesh does not cover the entire suture line because a desmoplastic response provides adequate support at the anastomosis.

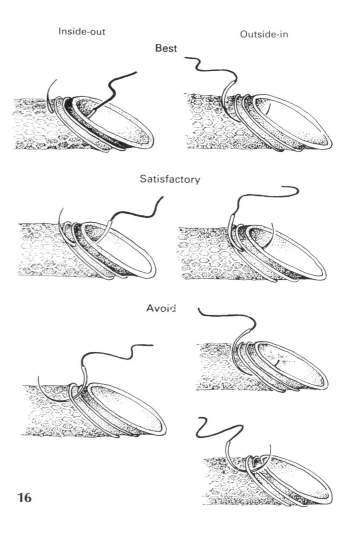

16

Tunnelling

Tunnels are established in the anatomical location for all popliteal reconstructions, as well as for bypasses to the proximal posterior tibial artery. Subcutaneous tunnels are established medially for many distal posterior tibial artery reconstructions, and laterally for most peroneal and anterior tibial artery reconstructions.

17 & 18

Tunnels are generally established before the patient is heparinized. This is performed with a slightly curved blunt instrument consisting of a metallic obturator and outer plastic sheath. The obturator is withdrawn after placement of the entire apparatus and the graft brought through the plastic sheath component with a long alligator-type forceps, the first anastomosis having usually been completed or initiated. The

graft is positioned slightly taut, and then the outer plastic tunnel is withdrawn over the graft and grasping forceps. Passing the graft through a tunneller is essential to avoid friction between the outer Dacron mesh and the host tissues which could cause damage to the graft. Once a subcutaneous graft has been seated, wound retractors must be positioned to avoid pressure on the graft, particularly above a lower leg exposure. Cloth or styrofoam padding is very helpful in this regard. It is also essential that tunnels be initiated and completed in the subcutaneous position, since it is possible to perforate the fascia blindly at the knee level and create a constriction by which the graft can be compressed. For this reason all subcutaneous tunnels are established with the aid of an auxiliary anterolateral incision in the lower third of the thigh. The incision is brought down to the fascia and the tunnel is initiated by finger dissection, pushing the subcutaneous layer off the fascia. The tunnelling instrument is then passed from this site upwards to the inguinal incision and downwards to the site of distal arterial exposure.

17

18

Intraoperative adjuncts

Heparin usage and monitoring

All patients are heparinized systemically at least 5 min before securing vascular control and performing the first anastomosis. We usually start with 2500–3000 u and add increments of 1000–2000 more units depending on the estimate of anticoagulation by the activated clotting time test. This test is useful to monitor adequacy of heparinization and need for reversal. Reversal of heparin anticoagulation, if required, is performed at the conclusion of all anastomoses and is accomplished with protamine sulphate in increments of 10–20 mg. Generally, none is required. During the operative period we irrigate the local anastomotic area with dilute heparin solution (50 mg per 500 ml). Dilute solution is also instilled into the distal circulation when the distal arteriotomy is established, but this should be done with the utmost caution and perhaps even omitted if the patient has extensive disease, particularly calcification.

Electromagnetic flowmeter recordings

Electromagnetic flowmeter recordings can be performed but are not essential. We have found that the information provides data suggesting the prognosis for early graft patency; it cannot be considered as an absolute monitor of the technical expertise with which the reconstruction was performed, nor can it

provide assurance that the disease will not progress. Nevertheless, if flow is augmented to at least twice the baseline value with papaverine hydrochloride, the prognosis for early graft patency and function is good for most of these patients (Dardik et al., 1978).

Completion arteriography

Completion arteriography is, in our opinion, mandatory before concluding the operation. It is performed simply by placing a No. 19 scalp vein needle either directly into the graft or into an adjacent artery, and then injecting a small amount of contrast medium as the X-ray cassette, placed under the distal anastomotic and run-off area, is exposed. This not only allows for the detection of any potential intraoperative defects, but also provides a definitive view of the run-off circulation for classification and gives some measure of the prognosis for the durability of graft function (Dardik et al., 1978). Run-off and pedal arch structure can be analysed and correlated with the subsequent fate of the graft and stability or progression of the atherosclerotic process. Separate injections are required for popliteal bypasses in order to demonstrate the distal anastomosis on one film and the pedal circulation on the other.

19

A simple, inexpensive device consisting of a double hydraulic syringe system and a holding fixture has been devised for intraoperative arteriography to avoid exposure of personnel

to repetitive radiation (Dardik et al., 1980). Completion angiography has thus become safer, less time-consuming and more reliable in obtaining high-quality angiographic studies.

19

Distal arteriovenous fistula

If reconstruction to a crural vessel is required, and a prosthetic graft material deemed necessary, we believe that an adjunctive distal arteriovenous fistula (dAVF) should be created in order to promote the likelihood for a reasonable result that would otherwise not be possible under these circumstances; that is, where haemodynamic factors by themselves will result in early bypass failure (Dardik, 1983). The theoretical basis for using distal arteriovenous fistulae as adjuncts to crural reconstructions in order to maintain graft patency and distal perfusion is based upon the need to reduce the vascular overload being presented to the distal circuit and, at the same time, to keep graft flow over the critical thrombotic threshold level (Dardik, 1985).

20

Establishing a vent (dAVF) results in an increased flow in the graft, most of which is then directed into the high capacitance venous circulation. The amount of blood that can be accepted by the arterial run-off, albeit limited, will perfuse distally and reverse the ischaemic state.

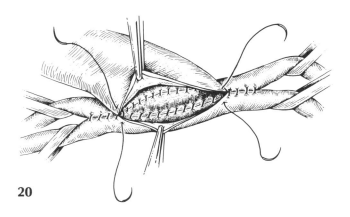

20

Postoperative management

Knee immobilization is employed routinely to prevent inadvertent flexion of the hip and knee, particularly as the patient awakens and is unable to follow instructions to keep his extremities straight. We employ the immobilizer for approximately 4 days but suggest that the patient continue using it during the entire period of hospitalization and even for another week at home. It is not required while walking. Weight-bearing and walking are usually instituted after the 3rd postoperative day; crural reconstructions are postponed for an additional day. The progress of those patients with gangrenous foot lesions will obviously determine the rate at which weight-bearing and walking will progress.

Reoperative surgery

Early thrombosis, usually due to technical mishap or poor run-off, is best managed on the basis of the post-reconstruction completion arteriogram. Those with poor run-off must be considered as distinct failures. The only possibility of graft salvage in these cases depends on the ability to use one of several adjunctive techniques including angioplasty, sequential bypass or distal adjunctive arteriovenous fistula. Cases which have failed as a result of technical error or otherwise unanticipated postoperative thrombosis should be returned immediately to the operating room for thrombectomy and correction of the underlying cause of failure. We usually explore the graft distally and, after heparinizing the patient, remove thrombus via an opening in the graft that can, if necessary, be extended across the anastomosis. If all thrombus cannot be easily removed in this manner, we do not hesitate to open the upper wound and either massage the thrombus to release it or open the graft at this level for extraction of all thrombus. The most important aspect of umbilical vein graft thrombectomy is extreme gentleness. It is best to try to extrude all thrombus by gentle external massage or direct irrigation of the graft via proximal and distal arteriotomies before proceeding to balloon catheter extraction. Over-inflation of balloon catheters must be avoided. While passing balloon catheters it is also important to make sure that there is no friction between the catheter and the inner vessel wall. This can be avoided by intermittent gentle irrigations of the graft lumen with heparinized solution. Incisions for exploring the grafts are vertical at the proximal and distal anastomotic areas and can usually be closed primarily. In the body of the graft, patching is usually required for vertical incisions. Transverse incisions can be employed but provide limited exposure.

21

Vein patch angioplasty should also be employed at the distal anastomosis if the arteriotomy is carried across the anastomosis into the host run-off artery.

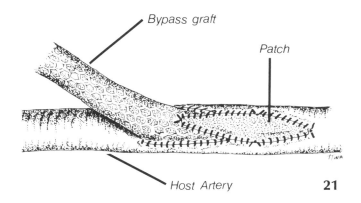

Bypass graft

Patch

Host Artery   **21**

If there is any concern about the structural integrity of the graft or if there is difficulty with the dissection, one should not hesitate to replace the graft with a new one. Late graft closures present a slightly different problem, in that the dissection may be very difficult, particularly at anastomotic areas. Lytic therapy may be employed in selected cases but success is a function of the run-off as well as the time interval between thrombosis and initiation of lytic therapy (Dardik *et al.*, 1984). When surgery is required, manoeuvres similar to those described for early thrombectomy are performed but it is often necessary to abandon the procedure and proceed directly with replacement of the graft either in the same site or at a different level. Ultimate success for either thrombectomy or placement of a new graft in patients suffering late closures will of course depend upon the cause of graft closure. In most instances, the cause is progressive downstream obstruction, and construction of an adjunctive arteriovenous fistula should be considered. For remediable lesions, such as anastomotic stenosis or inflow lesions, an aggressive approach is indicated and appropriate.

Conclusions

The glutaraldehyde-stabilized umbilical vein graft has enabled surgeons to use an on-shelf material that can be reliably employed for reconstruction of the small vessels of the leg as well as of medium-size vessels. Because of this, operating time can be decreased, as can surgical dissection. Patients lacking suitable autologous saphenous veins, as well as those with limited life expectancy or requiring expeditious performance of the operation, can be considered as potential candidates for this graft. Precise surgical technique is required to avoid injury to this material which should only be used by surgeons truly expert in vascular methodology. It is not for the novice or 'occasional' vascular surgeon. The glutaraldehyde-stabilized umbilical vein graft can function well as a vascular conduit at all levels in the lower extremity, provided that the surgeon employs the highest level of judgement for managing the disease process on an individual patient basis.

References

Dardik, H. (1985). The use of an adjunctive arterioenous fistula in distal extremity bypass grafts with outflow obstruction. In *The Ischemic Leg*. Kempczinski, R. F., ed. Chicago, Illinois: Year Book Medical Publishers.

Dardik, H., Dardik, I., Sprayregen, S., *et al.* (1975). Patient selection and improved technical aspects in small-vessel bypass procedures of the lower extremity. *Surgery* **77**, 249.

Dardik, H., Ibrahim, I. M., Koslow, A., *et al.*, (1978). Evaluation of intraoperative arteriography as a routine for vascular reconstructions. *Surgery, Gynecology and Obstetrics* **147**, 853.

Dardik, H., Ibrahim, I. M. and Dardik, I. (1979). The role of the peroneal artery for limb salvage. *Annals of Surgery* **189**, 189.

Dardik, H., Smith, M., Ibrahim, I. M. and Dardik, I. (1980). Remote hydraulic syringe actuator: Its use to avoid radiation exposure during intraoperative arteriography. *Archives of Surgery* **115**, 105.

Dardik, H., Sussman, B., Ibrahim, I. M., Kahn, M., Svoboda, J., Mendes, D. and Dardik, I. (1983). Distal arteriovenous fistula as an adjunct to maintaining arterial and graft patency for limb salvage. *Surgery* **94**, 478.

Dardik, H., Sussman, B., Kahn, M., *et al.* (1984). Lysis of arterial clot by intravenous or intraarterial administration of streptokinase. *Surgery, Gynecology and Obstetrics* **158**, 137.

Dardik, H., Miller, N., Dardik, A., *et al.* (1988). A decade of experience with the glutaraldehyde-tanned human umbilical cord vein graft for revascularization of the lower limb. *Journal of Vascular Surgery* **7**, 336.

Hufnagel, C. (1979). Heparin bonding in grafts. In *Graft Materials in Vascular Surgery*. Dardik, H., ed. Miami, Florida: Symposia Specialists.

Adjuvant arteriovenous fistula at the distal anastomosis of a femorotibial bypass graft

P. L. Harris MD, FRCS

Consultant in Vascular Surgery, Broadgreen Hospital, Liverpool, UK;
Lecturer in Clinical Surgery, University of Liverpool, Liverpool, UK

Introduction

An arteriovenous fistula is constructed at the distal anastomosis of a long prosthetic femorotibial graft in order to increase the velocity of blood flow through the graft above the thrombotic threshold level.

Indications

(1) Patients with critical ischaemia whose only alternative is a major amputation.
(2) Prosthetic grafts inserted into a single tibial vessel.
(3) Poor run-off due to disease in the distal tibial or pedal vessels, determined by:

    (a) pedal angiography pre- or intraoperatively;
    (b) direct observation of vessels at operation;
    (c) objective assessment of peripheral resistance or impedance;
    (d) failure of the bypass graft despite adequate inflow and perfect operative technique.

Special requirements

(1) Some arterial run-off is essential; the procedure is of no value if the venous system alone is perfused.
(2) The deep venous system should be patent and free from post-phlebitic damage.
(3) The construction of a fistula using superficial veins is associated with a high incidence of impaired wound healing and skin necrosis due to localized venous hypertension and should be avoided.
(4) Unrestricted inflow to the graft is essential. Aorto-iliac stenosis must be identified by appropriate non-invasive tests or biplanar angiography and must be corrected before or concurrently with the femorodistal bypass procedure.
(5) Adjuvant arteriovenous fistula is not advisable for patients with severely impaired myocardial function.
(6) The use of loupe magnification (x 2.5) is recommended.
(7) Heparin anticoagulation is essential during surgery and oral antiplatelet therapy postoperatively.

The operation

Common ostium fistula

1

The selected tibial artery and its largest concomitant vein are approached as described in the chapter on 'Sites and approaches for tibial anastomoses'. A suitable length of these vessels is dissected and controlled with narrow latex slings. Clamps must not be applied to these vessels.

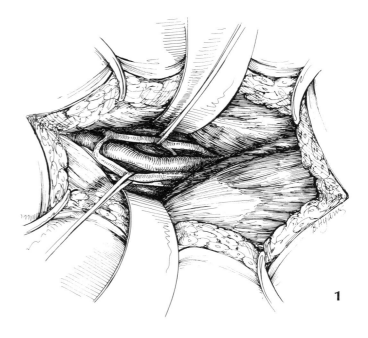

2

Longitudinal incisions approximately 15 mm in length are made in the artery and vein. Small catheters (not shown) are inserted into the artery distally and the vein proximally to control bleeding, permit perfusion of heparinized solutions, and to stent the anastomoses during construction. The adjacent walls of the vessels are sutured together using a double ended 7/0 polypropylene suture.

3

The distal end of the prosthetic graft is anastomosed to the 'common ostium' using 7/0 polypropylene sutures. Human umbilical vein is shown in the illustration as an example.

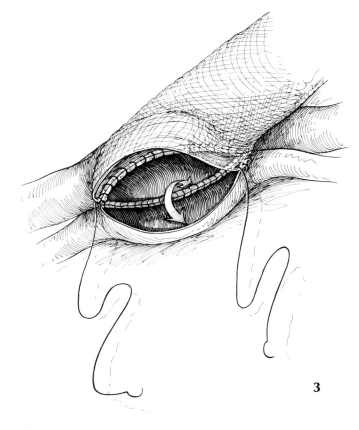

3

4

By reducing the length of the venotomy relative to that of the arteriotomy and constructing the fistula as shown, it is possible to simplify the graft to artery anastomosis at the toe and heel.

This slight modification of technique may help to reduce the risk of technical error at these critical points.

4

5

On completion the presence of a palpable thrill over the anastomosis indicates satisfactory functioning of the arteriovenous fistula. It is helpful to record bloodflow through the graft with an electromagnetic flow probe to assess the effect of the fistula. A mean flow greater than 200 ml per min is to be expected. Experimental studies indicate that less than 20% of the total flow through the graft passes distally into the artery, the remainder being shunted into the veins. There is no evidence that a fistula constructed at this site ever results in a 'steal' of blood from the distal arterial circulation in clinical practice.

5

6

Alternative method

Pre-anastomotic fistula

6

Construction of a side-to-side arteriovenous fistula at a point 0.5–1 cm upstream of the graft-to-artery anastomosis, as shown, has the following potential advantages:

(1) The intervening section of artery acts as a resistance which limits the volume of the shunt. The optimum size of shunt is one which results in a sufficient increase in blood flow through the graft to allow the thrombotic threshold to be exceeded with a small margin of safety. The 'common ostium' type of shunt sometimes results in flows considerably in excess of this with possible detrimental effects.
(2) The construction of the graft to artery anastomosis and the fistula separately is less complicated and therefore subject to fewer technical errors.
(3) The simpler form of construction may improve the flow characteristics at the graft-to-artery junction with less turbulence.

In practice the patency rates of grafts with common ostium and pre-anastomotic adjuvant fistula are similar.

References

Harris, P. L. and Campbell, H. (1983). Adjuvant distal arteriovenous shunt with femoro-tibial bypass for critical ischaemia. *British Journal of Surgery* 70(6), 377.

Dardik, H., Sussman, B. and Ibrahmin, M. *et al.* (1983). Distal arterio-venous fistula as an adjunct to maintaining arterial and graft patency for limb salvage. *Surgery* 94(3), 478.

Percutaneous transluminal angioplasty

James McIvor   MBChB, FRCR, FFR, FDSRCS
Consultant Radiologist, Charing Cross Hospital;
Senior Lecturer (Radiology), Institute of Dental Surgery, London, UK

Introduction

Percutaneous balloon dilatation of atheromatous lower limb arteries was first described by Grüntzig and Hopff (1974). A double-lumen catheter with an inflatable cylindrical polyvinyl balloon near its tip was passed through the stenotic segment and the balloon was inflated on several occasions before being withdrawn.

Ten years earlier Dotter and Judkins (1964) had described a technique for dilating stenotic arteries with a series of catheters of increasing diameter. Although there were some successes, the incidence of complications at the puncture site which required an arteriotomy, and at the site of the lesion, was high and the technique was not widely accepted.

The technical advantages of the Grüntzig balloon were twofold. First, the deflated balloon could be applied tightly to the shaft of a normal-sized arterial catheter (e.g. Fr 7, 8) and introduced percutaneously over a guide-wire without resorting to arteriotomy. Secondly, the inflated balloon applied a dilating force but no shearing force to the stenotic lesion.

Argon lasers have been used to treat occluded and severely stenotic femoral and popliteal arteries (Cumberland *et al.*, 1986; Ginsburg *et al.*, 1985). Extravasation of contrast medium indicated laser perforation in 4 out of 31 cases described in these two series, but there were no complications requiring surgery. The laser produces a channel measuring only 2–3 mm in diameter, so balloon angioplasty is usually necessary to dilate the lumen further.

1

There have been considerable improvements in the manufacture of balloon catheters since then, the most important being the replacement of polyvinyl by polyethylene as a balloon material because it is stronger and less likely to deform or rupture. Modern angioplasty catheters are radiopaque and also have metallic markers at both ends of the balloon which allow it to be accurately positioned within the stenotic segment at fluoroscopy before inflation. The diameters of currently available balloons vary from 3 to 12 mm and the lengths from 2 to 10 cm. The thickness of the catheter shaft varies from Fr 5 for small balloons to Fr 9 for the larger balloons.

1

2

Mechanism

Animal experiments and the examination of human arteries at post-mortem have increased our understanding of the mechanism of angioplasty in atheroma. Two processes appear to contribute to dilatation. First, the endothelial lining is damaged and fissures extend from the arterial lumen into the atheromatous plaque; and secondly, there is rupture or stretching of the media. During the following weeks and months the exposed atheromatous plaque epithelializes and contracts, further increasing the size of the arterial lumen.

2

Indications

In general, transluminal angioplasty should be confined to candidates for arterial surgery, and assessment of patients before angioplasty should be as careful as assessment before surgery.

The technique is of proved value in the treatment of atheromatous narrowing and occlusion of the iliac, femoral and popliteal arteries (Zeitler *et al.*, 1983; Cumberland, 1983) and in atheromatous narrowing· of the coronary arteries (Grüntzig, 1981; Cumberland, 1983). The immediate patency rates and the patency rates 2 and 5 years later are roughly similar to the patency rates after surgery, but no controlled trials have been carried out.

The technique is also valuable in treating renal artery stenosis, particularly if it is due to fibromuscular hyperplasia (Tegtmeyer *et al., 1984;* Martin *et al., 1986*) and it has been successfully used to dilate arterial narrowing in transplanted kidneys.

Successful dilatation of atheromatous lesions in other sites including the aorta (Kumpe, 1981) and its larger branches such as the axillary (Cumberland, 1983), subclavian (Beckman and Kim, 1980), coeliac (Saddekni *et al.*, 1980) and mesenteric (Novelline, 1980) arteries has been reported. Angioplasty has also been used to treat arterial narrowing due to therapeutic radiation, Takaysus' arteritis and surgery (Saddekni *et al.*, 1980).

There have been a few reports of successful dilatation of narrowing after venous anastomosis, such as splenorenal and mesocaval shunts (Cope, 1980; Novelline, 1980).

The success rate of second angioplasty procedures after complete or partial failure on the first attempt is roughly similar to the success rate of first attempts, but it is usual to leave an interval of 6 weeks between procedures to allow for epithelial regeneration.

Drug therapy

Although no control studies have been conducted it is customary to administer acetylsalicylic acid (aspirin) 300 mg for 1 day before angioplasty and to continue the treatment for 3–6 months afterwards.

It is also usual to administer 5000 u of heparin through the angioplasty catheter before inflating the balloon, with the aim of reducing the chances of thromboembolism. Although the therapeutic value of heparin is not proven in this respect, the risk of a single dose is extremely low and the potential benefit is high. The value of long-term heparin is more doubtful, unless there is evidence of distal embolization at the time of angioplasty, when it is usual to continue the drug for 7–10 days.

Access to vascular tree

3

The Seldinger technique may be used to obtain access to the femoral artery, femoral vein or axillary artery. The brachial artery and antecubital vein can be entered using a cut-down procedure. The details of the introduction of the catheter are given below.

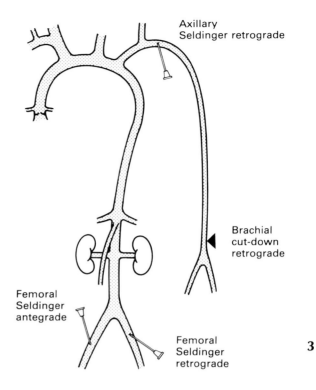

Axillary
Seldinger retrograde

Brachial
cut-down
retrograde

Femoral
Seldinger
antegrade

Femoral
Seldinger
retrograde

3

Procedure

4

After needle puncture (*a*), a standard guide-wire with a soft flexible tip is inserted (*b*). The tract is dilated through soft tissues and arterial wall (*c*) and the angioplasty catheter is passed over the guide-wire (*d*).

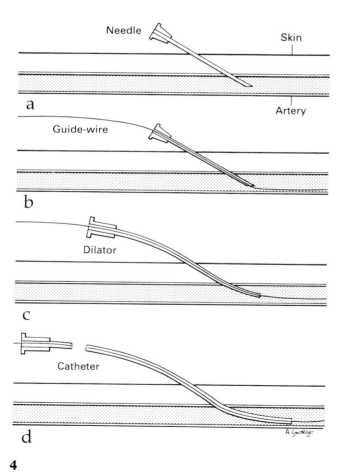

4

5

A standard guide-wire may be held up by plaque at the site of stenosis (a) as may a J-wire (b). In this case a J-wire with a moveable core, which allows the length of the flexible tip to be varied, can be used. In (c) the moveable core has been withdrawn and the guide-wire advanced to form a loop. Then the angioplasty catheter is passed over the wire and through the stenosis (d).

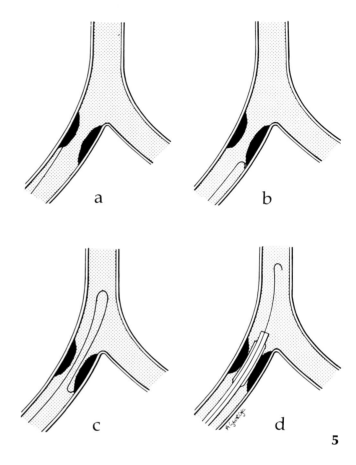

5

6

Selective catheterization using the wire exchange technique

Most angioplasty catheters have straight but flexible shafts and cannot be passed directly into branches of the aorta as can selective arterial catheters, which have preformed curves. In the wire exchange technique, the artery is first catheterized using an arterial catheter with a preformed curve, and a long (200 cm) exchange guide-wire is passed through the catheter and the stenosis. The arterial catheter is removed, leaving the guide-wire behind, and the angioplasty catheter is passed over the wire into the artery and through the stenosis.

6

313

7

Selective catheterization using a coaxial system

A large (Fr 8) catheter with a preformed bend near its tip is passed into the orifice of the artery which is to be dilated and a smaller (Fr 4) angioplasty catheter is passed through the large catheter and the stenotic segment. This technique is in general use for coronary artery angioplasty (as shown here) and is often used for renal artery angioplasty.

7

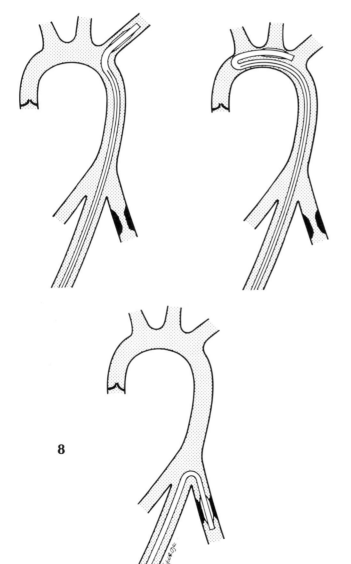

8

8

Selective catheterization using an angioplasty catheter with a preformed curve (e.g. Sidewinder or Shepherd's Crook)

Angioplasty catheters with preformed curves can sometimes be passed into the stenotic artery without resorting to the wire exchange technique or to a coaxial system.

In deciding which dilatation catheter to select, the most important single feature is the diameter of the inflated balloon. This should measure the same diameter as the 'normal' artery on the arteriogram films. The length of the balloon should, if possible, exceed the length of the stenosis by about 50%.

9

Angioplasty, like surgery, is most effective when used to treat a single, short stenotic segment. However, stenotic lesions that exceed the length of the angioplasty catheter can be treated by dilating one segment at a time, beginning with the end furthest from the puncture site so that neither the catheter nor the guide-wire is ever advanced through a recently dilated artery.

9

10

Multiple stenoses can be managed in the same way by dilating one segment at a time, beginning with the lesion furthest from the puncture site. The tip of the guide-wire or the catheter should *never* be advanced through a recently dilated stenotic segment, owing to the risk of dissection.

10

11

Complete occlusions of the iliac, femoral and popliteal arteries can often be recanalized by advancing a soft-tipped guide-wire through the occluded arterial lumen followed by a thin straight catheter, and finally by the angioplasty catheter. The recanalized segment is then dilated beginning at the end furthest from the puncture site. The chances of success depend to some extent on the length of the occlusion, and it has been suggested that recanalization should be limited to iliac occlusions of less than 6 cm and to femoropopliteal occlusions less than 10 cm.

11

12

12

Multiple balloons may be used to dilate stenotic segments in large arteries where the lumen is wider than the diameter of a single balloon (current maximum 12 mm). For instance, the aorta can be dilated with two catheters, which are passed upwards from the femoral arteries and inflated simultaneously, or even with three catheters, the third being passed down from the axillary artery.

13

Severe narrowing of both common iliac arteries is sometimes treated by simultaneous dilatation of both common iliac arteries using two angioplasty catheters.

13

14

14

Balloon inflation

The balloon should be inflated for several periods of 10–15 s with dilute ionic contrast medium containing 10–15 % iodine. Stronger concentrations of ionic media and even weak concentrations of non-ionic media should be avoided, as they are excessively viscous and cannot be completely aspirated from the angioplasty balloon at the end of the procedure.

For most balloons, the inflation pressure should be 3–4 atm (303–404 kPa) for the initial dilatations followed by 5–6 atm (505–606 kPa) if the balloon does not dilate fully on fluoroscopy. Some modern catheters can take pressures of 10–12 atm (1010–1212 kPa) without rupturing, but this pressure may increase the risk of serious arterial damage.

It is desirable to have a pressure gauge in the system, but if a gauge is not available the balloon should be inflated with a 10-ml syringe as pressures of 10 atm (101 kPa) are readily exceeded with smaller syringes.

Post-dilatation arteriogram

The arteriogram should if possible be repeated after dilatation to obtain a permanent record, and this can usually be carried out through the angioplasty catheter. If there is any possibility of further dilatation being attempted at the same session a guide-wire should be kept in position through the stenosis as the tip of a guide-wire or catheter should never be passed through a recently dilated artery owing to the risk of dissection.

The appearance of the post-dilatation arteriogram is often disappointing as the lumen of the recently dilated artery is often irregular and is slightly narrowed. However, a 30% narrowing is an acceptable result (except in the coronary arteries) as the lumen of the artery will almost certainly become wider and smoother during the following 6 weeks.

Complications

The most serious complication is sudden occlusion at the site of angioplasty; an incidence of 1–5% has been reported. Perforation is a much rarer complication which occasionally accompanies occlusion. The clinical significance of these technical disasters depends, of course, on the artery that has been damaged. Sudden occlusion of a coronary artery is a surgical emergency, and the possibility of this complication should restrict coronary angioplasty to centres with facilities for immediate cardiac bypass surgery. Even with these facilities coronary artery angioplasty has a mortality currently estimated at 1%. Occlusion of the renal, mesenteric or coeliac arteries usually requires immediate surgery, and occlusion of an upper or lower limb artery may require early surgery, but there has been no mortality reported with these complications.

Complications at the angioplasty site can be kept to a minimum by *never* passing the tip of the guide-wire or catheter through a recently dilated artery, as this is likely to cause dissection, and by accepting a less than perfect cosmetic result on the post-dilatation arteriogram.

Haematomas are not uncommon at the puncture site, particularly in hypertensive patients, and although arterial occlusion at the puncture site has been reported (Zeitler, 1978), the incidence is extremely low. Pain is common after angioplasty of the lower limb arteries and may follow renal artery angioplasty. Late aneurysm formation has been reported and may be a sequel to the use of balloon pressure higher than 10 atm (101 kPa).

Complications at the puncture site can be kept to a minimum by puncturing the femoral or axillary arteries as distally as possible, by using thin catheters, by applying prolonged digital pressure (for up to 30 min) over the puncture site after removing the catheter, and by immobilizing the limb for 12 h after the procedure.

References

Backman, D. M. and Kim, R. M. (1980). Transluminal dilatation for subclavian steal syndrome. *American Journal of Roentgenology* **135**, 995.
Cope, C. (1980). Balloon dilatation of closed mesocaval shunts. *American Journal of Roentgenology* **135**, 989.
Cumberland, D. C. (1983). Percutaneous transluminal angioplasty: A review. *Clinical Radiology* **34**, 25.
Cumberland, D. C., Tayler, D. I. and Procter, A. E. (1986). Laser-assisted percutaneous angioplasty: Initial clinical experience in peripheral arteries. *Clinical Radiology* **37**, 423.
Dotter, C. T. and Judkins, M. P. (1964). Transluminal treatment of arteriosclerotic obstruction. Description of a new technique and a preliminary report of its application. *Circulation* **30**, 654.
Ginsburg, M. D., Wexler, L., Mitchell, R. S. and Profitt, D. (1985). Percutaneous transluminal laser angioplasty for treatment of peripheral vascular disease. *Radiology* **156**, 619.
Grüntzig, A. R. (1981). Percutaneous transluminal coronary angioplasty. *Seminars in Roentgenology* **16**, 152.
Grüntzig, A. and Hopff, H. (1974). Percutaneous canalisation chronischer arterieller verschlusse mit einem neuen dilationskatheter. Modifikation der Dotter Technik. *Deutsche Medizinische Wochenschrift* **99**, 2502.
Kumpe, D. A. (1981). Percutaneous dilatation of an abdominal aortic stenosis: Three balloon technique. *Radiology* **141**, 536.
Martin, L. G., Casarella, W. J., Alspaugh, J. P. and Chuang, V. P. (1986). Renal artery angioplasty: Increased technical success has decreased complications in the second 100 patients. *Radiology* **159**, 631.
Novelline, R. A. (1980). Percutaneous transluminal angioplasty: newer applications. *American Journal of Roentgenology* **135**, 983.
Saddekni, S., Sniderman, K. W., Hilton, S. and Sos., T. A. (1980). Percutaneous transluminal angioplasty of non-atherosclerotic lesions. *American Journal of Roentgenology* **135**, 975.
Tegtmeyer, C. J., Kellum, C. D. and Ayers,C. (1984). Percutaneous transluminal angioplasty of the renal artery. Results and long-term follow-up. *Radiology* **153**, 77.
Zeitler, E. (1978). Complications in and after PTA. In *Percutaneous Vascular Recanalisation*. Zeitler, E., Grünzig, A., Schoop, W., eds. New York: Springer Publishing Co. Inc. pp. 120–125.
Zeitler, E., Richter, E. I., Roth, F. J., and Schoop, W. (1983). Results of percutaneous transluminal angioplasty. *Radiology* **146**, 57.

Peroperative transluminal angioplasty

Thomas J. Fogarty MD, FACS
Chief, Cardiovascular Section, Sequoia Hospital, Redwood City, California, USA

Albert K. Chin MD
Cardiovascular Research Staff, Sequoia Hospital, Redwood City, California, USA

James C. Finn MD
Stanford University Medical Center, Stanford, California, USA

Introduction

The concept of balloon catheter treatment of atherosclerotic narrowing was conceived by Dotter and Judkins in 1964, and rendered practical by Gruntzig, Senning and Siegenthaler in 1974. The use of balloon dilatation as an adjunct to surgical reconstruction has been described in various reports. Transluminal angioplasty has been applied as a percutaneous procedure, preceding a staged formal reconstruction (Porter *et al.*, 1973); or as an intraoperative procedure (Motarjeme, Keifer and Zuska, 1981; Pfeiffer and String, 1986). In these adjunctive procedures, a standard angioplasty catheter was passed in a coaxial fashion over a spring guidewire. In 1981, Fogarty *et al.* devised a linear extrusion dilatation catheter that did not require prior guidewire placement nor extensive radiographic control. This instrument simplified the procedure of intraoperative balloon angioplasty. Its mechanism of action decreased the shear force exerted on the endothelium and reduced the possiblity of arterial dissection during balloon placement (Kinney *et al.*, 1985).

1a & b

Intraoperative balloon angioplasty is applied as an adjunct to vascular reconstructive procedures, or as a primary operative procedure. Adjunctive balloon angioplasty is performed for two indications: (1) to reduce the magnitude of a surgical procedure, and (2) to enhance the flow through a standard graft. Thus, iliac artery dilatation may allow the placement of an otherwise contraindicated femorofemoral graft in a patient too debilitated to undergo aortofemoral reconstruction. A patient scheduled to receive a femoropopliteal graft may undergo adjunctive dilatation of an ipsilateral iliac lesion, improving the inflow to that graft while averting a lengthy abdominal procedure. Primary intraoperative balloon angioplasty is performed in situations in which percutaneous transluminal angioplasty may be difficult or contraindicated. Intraoperative dilatation of carotid fibromuscular lesions is an example of this. The ability to backflush the artery after dilatation is important in this situation.

Transluminal angioplasty is contraindicated in ulcerated or thrombosed lesions, and lesions located at critical bifurcations. The potential for embolism is great during balloon angioplasty of the first group, and dilatation of a lesion in a bifurcation may lead to occlusion of the uninvolved branch. Severe stenoses greater than 10 cm in length represent a relative contraindication, since these lesions have low dilatation success rates.

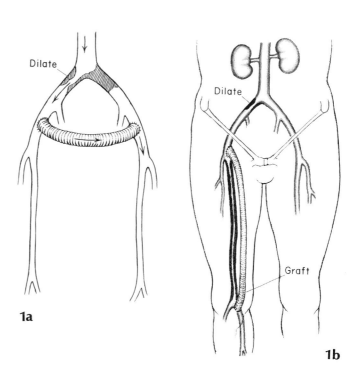

2

Coaxial dilators, coaxial balloon catheters and linear extrusion catheters represent the three types of dilatation instruments available for use. Coaxial dilators and coaxial balloon catheters require placement of guidewire prior to advancement of the catheter through the stenotic region. In severe stenoses, the shear force between the catheter and the plaque surface may be great, increasing the chance for plaque dislodgement, distal embolization and arterial dissection. The linear extrusion catheter does not require prior guidewire placement. The soft balloon portion insinuates itself through the lesion without the need for extensive fluoroscopic guidance, facilitating its use in the operative suite.

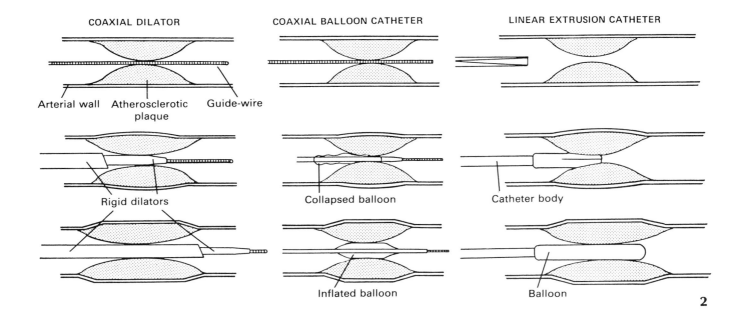

COAXIAL DILATOR   COAXIAL BALLOON CATHETER   LINEAR EXTRUSION CATHETER

Arterial wall   Atherosclerotic plaque   Guide-wire

Rigid dilators   Collapsed balloon   Catheter body

Inflated balloon   Balloon

2

3

The principle of linear extrusion involves unrolling of an inverted balloon through the residual arterial lumen. The balloon seeks out the path of least resistance, dilating the proximal plaque front sufficiently to allow the remainder of the balloon to proceed through the stenosis. There is little chance for this system to cause arterial perforation. No sliding occurs between the balloon and the arterial wall; instead, the force exerted by the balloon remains perpendicular to the contours of the plaque, resulting in effective dilatation.

3

Procedures

4

The following illustrations are based on the example of increasing inflow to a femoropopliteal bypass graft. A moderate stenosis in the upper external iliac artery, too high to patch over without making a separate incision and entering the abdominal cavity, will be dilated through the arteriotomy at the proximal anastomotic site. Both graft flow and graft survival can be enhanced. Numerous long-term clinical studies have shown that the durability of such dilatations approaches that of full reconstructions (Malone, Moore and Goldstone, 1975; Brewster and Darling, 1978; Spence *et al.*, 1981; Van Andle, 1980; Gallino *et al.*, 1984).

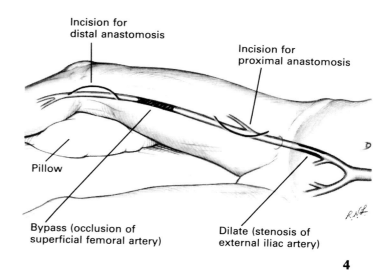

Incision for distal anastomosis

Incision for proximal anastomosis

Pillow

Bypass (occlusion of superficial femoral artery)

Dilate (stenosis of external iliac artery)

4

5

Occluder pads are applied to the exposed superficial femoral artery and profunda femoris. Along with occluding the lumen, they allow traction on the arteries via their silicone tapes. They are applied by passing one end of the tape under the artery and latching it to the pad, which is held by a clamp. A Velcro covering assists placement by reducing slippage on the artery. A Fogarty Hydragrip clamp is placed across the common femoral artery.

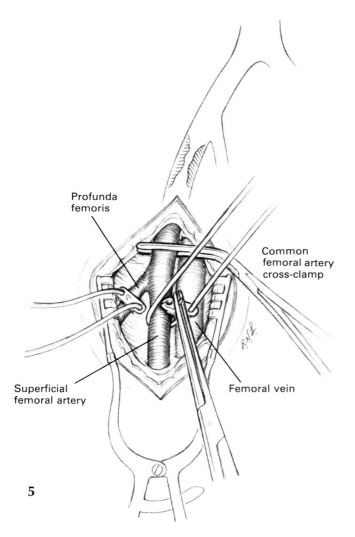

Profunda femoris

Common femoral artery cross-clamp

Superficial femoral artery

Femoral vein

5

6

Calibration of the distance to the lesion from the arteriotomy and of the diameter of the uninvolved artery adjacent to the plaque is the first step in intraoperative angioplasty. This is performed with a latex balloon catheter, which is inserted through the arteriotomy in a partially inflated state. Sterile saline is used to purge the catheter of air and to inflate the balloon. The calibrator is advanced to the level of stenosis at which point resistance to further advancement is encountered. The lesion should never be forcibly or repeatedly probed. The distance to the arteriotomy is read off the depth markings on the calibrator body.

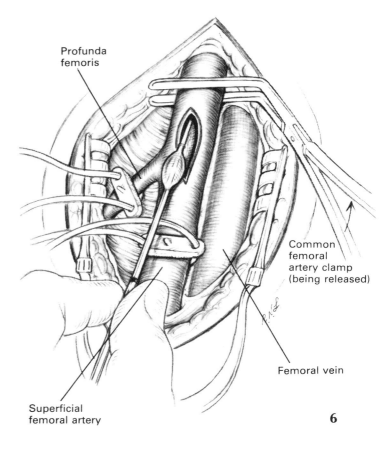

Profunda femoris

Common femoral artery clamp (being released)

Femoral vein

Superficial femoral artery

6

7

The diameter of the adjacent uninvolved artery is next assessed by slowly inflating the calibrator balloon while gently moving the catheter back and forth. Resistance to movement confirms that the balloon has engaged the arterial wall. The size of the balloon now represents the intraluminal diameter. The total volume of fluid injected is noted and the balloon deflated and removed. Care should be taken not to over-inflate the calibrator balloon during this procedure as damage to the arterial wall and overestimation of luminal diameter may result.

Balloon calibrator

7

8

The latex balloon is now reinflated outside the artery with the volume previously noted. A balloon calibrator scale is used to measure its inflated diameter. This estimate of uninvolved segment diameter is noted and the linear extrusion catheter with a maximum balloon diameter closest to this size is chosen.

2 mm diameter

12 mm diameter

8

9

The Fogarty-Chin Peripheral Dilatation Catheter has three ports: inflation, vent and infusion. Air is purged by injecting saline or dilute contrast media through the inflation port until liquid issues from the vent port, at which time it is closed.

The infusion line should also be purged by injection. The adjustable sliding silicone marker is set to a distance from the body tip 1 cm less than the length measured during calibration (i.e. the arteriotomy-lesion distance).

Depth markers

Distal infusion point

Adjustable marker

Radiopaque tip

Vent port (closed)

Infusion port

Inflation port (open)

9

10a & b

The catheter is advanced through the arteriotomy until the silicone marker reaches the incision. This should place the body tip 1 cm short of the leading face of the lesion. Note that the catheter tip should never be placed into or through the lesion. This is unnecessary and may damage the intima or create potential emboli. Although blood will return with release of the clamp, it will cease when the balloon is extruded.

10a

Inverted balloon

10 b

11

The smallest syringe that will accommodate the average recommended injection volume should be used to inflate the balloon. Sterile saline or dilute contrast media is used to extrude the balloon through the inflation port. Note that if any portion of the artery that is dilated is visible during extrusion, it will be seen to blanch and enlarge, providing a monitor of extrusion progress. During initial balloon contact with the leading edge of the stenosis, the catheter body may tend to back out of the arteriotomy site. In this event, the body can be braced either by gently holding the silicone marker with forceps or by clamping the side of the marker with a right-angle clamp. In either case, care must be taken not to clamp or restrict any part of the catheter body itself.

11

12

The progress of extrusion through the stenosis can be monitored using a pressure gauge. It will be found that high pressures, even exceeding the maximum recommended inflation pressure, may be experienced prior to balloon eversion. This initial rise will not damage the balloon and should not alarm the surgeon. A mechanical assist inflation device or small-bore syringe may be used to help overcome these pressures. The pressure then drops upon extrusion until the balloon contacts the stenosis, at which time it will rise again. As the balloon negotiates the lesions. the inflation pressure will vary depending on the severity of that section of the lesion in which the balloon tip is currently located. At the end of extrusion, the pressure will uniformly rise and remain high until deflation. It should be noted that in the presence of a severe stenosis or marked angulation, the balloon is found to pass more easily (i.e. the peak inflation pressure is reduced) if the extrusion balloon is alternately inflated and then deflated.

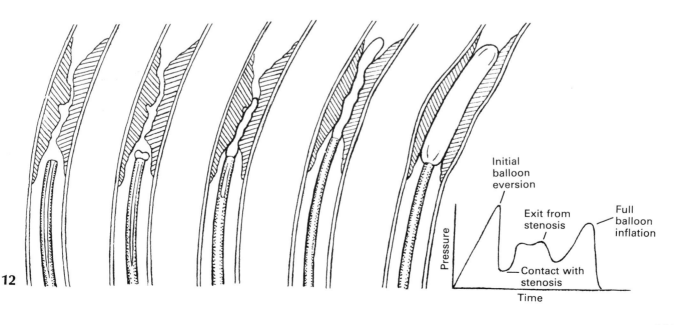

12

13

The angioplasty balloon may be left inflated to occlude the lumen as the distal anastomosis and most of the proximal anastomosis are performed. Prior to completing this anastomosis, the balloon is deflated by aspiration and removed. Generous flushing with blood is allowed to wash out air and any atherosclerotic debris that may have been loosened from the luminal wall during dilatation. Recalibration using a balloon catheter is not performed, due to the risk of intimal flap formation during repeat instrumentation of the dilated segment. Assessment of dilatation success is performed via the completion angiogram.

Complications

Complications that may occur with the use of the linear extrusion catheter include arterial injury, thrombosis and embolism. Balloon sizing is important, and the use of an inappropriately large balloon may cause vessel rupture. The linear extrusion balloon proceeds down the straightest pathway. At a bifurcation, selective cannulation is required for dilatation of a branch that angles away from the main trunk. Otherwise, inadvertent dilatation of the other branch may result. Thrombosis may occur if a column of blood stagnates in the dilated segment following balloon removal. In adjunctive iliac angioplasty, we recommend inflow occulsion with the dilatation balloon versus a clamp, during completion of the anastomosis. Arterial flow is established immediately following dilatation catheter removal. Distal embolization, a potential complication with the use of any intravascular catheter, is reduced by the unrolling mechanism of the linear extrusion catheter.

13

Conclusion

Transluminal angioplasty is a technique that may contribute significantly to the effectiveness of standard vascular reconstructive procedures. Balloon dilatation may be performed with little operative time and effort on the part of the surgeon. Its safety of application is increased when performed under controlled situations in the operating room. It is important that surgeons add new catheter technolgies to their therapeutic armamentarium, as these advancements will surely grow in the next few years.

References

Brewster, D. C. and Darling, R. C. (1978). Optimal methods of aortoiliac reconstruction. *Surgery* **84**, 739.

Dotter, C. T. and Judkins, M. P. (1964). Transluminal treatment of arteriosclerotic obstruction: description of a new technique and a preliminary report of its application. *Circulation* **30**, 654.

Fogarty, T. J., Chin, A., Shoor, P. M., Blair, G. L. and Zimmerman, J. J. (1981). Adjunctive intraoperative arterial dilatation: simplified instrumentation technique. *Archives of Surgery* **116**, 1391

Gallino, A., Mahler, F., Probst, P., *et al.* (1984). Percutaneous transluminal angioplasty of the arteries of the lower limbs: a 5 year follow-up. *Circulation* **70**, 619

Gruntzig, A., Senning, A. and Siegenthaler, W. E. (1979). Nonoperative dilation of coronary artery stenosis: percutaneous transluminal coronary angioplasty. *New England Journal of Medicine* **301**, 61.

Kinney, T. B., Fan, M., Chin, A. K., Finn, J. C., Hayden, W. G. and Fogarty, T. J. (1985). Shear force in angioplasty: its relation to catheter design and function. *American Journal of Radiology* **144**, 115.

Malone, J. M., Moore, W. S. and Goldstone, J. (1975). The natural history of bilateral aortofemoral bypass grafts for ischemia of the lower extremities. *Archives of Surgery* **100**, 1300.

Motarjeme, A., Keifer, J. W. and Zuska, A. (1981). Percutaneous transluminal angioplasty as a complement to surgery. *Radiology* **141**, 341.

Pfeiffer, R. B. and String, S. T. (1986). Adjunctive use of the balloon dilatation catheter during vascular reconstructive procedures. *Journal of Vascular Surgery* **3**, 841.

Porter, J. M., Eidemiller, L. R., Dotter, C. T., Rosch, J. and Vetto, R. M. (1973). Combined arterial dilatation and femorofemoral bypass for limb salvage. *Surgery, Gynecology and Obstetrics* **137**, 409.

Spence, R., Freiman, D. B., Gatenby, R., *et al.* (1981). Long term results of transluminal angioplasty of the iliac and femoral arteries. *Archives of Surgery* **116**, 1377.

Van Andle, G. J. (1980). Transluminal iliac angioplasty: long term results. *Radiology* **135**, 607.

Atherectomy

Thomas J. Fogarty MD, FACS
Chief, Cardiovascular Section, Sequoia Hospital, Redwood City, California, USA

Albert K. Chin MD
Cardiovascular Research Staff, Sequoia Hospital, Redwood City, California, USA

Introduction

The concept of transluminal atherectomy represents an advancement in the technique of endovascular therapy. Atherectomy involves plaque removal versus plaque displacement, and it addresses the problem of restenosis that occurs following balloon dilatation. Fibroelastic lesions that do not achieve permanent dilatation upon balloon angioplasty may be successfully treated with transluminal atherectomy. The intimal flap formation and medial dissection that typically occur during angioplasty (Block et al., 1981; Chin et al., 1984) are avoided with atherectomy. The resultant smooth-walled lumen will hopefully decrease the restenosis rate following this procedure.

1

The atherectomy device, devised by Simpson, has undergone clinical use since 1985 (Simpson *et al.*, 1988: Schwarten *et al.*, 1988). This catheter contains a guidewire tipped cylinder with a section cut out of one side and a nonelastomer balloon attached to the other side. The open side of the cylinder is moved adjacent to the plaque and the balloon inflated to push the cylinder against the atheroma. A tubular cutter, cable-driven to 2000 revolutions per min, is advanced forward within the cylinder to slice a segment of plaque and impact it in the distal portion of the cylinder.

① Guidewire Tip	⑦ Motor Driven Cable
② Cylindrical Housing	⑧ Cutter Advance Lever
③ Cutaway	⑨ Handpiece and motor
④ Tubular Cutter	⑩ Flush port
⑤ Nonelastomeric Balloon	⑪ Balloon Inflation Port
⑥ Distal Housing Chamber	⑫ Motor Switch

1

2

2

Unlike balloon angioplasty, which enlarges the lumen by distending the vessel in a fusiform fashion, atherectomy recanalizes the artery through direct removal of the offending atheroma. The atherectomy catheter is employed in discrete lesions less than 10 cm in length. Removal of extended lengths of disease may become tedious, as multiple catheter withdrawals are required to remove plaque sections impacted in the cylindrical housing. Atherectomy may be used as an adjunct to standard vascular reconstructive procedures, treating inflow or outflow lesions about a newly placed graft. It may also be performed as a primary operative procedure in situations requiring increased arterial control, such as obese patients, in which percutaneous placement of the device may be hazardous.

Procedure

3

For superficial femoral artery atherectomy, a groin incision is used to isolate the common femoral, superficial femoral and profunda femoris arteries. Following systemic anticoagulation with 5000 u of heparin, a Fogarty Hydragrip clamp is applied to the common femoral artery. The profunda femoris artery is occluded using an occluder pad, and a Fogarty Hydragrip clamp with double Hydrajaw inserts is applied to the superficial femoral artery. An arteriotomy is made in the superficial femoral artery and an #11 French sheath containing a haemostatic valve is carefully placed down the vessel upon release of the soft-jawed clamp. An arteriogram is performed through the sheath, using image intensification fluoroscopy, and a needle is used to mark the site of stenosis.

3

4

4

Under fluoroscopic guidance, a #11 French atherectomy catheter is passed through the haemostatic sheath, with the opening of the cylinder oriented towards the raised lesion and the tubular cutter fully advanced. The balloon opposite the opening is inflated to 10 p.s.i. and the tubular cutter retracted proximally.

5

The balloon pressure is increased to 30 p.s.i. and the motor unit is activated by pressing the button switch on the handle. While maintaining rotation of the motor unit, the tubular cutter is advanced forward using the slide on the handle. A selection of plaque is shaved off and impacted in the distal housing.

5

6

Following a single pass of the tubular cutter, the balloon is deflated. This is accomplished by drawing a vacuum on the syringe connected to the balloon inflation port.

6

7

The atherectomy catheter is rotated under fluoroscopic guidance to align the opening in the cylinder with remaining areas of plaque. After the desired position is achieved, atherectomy is repeated using the previous steps:

1. balloon inflation to 10 p.s.i.;

2. proximal retraction of the tubular cutter;
3. balloon pressure increase to 30 p.s.i.;
4. activation of the motor drive;
5. distal advancement of the tubular cutter; and
6. balloon deflation.

7

8

Atherectomy should be continued until a satisfactory fluoroscopic image of the stenosis site is obtained, or until repeated advancement of the tubular cutter produces no additional plaque shavings. Aggressive removal of the lesion is necessary to reduce the incidence of restenosis. Patients with a residual stenosis <30% had an 18% recurrence rate compared with a 52% recurrence rate for residual stenoses >30% (Simpson et al., 1988). When it becomes difficult to advance the tubular cutter, due to the filling of the distal housing with plaque shavings, the atherectomy catheter is removed from the vessel. The number of cutter passes required to fill the distal housing ranges from 4 to 8. While removing the catheter, the tubular cutter should be held in the advanced position to insure that no plaque shavings escape from the distal chamber. Using a small pair of forceps, the distal chamber is emptied of plaque shavings.

8

Conclusion

Atherectomy is an endovascular procedure that is simple to perform and adds little to the operative time. Its indications for use mirror those of balloon angioplasty. However, atherectomy, which employs a plaque removal process, attempts to improve the functional result of revascularization by leaving a smooth luminal surface. It is hoped that this second-generation catheter device will result in increased patency of treated vessels.

References

Block, P. C., Myler, R. K., Stertzer, S., *et al.* (1981). Morphology after transluminal angioplasty in human beings. *New England Journal of Medicine* **307,** 382.

Chin, A. K., Kinney, T. B., Rurik, G. W., Shoor, P. M. and Fogarty, T. J. (1984). A physical measurement of the mechanisms of transluminal angioplasty. *Surgery* **95**(2), 196.

Schwarten, D. E., Katzen, B. T., Simpson, J. B. and Cutcliff, W. B. Simpson catheter for percutaneous transluminal removal of atheroma. *American Journal of Radiology* **150**, 799.

Simpson, J. B., Selmon, M. R., Robertson, G. C. *et al.* (1988). Transluminal atherectomy for occlusive peripheral vascular disease. *American Journal of Cardiology* **61**, 96G.

Above-knee amputation

Hero van Urk MD

Chief, Vascular Surgery, University Hospital, Erasmus University, Rotterdam, The Netherlands

Introduction

Although the ratio of above-knee amputations to below-knee amputations has changed over the last decades in favour of the latter, the actual number of above-knee amputations has not decreased dramatically.

Whenever possible, an above-knee amputation should be avoided if it is possible to perform either a below-knee or through-knee amputation. The functional results of rehabilitation of patients with a below-knee prosthesis is infinitely better than those with an above-knee prosthesis.

In almost all cases where this operation is indicated, the superficial femoral artery is occluded, leaving the profunda femoral artery (or its remaining branches) as the only remaining blood supply for the thigh muscles. Usually, this arterial supply is further compromised, resulting in insufficient oxygenation of the distal part of the muscles. Hence the principle of preserving as much leg length as possible no longer applies once the decision to perform an above-knee amputation has been taken.

1

Conventional knee mechanisms extend 8–10 cm into the thigh portion of the prosthesis. Therefore, if a thigh amputation is performed too far distally, this may cause problems with prosthetic fitting and unequal knee height. This difficulty has caused some reluctance on the part of surgeons to perform through-knee amputations, but the most recent prosthetic techniques have overcome this. Nevertheless, a too distal diaphyseal amputation may result in an excessively long stump, which is of no benefit to the patient; such a stump end has poor weight-bearing abilities, in contrast to the mid-diaphyseal or through-knee amputation.

On the other hand, an amputation which leaves the limb too short, is equally to be avoided. About 10 cm below the minor trochanter is the upper limit of an amputation. A shorter stump will lead to a flexion–abduction contracture, which poses a problem both cosmetically and functionally. Disarticulation in the hip is preferred in such cases, usually after a high above-knee amputation has failed to heal properly.

1

The operation

2

The patient is placed in the supine position. Usually, general anaesthesia is preferred, but epidural anaesthesia or a regional block can be given to elderly patients with a critical medical condition.

If gangrene of the foot or lower leg is present, the foot can be packed in a plastic bag. In cases of wet gangrene, the author prefers to administer antibiotics intravenously the evening before the operation. If there is dry necrosis or rest pain only, antibiotics are started just after induction of anaesthesia and continued for 24 h postoperatively.

After suitable skin preparation and draping, the intended skin incision is marked with a sterile marker pen, having the dorsal flap slightly shorter than the anterior flap. The apex of the angle between the anterior and posterior flaps is approximately at the level of transection of the shaft of the femur. On both sides this point is in the mid-medial and mid-lateral line of the thigh or slightly more to the dorsal side.

2

3

3

An incision is made through the subcutaneous tissue and the fascia femoris. If still intact, the greater saphenous vein is transected and ligated. In cases where an *in situ* saphenous vein bypass has previously been performed, this conduit is likely to be thrombosed, but, if not, special care should be taken to avoid blood loss from this source.

After completion of the skin and fascia incisions, the skin usually retracts somewhat on both sides. The muscle incision should be in the same line as the skin incision, because of the tendency of muscles to retract even more than skin.

The anterior and lateral muscles are divided first. When the medial muscles are incised, care should be taken to locate the superficial femoral vessels first. After separate ligation of artery and vein, the deep femoral artery and the sciatic nerve are exposed. In order to minimize neuroma formation, the sciatic nerve is identified anteriorly to the hamstring muscles and is pulled down and divided after ligation of the arteria concomitans. The author prefers not to ligate the sciatic nerve itself, because this is thought to cause more neuroma formation and/or phantom pain.

There seems to be no guaranteed method of avoiding neuroma formation, but the nerve should always be allowed to retract well upwards between the surrounding muscles. It may be of some value for pain relief in the immediate postoperative period to inject the nerve with a local anaesthetic like Marcaine® (bupivacaine).

4

When all muscles have been divided and all bleeding points are clamped and ligated proximally, the periosteum of the femur is incised circumferentially. The periosteum is then pushed upward 3–4 cm. The femoral shaft is divided with a saw, the level of the bony amputation being 4–5 cm more proximal than the musculocutaneous flap.

After the muscle flaps have been bevelled, accurate haemostasis is obtained. In diabetic patients with calcified small vessels, all bleeding points need to be ligated, preferably with absorbable material, because electro-cautery may not be sufficient in such cases.

4

5

The wound is then closed by approximating – with minimal tension – the anterior fascia to the posterior fascia, using interrupted sutures. One or two suction drains are left deep in the wound. No subcutaneous sutures are necessary and the skin is closed in one layer, preferably with interrupted monofilament nylon sutures.

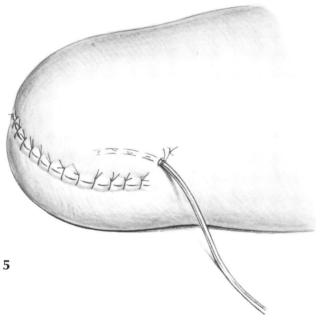

5

Postoperative care

6

Sterile dressings are applied, followed by synthetic orthopaedic padding and, finally, a cotton stretch bandage. This dressing can be left in place for several days unless the patient complains of increasing pain, which may be caused by swelling of the stump.

In some clinics, elevation of the stump on a pillow for the first 24–48 h is advised. The author prefers to keep the stump flat on the bed to prevent a flexion contracture. Exercises can be started after the first few postoperative days. Lying in a prone position for several short periods during the day may be helpful in the prevention of a flexion contracture.

Cotton elastic bandages are applied and regularly changed in order to aid shrinkage of the stump. In contrast with below-knee amputations, no temporary plaster cast is used; instead, a prosthesis is fitted directly when the stump is free of oedema after application of the elastic dressings. Unfortunately, only a small proportion of vascular patients are able to follow a complete rehabilitation programme, and the number of elderly patients who are eventually able to walk again is disappointing.

6

Through-knee amputation

Kingsley Robinson   MS, FRCS
Consultant Surgeon, Westminster Hospital, London, UK

Introduction

The through-knee amputation is the quickest major lower-limb amputation that can be performed as no bony structure needs to be divided and ligation of the single large popliteal artery and its accompanying veins controls nearly all the bleeding that can be encountered. Only the long saphenous vein usually requires an additional ligature. The large size of the femoral condyles means that ample skin must be provided for adequate and lax skin cover, otherwise skin necrosis can be produced by tension across the edges of the articular surface. It is also important that the patella retains its normal position on the front of the knee rather than being drawn down where it may be subjected to weight-bearing stresses and produce extreme discomfort. The procedure is so atraumatic and speedy that it can be carried out as a debriding procedure prior to a definitive higher amputation. The absence of noise, because no saw is required, is a great asset when operating on patients under regional anaesthesia.

1

Lateral and medial sagittal flaps centred on the tibial tubercle anteriorly and the fold at the flexion line in the popliteal fossa constitute the most satisfactory skin flaps. The classical skin flap is a long anterior flap with a transverse scar across the popliteal fossa, and if this incision is used the patient is best placed prone with the distal part of the leg flexed to provide access to the anterior structures. This is an unsatisfactory position for the severely ill patient with vascular disease and a supine position with the hip flexed is entirely satisfactory if sagittal flaps are utilized. The skin incision is cut at one with the subcutaneous fat but the fascia lata and aponeurotic fibres of the lower leg muscles need not be incised.

1

2

2

The skin flaps are elevated by brushing upwards with a wet swab and the patella tendon is defined and its insertion into the tibial tubercle. At this stage the long saphenous vein will be ligated with fine catgut or vicryl, care being taken to avoid inclusion of the saphenous nerve.

3

Retraction on the medial and lateral flap will be necessary to obtain exposure of the tibial plateau. The patella tendon is then divided, erasing it from the patella tubercle to obtain a maximum length and held in a tissue forcep. The patella tendon can be elevated to provide additional retraction and exposure of the fat pad that is anterior to the synovial membrane covering the cruciate ligaments. The joint capsule is incised transversely to each side of the patella tendon exposing the condyles of the femur and if correctly placed the genicular cartilages should be left attached to the tibial plateau. Further flexion of the knee allows clear exposure of the cruciate ligaments. The hamstring tendons and the medial ligament of the knee joint can then be divided as can the lateral ligaments and biceps femoris tendon, allowing further flexion when the cruciate ligaments themselves can be divided leaving as much length as possible attached to the femur.

4

The posterior part of the knee joint capsule can then be incised. Access to the popliteal artery and its veni comitans can either be obtained through the back of the knee joint capsule with some traction on the tibia or, alternatively, a finger can be hooked around the medial head of the gastrocnemius which can then be erased from the point of origin above the femoral condyle when the popliteal artery has been ligated and divided. The two elements of the sciatic nerve can also be transected under tension with the proximal end allowed to retract as far as possible. The lateral head of the gastrocnemius can also be divided.

3

4

5 & 6

When all these structures are completely divided the specimen is freed. The hamstring tendons and biceps tendons are marked with artery forceps and preserved and haemostasis secured. Myoplasty is effected by anchoring the biceps femoris tendon and the semimembranosis gracivis and semi-tendonosis tendons being attached to the residue of the cruciate ligaments. These sutures have to hold the tendons against considerable tension when the muscles are active and must be at least 1 chromicatgut or 0 vicryl. At this stage the patellar tendon is also sutured into the intercondylar notch securely attached to the residue of the cruciate ligaments, and care must be taken not to pull the patellar tendon down too far and to allow it to remain in its anatomical position in relation to the anterior surface of the femoral condyles. At this stage there should be an appreciable excess of skin in the flaps and the skin can usually be closed in a single layer. In case of continuing synovial fluid production a Redivac drain is best placed across the condyles and, leaving the stump well above the condylar area, the skin is closed as a single layer of subcutaneous fat using vertical interrupted mattress sutures.

5

6

7

7

When the suture line is complete it will be found that the scar lies entirely within and above the femoral intercondylar notch and the skin area related to the inferior surface of the femoral condyles is free of any sutures or scar tissue. This allows the stump to be used for terminal weight-bearing, a great advantage in prosthetic design as ischial weight-bearing can be avoided. Many patients with bilateral through-knee amputations learn to crawl on the stump ends and may be mobile without any prosthesis at all. If the patient finds this mode of progression satisfactory, provision of knee bootees can be of some value.

Posterior flap below-knee amputation

Charles N. McCollum MD, FRCS

Reader in Surgery, Charing Cross and Westminster Medical School, London, UK
Consultant Surgeon, Charing Cross Hospital, London, UK

Introduction

In modern practice, over 80% of all lower limb amputations are for peripheral vascular disease with the vast majority performed by vascular surgeons. These amputations are usually necessary because the severity of distal disease prevents arterial reconstruction, acute or severe ischaemia is prolonged, or our reconstructions fail. Nevertheless, the purpose is to relieve pain and to restore mobility to a patient who would otherwise have been immobilized either by pain or by developing gangrene. Amputation surgery therefore requires to be of the highest standard with gentle handling of ischaemic tissues to achieve primary healing. The type of amputation will be tailored to the individual needs of the patient and to their ability to regain full mobility. The surgeon must work in close cooperation with his limb-fitting service, as there is little point in achieving excellent primary healing rates if the resulting stump will only accommodate a difficult or clumsy prosthesis.

In major lower limb amputation, below-knee amputation has substantial advantages for rehabilitation over both through-knee and above-knee amputation. Only 20 years ago it was rarely performed in arterial disease because the anterior flap suffered necrosis and the amputation had to be revised to above-knee. The use of a longer posterior flap was advocated by Kendrick in 1956, but the modern posterior flap technique was popularized a decade later by Burgess (1968; Burgess *et al.*, 1971). Although the proportion of below-knee to above-knee amputations was 6:1 in Kendrick's series, the tragedy of vascular surgery over the following 20 years was that this ratio was progressively reversed, with many vascular surgeons rarely performing below-knee amputation.

Selection for below-knee amputation

Where an amputation is essential, or arterial reconstruction is not possible or has failed, it requires to be performed in such a way as to ensure the greatest chance of the patient returning to full mobility and independence and with the objective of achieving primary healing. Perhaps one reason that above-knee amputation became so frequent was that primary healing could almost be guaranteed. In below-knee amputation, particularly when operating in an ischaemic calf, the technique is critical to achieve primary healing. On our vascular surgical service, above-knee amputation is now reserved for those patients with crippling disability, such as hemiplegia, where mobilization is impossible. As a result, we have only performed 24 such procedures over the last 5 years, with 6 of these being revisions of below-knee amputations. Over the same interval, we have performed 61 below-knee amputations with an in-hospital mortality of 6.5% and revision to above-knee in just under 10%. These results can be achieved even where there is no recordable arterial pressure at the ankle by Doppler as the long posterior flap is based on the collateral blood supply to the calf.

Blood supply to the posterior flap

1

In the majority of patients for amputation, the popliteal artery and the posterior calf arteries are completely occluded, otherwise arterial reconstruction would be possible. An example of a typical arteriogram in a patient where distal reconstruction may not be possible is shown in *Illustration 1* where the superficial femoral artery is patent down to the mid-popliteal with complete occlusion of the distal popliteal and all calf arteries. An almost invariable feature of such cases is a fan of collaterals, including the sural artery, arising with its apex in the suprageniculate vessels. These collaterals fill either from thigh collaterals if the suprageniculate popliteal is occluded or from the suprageniculate arteries themselves. They then ramify distally, posterior to the gastrocnemius with branches entering the gastrocnemius. These vessels may represent the main source of supply of the lower limb as there are very few collaterals passing down in the tissues anterior to the knee. Clearly collateralization to the anterior skin will be poor, as there is no easy communication between the posterior compartment of the calf and the peroneal or anterior compartments, other than in collaterals within the skin itself.

As these posterior calf collaterals may also be the main source of supply for the lower leg, including the soleus muscle and the anterior and peroneal compartments, there may be considerable 'steal' of blood from the posterior calf compartment. The available blood supply to the posterior flap is, therefore, improved on amputation of the lower leg, providing all tissue anterior to the gastrocnemius is removed. It is for this reason that I emphasize that the soleus muscle should be completely removed up to a level just above the division of the bone.

Preoperative preparation

As the mean age of these patients is over 70 and the early postoperative mortality in the range of 7–14%, these patients require careful assessment for anaesthesia and close postoperative supervision (Hayes and Middleton, 1981; Harrison, Southworth and Callum, 1987; Sethia *et al.*, 1986; Robinson, Hoile and Coddington, 1982). Associated cardiovascular or respiratory disease and diabetes add to the risks. Often, these patients have become debilitated and malnourished through prolonged opiate therapy for rest pain, or may have already undergone arterial reconstruction or previous attempts at conservative amputation. Despite this, amputation should not be delayed, because the patients will usually continue to deteriorate with pain, spreading infection or gangrene.

Once the decision to amputate has been made the leg should be elevated to reduce tissue oedema and antibiotics started if there is evidence of infection or gangrene. Diabetes should be carefully controlled by soluble insulin infusion and the patient rehydrated. Where malnutrition is a problem, fine-bore gastric feeding may be started, even though amputation should be scheduled within 24 h. The level of amputation is carefully explained and consent obtained for below-knee amputation only, unless there is spreading gangrene and the viability of the calf muscles is in doubt.

1

Selecting amputation level

Much has been written about methods of assessing tissue perfusion for the selection of the most distal amputation site likely to heal. This is critical, as the more distal the amputation the greater the proportion of patients who achieve complete rehabilitation, whereas the more proximal the amputation the higher the chances of primary healing. Methods described to measure this objectively include Doppler segmental pressures, pulse volume recording, zenon-133 clearance studies, photoplethysmography, muscle pH measurements, thermography and $TCPO_2$ measurements. Of these, transcutaneous oxygen tension measurement appears the most promising, with the potential that laser Doppler may be equally valuable in the future. Planning is still difficult, as healing may occur in the face of low $TCPO_2$ levels unless skin heating to overcome vasospasm or high inhaled oxygen concentrations are administered (Spence and McCollum, 1985; Franzech et al., 1982; Rattiff et al., 1984). Furthermore, in below-knee amputation, it is impossible to predict how much the $TCPO_2$ of the skin flap will improve once the distal tissue dependent on the same collaterals has been removed, although some improvement in the flap has been acknowledged (Katsamouris et al., 1984). For most vascular surgeons, there is still no clear indication as to which technique should be used routinely because development has not yet reached the standard that they can be applied generally. From our own results, clinical judgement alone may be used, because reamputation at a higher level was required in less than 10% of patients despite performing below-knee amputations on all patients with viable posterior calf skin. When an adequate posterior flap cannot be fashioned due to ulceration or gangrene, the 'skin flap' technique may be appropriate, but in my opinion requires a better blood supply (Robinson, Hoile and Coddington, 1982).

The operation

In most cases, general anaesthesia is used, although epidural or spinal local anaesthesia may be appropriate for individual cases. Prophylactic antibiotics are given before incision, or earlier for spreading infection.

2

The skin is marked 8–12 cm below the tibial tuberosity where the anterior skin incision is made and the bone divided. The medial and lateral limits of the anterior incision are then marked, as this will form the base of the posterior flap. This base should be more medially placed by only extending the anterior incision medially 1–2 cm posterior to the border of the tibia, but the lateral incision should extend just posterior to the line of the fibula. The posterior flap will be cut to size later in the procedure.

2

3

The anterior skin incision is made down to the tibia and through the anterior tibial compartment to the neurovascular bundle. Once this has been ligated the fibula can easily be cleaned of its periosteum and divided using rib shears 3–4 cm above the proposed level of tibial division.

3

4

4

Using minimal retraction, so as not to disturb the precarious blood supply to the anterior skin, the periosteum on the tibia is then divided and elevated on its anterior surface, only far enough for the anterior bevel on the tibia to be cut. The tibia is then divided transversely and grasped firmly so that it can be pulled gently forward and the cut end of the fibula brought forward from the bulk of the muscle.

5

The posterior flap is cut with long medial and lateral incisions and rapid separation of the calf muscles from the posterior surface of the tibia and fibula. The posterior flap is divided distally to provide excessive length so that it may subsequently be trimmed to fit with absolutely no tension. The cut end of the tibia is rounded by filing and all sawdust and filings rinsed away with saline.

5

6

6

The plane between the gastrocnemius and the soleus is easily identified on the medial aspect of the flap and can simply be developed by blunt dissection. This plane is virtually avascular, demonstrating that the posterior flap is supplied by the sural arterial and not from the tibial vessels. The soleus is firmly adherent to the tendon of the gastrocnemius in the lateral part of the flap, but this may easily be divided leaving no soleus on the flap.

7

Once fully mobilized, the soleus is pulled distally and divided transversely at the level of the tibia, ligating the posterior tibial vessels and securing haemostasis at this stage. This procedure greatly reduces the bulk of the posterior flap so that the flap may be shortened without undue tension, improving the shape of the stump, preventing 'dog ears' and reducing the disproportion in thickness between the anterior and posterior tissues.

7

8a

8a & b

The gastrocnemius tendon and deep fascia are divided first and sutured anteriorly, ensuring complete muscular cover of the bone end. Only then is the skin folded up and divided to an exact fit with no tension.

8b

9

Three or four 4/0 prolene sutures are loosely placed, but the main skin aposition is achieved with 0.5-inch wide steri- or suture-strips. I routinely use a redivac drain and the stump is then wrapped in a generous layer of wool, held in place by a gentle crêpe bandage applied to exert as little pressure as possible on the stump.

9

Postoperative care and rehabilitation

The patient is encouraged to mobilize the knee from the first postoperative day, with elevation initially and vigorous physiotherapy to ensure complete extension of the knee joint. As the suture strips maintain skin aposition the skin sutures may be removed after 5 or 6 days. The suture strips are left until wound healing is adequate, which may be anything between 8 and 20 days. Physiotherapy ideally starts prior to amputation and is designed to relieve any contractures that may be developing as a result of rest ischaemia. The emphasis is on the rapid recovery of a full range of movement in the knee joint so that the patient can 'drive' a patella tendon-bearing prosthesis. In this respect, knee extension must be complete so that mobilization with a pneumatic limb starts in the second week and a temporary prosthesis may then be fitted within 3–4 weeks.

References

Burgess, E. M. (1968). The below knee amputation. *Bull. Pros. Res. BRP* **10**, 9.

Burgess, E. M., Romano, R. L., Zettl, J. H. and Schrock, R. D., Jr (1971). Amputations of the leg for peripheral vascular insufficiency. *Journal of Bone and Joint Surgery* **53A**, 874.

Franzech, U. K., Talke, P., Bernstein, E. F. *et al.* (1982). Transcutaneous PO$_2$ measurements in health and peripheral arterial disease. *Surgery* **91**, 156.

Harrison, J. D., Southworth, S. and Callum, K. G. (1987). Experience with "skew-flap" below knee amputation. *British Journal of Surgery* **74**, 930.

Haynes, I. G. and Middleton, M. D. (1981). Amputation for peripheral vascular disease: Experience of a district general hospital. *Annals of Surgery* **63**, 342.

Katsamouris, A., Brewster, D. C., Megerman, J., Cina, C., Clement Darling, R. and Abbot, W. M. (1984). Transcutaneous oxygen tension in selection of amputation level. *American Journal of Surgery* **147**, 510.

Kendrick, R. R. (1956). Below knee amputation for arteriosclerotic gangrene. *British Journal of Surgery* **44**, 13.

Malone, J. M. and Godstone, J. (1986). Lower extremity amputation. In *Vascular Surgery: A Comprehensive Review*, 2nd ed. Moore, W., ed. London and San Diego: Grune and Stratton.

Rattiff, D. A., Clyne, C. A. C., Chant, A. D. B., *et al.* (1984). Prediction of amputation wound healing: The role of transcutaneous PO$_2$ assessment. *British Journal of Surgery* **71**, 219.

Robinson, K. P., Hoile, R. and Coddington, T. (1982). Skew flap myopastic below-knee amputation: A preliminary report. *British Journal of Surgery* **69**, 554.

Sethia, K. K., Berry, A. R., Morison, J. D., Collin, J., Murie, J. A. and Morris, P. J. (1986). Changing pattern of lower limb amputation for vascular disease. *British Journal of Surgery* **73**, 701.

Spence, V. A. and McCollum, P. T. Evaluation of the ischaemic limb by transcutaneous oxymetry. In *Diagnostic Techniques and Assessment Procedures in Vascular Surgery*. Greenhalgh, R. M. ed. London and San Diego: Grune and Stratton.

Skew-flap below-knee amputation

Kingsley Robinson MS, FRCS

Consultant Surgeon, Westminster Hospital, London, UK

Introduction

This technique is designed to make the best use of the blood supply to the below-knee skin in patients with peripheral vascular disease to form a stump which is shaped to be suitable for prosthetic use at the conclusion of the surgical operation, and which has a standardized technique that is reproducible in the hands of different surgeons, so that a stump with the same characteristics can be consistently produced.

1

The length of the stump is determined by the line of bone section which is measured from the articular surface of the tibial plateau and according to the patient's build is between 10 and 14 cm below this level. The level should be judged to be just above the maximum convexity of the calf muscle mass and not shorter than a point that allows 4 cm of stump to protrude beyond the hamstring tendons when the knee is flexed to 90°. The line of bone section is drawn on the skin overlying the tibia and a circumferential equator line is extended around the limb at this point. It is important to use a fully waterproof marking device, and if the skin marking is performed in the anaesthetic room, a waterproof fibre-tip cartridge writer is ideal and the skin can be subsequently prepared with a spirit-based antiseptic without removing the marks. A point 2 cm lateral to the subcutaneous tibial crest is marked on the equator line and a vertical mark parallel to the axis of the limb is extended upwards for 2 cm. This point represents the junction of the anteromedial and posterolateral skin flap. To identify the diametrically opposite point on the back of the limb a tape is passed around the equator line and cut to that length. This tape folded in half will then indicate the posterior junction of the flaps. If the same tape is then folded to obtain a quarter length, this will indicate the midpoints of each flap along the equator line from which the quarter circumference length can be drawn on the skin to indicate the length of the skin flap at its maximum extent. A semicircular line then connects the three marks to form the skew flaps. The skin is incised together with the subcutaneous fat, the periosteum over the tibia and the anterior tibial compartment and peroneal compartment fascia.

1

2

2

When the skin incision has been completed and the skin retracted, the long saphenous vein and the short saphenous vein need to be secured with artery forceps and ligated with fine catgut or vicryl 3/0, while the saphenous nerve and sural nerve are separately divided under some tension to allow the ends to retract. Very few bleeding points require attention at this stage and the skin flaps can be elevated to expose the anterior aspect of the tibia and the peroneal and anterior tibial muscle compartments. The tibial periosteum and the anterior tibial muscles are divided along the line of the equator mark on the skin, the upward extension of the skin incision providing access to the anterior tibial compartment with moderate retraction.

3

The dissection is carried through the anterior tibial peroneal muscles, a few muscle fibres at a time, either with a scalpel or diathermy point, until the anterior tibial nerve and the musculocutaneous nerve are revealed in each compartment, allowing them to be drawn down under tension and cut transversely with a scalpel so that they can retract clear of the area of the stump end. The anterior tibial artery and its venae comitans are revealed close to the interosseous membrane and can be divided between haemostats and ligated with a fine vicryl or catgut suture. The anterior surface of the fibula and the lateral surface of the tibia are now exposed together with the interosseous membrane. The latter is divided in the line of the dissection and a periosteal elevator is used to clear all surfaces of the tibia at this same level. The fibula can similarly be cleared and retraction will expose an adequate length to allow the fibula to be divided 2 cm proximal to the line of bone section marked on the skin.

3

4

The fibula is divided first. Bone forceps should not be used for this purpose because the fibula will fragment into sharp pieces and may split along its whole length. A Gigli saw is convenient for dividing the bone, although a cantilever power-saw is much easier to manage. Sometimes the nutrient vessels of both the fibula and tibia are encountered at this level and may produce some bleeding that has to be controlled with a pack until better access is obtained after the bones are divided. Once the fibula is divided, the tibia can be transected.

4

5

The tibia is most conveniently cut with a cantilever power-saw while copious irrigation is maintained to avoid any heat damage to the bone ends and to remove the bone dust and fragments. The cantilever power-saw will permit a gentle anterior curve to be described as the bone is transected, but if a hand saw is used, a sloping cut is made through the anterior half of the bone and then a transverse cut through the remaining half to produce a partial bevel which can then be rounded by subsequent filing. Once the tibia is completely divided, the distal fragment is stabilized by inserting a sharp bone hook into the medullary cavity and applying some traction.

5

6

6

While downward traction is maintained on the distal fragment of the tibia, the tibialis posterior muscle is clearly visible and can be divided a few fibres at a time until the neurovascular bundles and the posterior tibial nerve are revealed beneath it. The most convenient technique to handle the neurovascular bundles is the application of a large artery forcep of the Robert's type with enough length being allowed for a second forcep to be applied behind the first so that the posterior tibial nerve can be extricated, and both the peroneal and posterior tibial arteries and their venae comitans can then be separately secured and the temporary proximal forcep removed. The posterior tibial nerve, the largest encountered in the dissection, is drawn down strongly and cut across with the scalpel and allowed to retract well away. Some bleeding from its concomitant artery may be encountered and this is never a problem. The skin flaps are separated from the distal part of the limb by a blunt dissection and drawn down to allow access to the full thickness of the gastrocnemius soleus muscle mass which is extricated from the distal portion of the limb, the very distance at least equal to the vertical thickness of the formed stump. If the assistant presses firmly across the upper part of the calf muscles, a degree of control of the remaining vessels is obtained and the gastrocnemius muscle mass can be transected at the chosen distal level with a minimum of blood loss.

7

At this point the myoplastic flap to be formed from the gastrocnemius soleus mass is formed. The muscle tongue is pulled out with tissue forceps and a slope is cut from the line of bone section to the distal end of the flap leaving only aponeurosis for the last few millimetres. This will transect the soleal venous sinuses and numerous small arteries which will require individual transfixion and underrunning with sutures to obtain full haemostasis. The use of diathermy ligaclips and simple ligatures is rarely successful and an underrunning suture will save a considerable amount of time.

7

8

Once haemostasis is obtained and the tapering flap has been constructed, the dimensions of this are then checked by folding it forward to approximate its distal end to the anterior tibial periosteum and the anterior tibial fascia. This will demonstrate how much bulk the folded muscle mass will produce at the medial and lateral aspects and, following accurate trimming of the distal end of the flap, the sides of the muscle mass must then be reduced to make sure that there is no widening when the muscle flap is folded over.

8

9 & 10

A large scalpel is used to trim away the excess muscle tissue and the trimming process may have to be extended above the line of bone section into the peroneal muscle group and on the medial side of the gastrocnemius. Some further venous sinuses may require underrunning and ligation. At this stage attention is paid to the bone ends which are then carefully shaped with a coarse rasp and then a fine bone file to produce a rounded corner with a smooth surface in all dimensions. Similar attention must also be paid to the fibula end so that there is no excess scar tissue formed by trauma due to movement of bone fragments in the muscle tissue. A careful wash out is required to remove all the calcium fragments and a suction drain is placed in relation to the bone ends and passed through the skin laterally and secured with a stitch. The myoplastic flap is now finally folded over.

9

10

11

The folded flap is carefully opposed to the anterior tibial fascia and the anterior tibial periosteum. A continuous suture of '1' chromic catgut or '0' vicryl is used to run along the whole anterior aspect of the stump and to complete the myoplasty. The skin flaps remain partially attached to the gastrocnemius soleus mass and a small degree of separation may be required to allow them to come into comfortable apposition and the skin and subcutaneous fat are sutured with interrupted stitches – usually vertical mattress sutures of 3/0 nylon – to approximate the skin edges along the line of the skew flaps. It is recommended that the anterior and posterior sutures are inserted first and then a central stay stitch to allow any fine adjustment in the alignment of the flaps to be obtained before closure is complete. The application of steristrips to the skin between each interrupted suture may relieve tension loading on the sutures.

11

12

12

At completion, the stump is usually well-rounded, parallel-sided and symmetrical, with the suture line just clear of the anterior tibial crest and the tibia and fibula bone ends. The soft tissues are not excessive or redundant and the patient may be allowed to apply stress to the stump between 2 and 4 days from the completion of the operation. Definitive stump bandaging is not recommended and our current practice is to use finely fluffed cotton gauze without any cotton wool or padding applied to the stump, and a spiral of 4″ crêpe bandage keeps the fluffed gauze in place without applying any pressure or constriction to the stump itself. At the first dressing change, a netalast elastic net is used to retain the dressing, and as soon as possible the dressing is discarded altogether.

Toe and foot amputations

Frank J. Veith   MD

Professor of Surgery and Chief of Vascular Surgical Services, Albert Einstein College of Medicine and Montefiore Medical Center, New York, USA

Sushil K. Gupta   MD

Associate Professor of Surgery and Associate Chief of Vascular Surgery, Albert Einstein College of Medicine and Montefiore Medical Center, New York, USA

Enrico Ascer   MD

Associate Professor of Surgery, Albert Einstein College of Medicine, New York, USA;
Vascular Surgeon in Charge, North Central Bronx Hospital, New York, USA

Kurt R. Wengerter   MD

Assistant Professor of Surgery and Assistant Attending Vascular Surgeon, Albert Einstein College of Medicine and Montefiore Medical Center, New York, USA

Introduction

Performance of successful toe or partial foot amputation can be a critical part of limb salvage surgery in many patients who have gangrene and/or infection with or without ischaemia from arterial occlusive disease. These amputations within the foot include ablation of one or more toes, toe amputation with a portion of the adjacent metatarsal bone, partial (medial or lateral) transmetatarsal amputation, complete transmetatarsal amputation and a variety of unnamed or free-style partial foot amputations or debridements designed to remove necrotic or infected tissue and allow healing of enough of the foot to permit functional weight-bearing on the residual part of the extremity.

General principles

Before considering the specific techniques for these amputations within the foot, several principles must be emphasized. The first is that with normal or near-normal arterial circulation to the foot and adequate debridement or excision of infected and necrotic tissue, remarkable healing of the residual foot can be obtained. Moreover, even a small remnant of the foot can be effectively used for bipedal ambulation in sick, old patients, with one or more other disabilities. Salvage of less than half the foot with its plantar skin intact will permit more effective ambulation than a below-knee amputation if the patient has had a contralateral major amputation or a stroke. In this regard, we have found it possible to remove a major portion of the heel, including the Achilles tendon and the weight-bearing part of the os calcis, and still have the patient use the foot effectively in walking. Similarly, loss of the toes, metatarsals and most of the tarsal bones, leaving a foot remnant one-third the length of normal, does not preclude effective bipedal ambulation, which is not achieved in more than 30% of our patients undergoing below-knee amputation because of their frequent intercurrent disabilities.

A second principle relates to the importance of confirming adequate arterial circulation to permit successful performance of amputations within the foot. Simple toe amputations will occasionally heal with somewhat diminished ankle–brachial pressure indices and pulse volume recordings, but they almost never will when the ankle–brachial index is less than 0.6 and forefoot waves are flat or less than 5 mm in amplitude. Moreover, complex partial foot amputations and particularly some of the free-style transtarsal amputations to be described require near-normal arterial circulation to the foot. If a normal pedal pulse is not palpable or non-invasive tests do not indicate direct or straight-line arterial flow to the foot, the amputation within the foot should not be undertaken until arteriography and successful revascularization of the foot have been performed.

A third set of principles relate to the decision to close the skin primarily or leave the wound open. Although this decision requires careful judgement, there are certain guidelines which the surgeon should follow. If infection is evident or tissue viability is in question, the wound must be left open. Skin closure should never be under tension. Any wound that is closed must be reopened if wound edges become dusky or tension develops because of oedema. Open wounds are best kept moist with saline. This can be accomplished effectively by incorporating impermeable plastic within the saline-soaked dressing.

Fourthly, control of infection and normal or near-normal circulation are necessary for successful healing by secondary intention. Adequate debridement of infected and necrotic tissue is also essential and may require several trips to the operating room. Split thickness skin grafting can hasten healing once a clean granulating wound is obtained. Even on weight-bearing surfaces, such skin grafts can help to save feet.

Fifthly, there are no absolute barriers to debridement. Infected or necrotic tissue must be removed even if it requires exposure of joint interiors between the tarsal bones or even the ankle. With good circulation, adequate debridement and postoperative care healing can be achieved. A rongeur is a most useful instrument to perform adequate debridement of infected or necrotic tissues within the foot. This includes soft tissue, tendons, cartilage and bone.

A sixth and final principle is adherence to the use of minimally traumatic technique to handle all remaining tissue. Crushing of tissue and grasping of the skin with forceps must be avoided. Haemostasis should be complete but no adjacent tissue should be ligated or coagulated with blood vessels.

Specific amputations within the foot

1

Simple toe amputation

This is performed by making a circular incision in the skin of the toe as close to the proximal interphalangeal joint as possible, thereby assuring adequate skin length to permit closure by primary or secondary intention. The actual position of the skin incision is determined by the amount of remaining viable skin left on the toe. Care is taken to make the incision in viable skin. The soft tissues are then sharply divided down to the proximal phalanx. A flap of soft tissue is raised to provide access to the base of the proximal phalanx and the bone is divided using a bone-cutting forceps or rongeur without entering the metatarsal-phalangeal joint. If the skin is clearly viable and uninfected and closure without tension can be performed, a few monofilament sutures are placed in the skin to close the wound in a transverse plane. If any of these conditions cannot be fulfilled, the wound is left open to heal by secondary intention. If the metatarsal-phalangeal joint is entered, all of the cartilage, the entire proximal phalanx and much of the head of the metatarsal bone should be removed with a rongeur. Care is taken to remove all bone spicules and tissue fragments using the same instrument.

2

Removal of one or more toes with a portion of the corresponding metatarsal bone

If all the phalanges and all of the associated metatarsal bone are amputated, the procedure is often described as a 'ray' amputation. The 'ray' amputation is frequently required for quite severe osteomyelitis in association with diabetic gangrene. However, more frequently, the degree of infection dictates only that the head of the metatarsal needs to be excised with the toe, as is described here.

The skin incision is performed at the distal-most limit of viability. This incision is deepened to bone. The formation of flaps with so-called racquet handle incisions is kept to a minimum, but proximal extension of the incision is acceptable to provide proximal exposure of the metatarsal shafts. A periosteal elevator is used to expose the metatarsal-phalangeal joint and the distal portions of the metatarsal bones. These are transected in their midshaft with bone-cutting forceps or a vibrating saw. Sharp or projecting bone fragments are smoothed with a rongeur, and the same instrument is used to facilitate excision of deep soft tissue that may be non-viable or infected. The presence of dark thrombosed small blood vessels in the soft tissues indicates both infection and non-viability, and all such tissue must be excised. Haemostasis is obtained, and the wound edges are then loosely approximated or left open according to the principles already outlined.

2

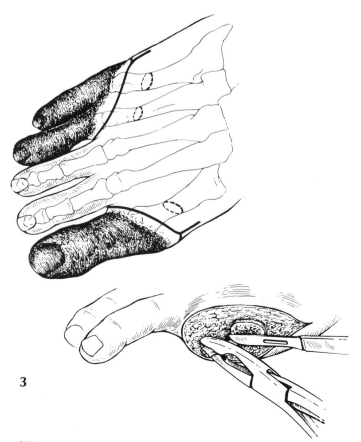

3

3

Partial (medial or lateral) transmetatarsal amputation

These procedures are useful when gangrene involves the proximal portions of one or two toes medially or laterally with or without involvement of the adjacent webspace or webspaces. Again the skin incision is made to preserve as much viable skin and soft tissue as possible. The incision is deepened to bone and the thickest possible flaps are raised using sharp dissection with a scalpel supplemented by a periosteal elevator. The metatarsal bone or bones are then transected through their shaft with bone-cutting forceps or a vibrating saw as far proximally as is necessary to permit the skin and soft tissue to fall together over the bone ends without tension. The interior of the wound is carefully inspected for bone spicules and tissues of questionable viability. These include remnants of divided tendon and joint capsule. All these elements which require debridement are sharply excised by grasping them with a rongeur and transecting them with this instrument or cutting them with a scalpel while they are held in tension by the rongeur. This particular technique with a rongeur is useful in all debridements and excisions of necrotic tissue within the foot. It is the most effective way to assure smooth bone ends and minimally traumatic removal of all tendonous and ligamentous remnants which tend to have a poor blood supply.

4

Transmetatarsal amputation

This operation is indicated when gangrene involves all the toes including one or more webspaces. It produces a very functional foot without the need for a prosthesis or special shoe. If only the distal portion of four or five toes are necrotic, several simple toe amputations are performed in preference to a transmetatarsal amputation. Although the resulting foot remnant after multiple toe amputations may be less pleasing aesthetically, it has the advantage of preserving the important weight-bearing and step-off functions of the metatarsal heads. In addition, leaving the webspaces intact preserves important collateral circulation to skin edges and maintains skin bridges which minimize tension on the suture line.

Transmetatarsal amputation is performed by making an incision through the distal-most viable skin. Because of its greater thickness and tolerance to weight-bearing, preservation of plantar skin is particularly important. Accordingly, if possible, the end of the foot remnant should be covered with a relatively longer plantar flap. However, if viable plantar skin is limited, closure can be achieved by leaving more of the dorsal skin. If closure of viable skin without tension or residual infection is not possible, the wound may be left open to heal by secondary intention with or without skin grafting. Although this may require a protracted hospital stay, the resulting foot remnant can provide excellent function. Occasionally, if a portion of the wound is questionable, the rest of it may be closed loosely by adhesive strips and the questionable part left open and treated with wet dressings.

After the plantar flap is developed superficial to the tendons of the toe flexors to the level of bone transection, the forefoot is plantar flexed and the dorsal incision is carried down to the metatarsal heads. With continued plantar flexion, all tendons are incised as far proximally as possible. The forefoot

4

is then dorsiflexed and the plantar tendons divided as far proximally as possible. The metatarsal shafts are then transected by already described techniques that will permit approximation of wound edges without tension. The rongeur–scalpel techniques described above are then used to provide smooth bone ends and to debride devitalized tissue and tendon ends. Haemostasis is secured and the wound approximated completely or partially, or left open depending on the pathology and principles already discussed.

5

5

Freestyle foot amputations (transtarsal amputations, heel amputations, excision of metatarsalphalangeal joint and excision of toe bones)

The first two of these procedures facilitate removal of necrotic or infected tissues that are more extensive than those treated by the standard procedures already described. The other two procedures preserve the soft tissue of the toes and permit excision of bones that are involved with osteomyelitis, thereby facilitating healing of toe or foot lesions. In all four instances excision of involved bone and soft tissue is accomplished by the rongeur–scalpel techniques already described and wounds are left open to heal by secondary intention with or without skin grafting. If transtarsal amputation is performed the Achilles tendon should be divided by dorsiflexing the foot remnant and cutting the stretched taught tendon with a No. 11 blade inserted alongside the tendon via a 3-mm skin incision.

Conclusions

All of these foot amputations can be valuable in preserving bipedal gait in patients with extensive gangrene and/or infection. In general, as much viable foot as possible should be preserved. Although multiple operations may be required and normal or near-normal arterial circulation is usually a prerequisite, the foot has a remarkable ability to heal and, by using the techniques described in this chapter, functional remnants of foot can be preserved despite the presence of surprisingly extensive gangrene and infection.

Acknowledgements

This work was supported in part by the Manning Foundation, The Anna S. Brown Foundation and the New York Institute for Vascular Studies.

Portacaval and splenorenal shunts for portal hypertension

Martin Birnstingl MS, FRCS

Consultant Surgeon, St Bartholomew's Hospital, London, UK

Introduction

The rationale for using portal-systemic shunting procedures for variceal haemorrhage is their effect in reducing pressure and flow in the gastro-oesophageal collateral veins. Unfortunately, total shunts, which are the most effective in producing permanent lowering of portal venous pressure, also tend to cause the highest incidence of portal-systemic encephalopathy (PSE). They also lead to progressive deterioration in liver function in patients with cirrhosis. However, the more selective shunts are not only difficult to construct, but also more likely to thrombose, and are therefore less reliable in securing permanent protection against recurrent variceal bleeding. These disadvantages have to be set against a probable lower incidence of PSE.

Direct portacaval shunts are appropriate for emergency procedures, where the shorter operating time and reliable decompression are advanges (Orloff *et al.*, 1974). The end-to-side procedure is usual, side-to-side portacaval anastomosis is used in the Budd-Chiari syndrome and occasionally in the presence of refractory ascites. Splenorenal shunts are used when the portal vein is unsuitable, for instance following congenital or neonatal thrombosis (extrahepatic portal obstruction).

The selective splenorenal (Warren) shunt is appropriate as an elective procedure in certain instances (Warren, Zepa and Fomon, 1967). It is tedious to perform and its claimed low incidence of PSE and improved maintenance of liver function are still unconfirmed by good follow-up studies. The author's preference is for end-to-side portacaval anastomosis as the most effective shunting procedure for variceal haemorrhage. A hospital mortality of 18% has been achieved in a series of 56 consecutive emergency operations (Birnstingl, 1980).

The mortality of elective shunt operations is of course much lower than this (2% in Orloff's series of 612 patients), although much influenced by the type and severity of the underlying liver disease. End-to-side portacaval anastomosis is the most likely to remain patent, most likely to stop the bleeding and to prevent later rebleeding and the easiest to perform quickly. It remains the best standard with which to compare other shunt operations.

In selecting patients for shunt operations the most important consideraions are the pathology of the underlying liver disease, which varies greatly in different countries, and the degree of impairment of liver cell function, assessed by a classification such as Child's (Child, 1954). In emergency shunts, the duration and severity of the current bleeding episode also influence survival.

Portacaval shunt

1

The patient is positioned lying on the left side with a 30° lateral tilt towards the right side. The knee is bent up and the right arm carried on a rest across the front of the neck. The long thoracoabdominal incision is preferred. This extends through the bed of the right 10th rib nearly to the midline. A long right subcostal incision is also fairly satisfactory, provided the liver is not too large.

A self-retaining retractor is inserted, the diaphragm partially divided and then sutured to the edge of the wound to improve access. An open or trucut needle biopsy of the liver is taken and the presence of portal hypertension confirmed, if necessary, with a saline manometer after tying a plastic cannula into a jejunal vein in the mesentery.

1

2

2

The lateral reflection of the peritoneum is divided along the margin of the second part of the duodenum to expose the inferior vena cava as far up as the caudate lobe of the liver. The peritoneum must be clamped and tied, and it is usually very vascular and thickened in portal hypertension. Oedema of the retroperitoneal tissues is also often striking. The front and both lateral aspects of the inferior vena cava must be displayed, taking care to avoid the right adrenal vein and inferior hepatic veins, when present.

The shunt will usually be positioned just above the entry of the right renal vein, which is clearly evident.

It is essential to identify the common bile duct and retract this forward and medially before searching for the portal vein, which lies behind the duct on a deeper plane and may be difficult to find. The portal vein is carefully exposed by very gentle dissection in the hepatoduodenal ligament.

3

A plastic sling is carried round the portal vein, which is gently freed nearly to the lower border of the liver, although its bifurcation is not always seen. Care must be taken not to tear the left gastric (coronary) vein which joins the left side of the portal vein. The portal vein is now securely tied just proximal to its bifurcation, using 2/0 linen thread or silk.

3

4

A straight vascular clamp is applied to the portal vein where it emerges from the pancreatic bed. Some areolar tissue may need to be divided at this point to prevent kinking of the vein. The portal vein is then cleanly divided at an appropriate level near to the bifurcation ligature.

4

5

5

A Satinsky partial exclusion vascular clamp is next applied to the front of the vena cava. The precise siting of the stoma needs great care, to prevent angulation or flattening of the portal vein. The best level is usually at or just above the right renal vein and it should be well towards the left side of the vena cava, at the junction of the anterior and left lateral aspects. With the vascular clamp in place, an opening is made in the vena cava and an ellipse of vein wall carefully removed with scissors.

6

6

A double-ended 4/0 polypropylene suture is used for the anastomosis. The suture is passed through the lower margin of the opening in the portal vein and the lower end of the caval incision and then tied. A single running, everting suture is then inserted from within the lumen of the two channels, since the back of the anastomosis is otherwise inaccessible. The illustration shows the posterior run completed and the beginning of the front run, which of course is constructed from the outside. Care must be taken not to pick up the earlier row of stitches since the stoma is rather flattened at this stage. The suture can either be continued as far as the initial knot and tied there as shown, or the unused needle can complete the anastomosis.

When the anastomosis is finished the Satinsky clamp on the vena cava is opened and, provided there is no leakage, it is withdrawn. Should any leak occur, the clamp is reapplied and additional interrupted sutures placed. Finally, the portal vein clamp is removed and the shunt should be seen to be open.

7

The shunt should be wide and there must be no suspicion of kinking, twisting or angulation of the portal vein. This is largely a matter of choosing the right site on the vena cava. Occasionally, a small wedge of pancreatic tissue or part of the caudate process of the liver must be excised to allow proper positioning, and this may require division of inferior hepatic veins (*see Illustration 2*).

The incision is closed in the usual way. An underwater seal pleural drain should be used for the thoracotomy, but the abdomen should not be drained as this may lead to serious protein loss if ascites develops during the postoperative period. Ascites can also be avoided by reduction of sodium intake in the intravenous fluid to a minimum.

7

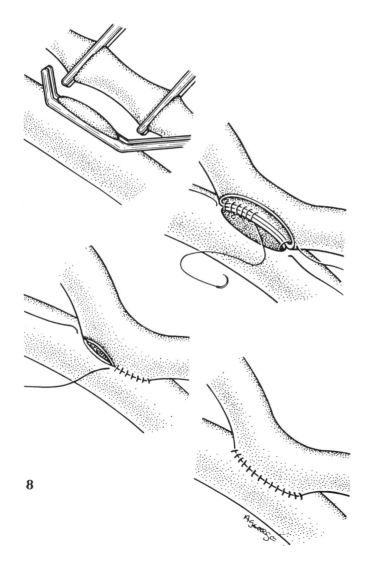

8

8

Side-to-side portacaval shunt

This shunt is seldom appropriate. The essential steps are similar to those in end-to-side anastomosis. It is often necessary to resect some of the caudate lobe of the liver and it is not always possible to approximate the two veins to allow a tension-free shunt. In such cases, the procedure is abandoned or an interposition graft of jugular vein or Dacron is used.

Splenorenal shunts

Selective distal splenorenal (Warren) shunt

9

The right gastric (coronary), left gastric, right gastroepiploic and splenic veins are ligated. The intention is to allow hepatic perfusion from the superior and inferior mesenteric veins, while diverting the flow from the gastro-oesophageal varices through the shunt. However, the fall in portal pressure produced by the shunt, combined with the increase in hepatic resistance due to the liver disease, produces a pressure gradient between the portal vein and the rest of the portal bed. The result is a gradual resumption of collateral flow towards the shunt, as shown by portal venography at various times after selective shunting (Rikkers *et al.*, 1978). In spite of obvious theoretical advantages and a low incidence of early PSE, selective portal shunting requires long-term evaluation before it can be recommended.

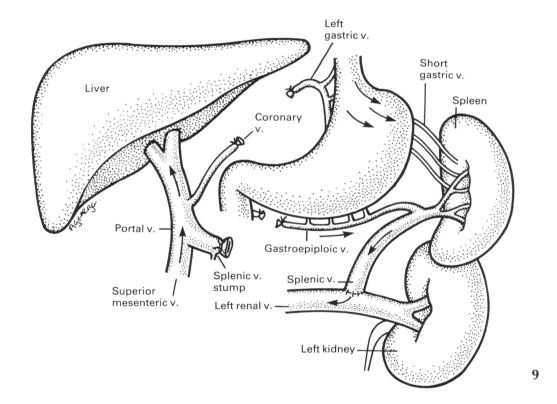

9

10

Before the operation it is important to have angiographic evidence of patency of the splenic vein. For the procedure, the patient lies prone and a midline upper abdominal incision is used.

The splenic vein can be exposed above or below the transverse mesocolon. The author prefers to retract the transverse colon upwards. The posterior parietal peritoneum is then opened along the lower border of the pancreas. Three or four 3/0 silk sutures are placed at intervals along the lower border of the pancreas and tied to provide slings to hold it forward.

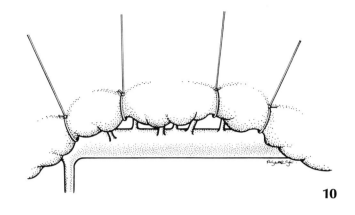

10

11

11

The splenic vein is identified and gradually mobilized, which necessitates the division of many small veins joining it from the pancreas. This is tedious and difficult, as they must be tied with 3/0 silk before division and they are easily torn.

12

When several centimetres of splenic vein have been freed, the vein is ligated and after applying a covered bulldog clamp, divided well to the right, close to the junction of the inferior mesenteric vein. The latter vein is a useful guide to the splenic vein if it proves difficult to find.

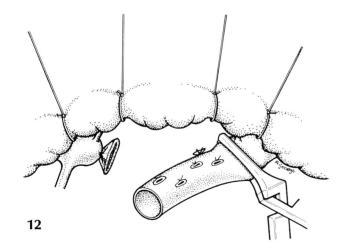

12

13

The left renal vein is identified in the retroperitoneal tissues and it may be necessary to divide a large adrenal vein. If the renal vein is difficult to find, the kidney can be felt and the hilum identified. The renal vein usually needs two straight vascular clamps. This has never caused detectable effects upon the kidney, presumably because of adequacy of collateral veins in the renal hilum.

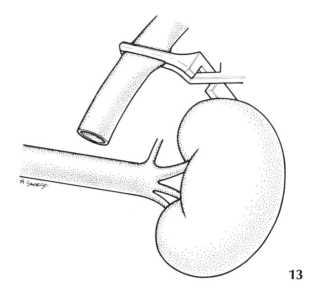

13

14

14

An ellipse of renal vein is removed at an appropriate site on its upper border and an end-to-side anastomosis constructed using a double-needle 5/0 polypropylene suture. Occasionally, positioning demands that the renal vein must be tied and the left end turned up and anastomosed to the side of the splenic vein. Ligation of the renal vein seems to cause no harm in such cases.

15

Central splenorenal shunt

This is a non-selective shunt, suitable when the portal vein is not available. The infrapancreatic site is more accessible than that used in the older approach which entailed splenectomy, followed by mobilization of the much smaller and branching distal part of the splenic vein.

Isolation of the splenic vein is performed as in the selective operation, but the vein is ligated towards the left and the central (right) end of the vein is used for the anastomosis, as shown. The right and left gastric and gastroepiploic veins are not ligated.

This shunt probably has a lower incidence of PSE than portacaval anastomosis, but the advantage is offset by less complete portal decompression and a tendency to shunt thrombosis leading to variceal bleeding. These disadvantages also apply to the mesocaval shunt, which for this reason is not described here.

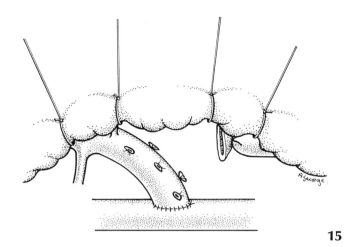

15

Conclusion

The complications of these procedures can be severe. Portal-systemic encephalopathy is a great concern and the problem of bleeding during surgery has been stressed. The high mortality rate of these procedures has to be weighed against the natural history of the condition without surgery.

References

Birnstingl, M. (1980). Surgical treatment of emergencies. In: *Medical and Surgical Problems of Portal Hypertension*. Orloff, M. J., Stipa, S. and Ziparo, V., eds. London and San Diego: Academic Press.

Child, C. G. (1954). *The Hepatic Circulation and Portal Hypertension*. London and San Diego: W.B. Saunders.

Orloff, M. J., Charters, A. C., Condon, J. K. *et al.* (1974). Emergency portocaval shunt for bleeding oesophageal varices. *Archives of Surgery* **108**, 293.

Rikkers, L.F., Rudman, D., Warren, W. D. *et al.* (1978). A randomized controlled trial of the distal splenorenal shunt. *Annals of Surgery* **188**, 271.

Warren, W. D., Zeppa, R. and Fomon, J. J. (1967). Selective transsplenic decompression of gastro-oesophageal varices by distal splenorenal shunt. *Annals of Surgery* **166**, 437.

Injection sclerotherapy for oesophageal varices

K. W. Reynolds MS, FRCS
Consultant Surgeon, Gastrointestinal Unit, Charing Cross Hospital, London, UK
N. A. Theodorou FRCS
Consultant Surgeon, Gastrointestinal Unit, Charing Cross Hospital, London, UK

Introduction

The terminal event in patients with portal hypertension and oesophageal varices is often exsanguination. The hospital mortality from acute variceal haemorrhage is reported to be as high as 67–75% (Palani *et al.*, 1981), depending on the underlying hepatic function and the adequacy of the initial treatment. Unfortunately, operative procedures designed to decrease the portal pressure in order to control haemorrhage in the acute phase have a high mortality and morbidity. Injection sclerotherapy has therefore been developed as a far simpler procedure in order to avoid the metabolic consequences of major abdominal surgery in these very ill patients.

Injection sclerotherapy was first performed in 1939 by Crafoord and Frenckner and the early practice of this technique was by ENT surgeons. MacBeth at Oxford in 1955 was the first British surgeon to draw attention to the relevant detailed anatomy of the varices and to establish the technique of sclerotherapy in the literature.

At present patients with oesophageal varices are not injected unless the varices have bled; bleeding occurs in only 30% of patients with oesophageal varices but 70% of these patients rebleed (Conn, 1974).

Aims of treatment

1. Initially to control the presenting bleeding with injection sclerotherapy and balloon tamponade, paying attention to adequate resuscitation, correction of clotting abnormalities and liver function.
2. Subsequently to enter patients into a long-term programme of elective sclerotherapy to prevent recurrent haemorrhage.

Preoperative management

1. The mainstay of management is *urgent* endoscopy under general anaesthesia. This allows early control of haemorrhage by injection sclerotherapy and balloon tamponade.
2. General anaesthesia is essential in the acute situation to provide adequate protection of the airway from aspiration of the gastric contents. It will also allow rigid oesophagoscopy if indicated and the safer, controlled passage of a Minnesota tube.
3. There must be minimal delay between admission and transfer of the patient to theatre while blood is taken for urgent estimation of haemoglobin, urea and electrolytes, clotting studies, cross-matching and, if appropriate, Australia Antigen status.
4. Intravenous lines are established with 5% dextrose. Resuscitation should be with blood and fluids which do *not* contain saline, because patients with poor liver function cannot handle sodium loads. Two units of fresh frozen plasma and a loading dose of vitamin K 10 mg i.v. are given.
5. The patient is transferred to theatre as soon as possible where, after control of haemorrhage, a central venous line and urinary catheter are passed to facilitate further resuscitation.

Anaesthesia

1. Endoscopy is performed under general anaesthesia with continuous ECG and blood pressure monitoring.
2. Anaesthesia is induced with thiopentone sodium, the patient intubated with an oral cuffed latex armoured tube and anaesthesia maintained with nitrous oxide, oxygen and intermittent suxamethonium.
3. Possible hepatotoxic inhalational agents (e.g. halothane) are avoided, and narcotic analgesics must be used with extreme caution.

The procedure

For all cases a fibre-optic diagnostic oesophagogastroduo-
denoscopy (OGD) should be performed to confirm the source
of the bleeeding and to exclude other upper gastrointestinal
pathology. Following this, sclerotherapy may be instituted in
the following manner.

1

Rigid oesophagoscopy

In major variceal haemorrhage the use of the rigid (Negus)
oesophagoscope has the advantage that individual varices may
in turn be allowed to prolapse into view while the remaining
variceal columns are compressed with the leading edge of the
instrument. In the presence of severe active bleeding this
allows a clear view of the prolapsed varix which may then be
injected with ethanolamine using a MacBeth needle. After
the injection of 2–3 ml of ethanolamine, the scope is advanced
and axially rotated. This allows compression of the injected
varix while another column is allowed to prolapse into view.
A total of 8–10 ml of ethanolamine are injected as near as
possible to the cardio-oesophageal junction and at the end of
the procedure tamponade is instituted by means of a Minnesota tube.

2

Fibreoptic endoscopy

This is performed with a forward-oblique viewing endoscope.
A full upper gastrointestinal endoscopy is performed on each
occasion to note any other possible source of bleeding. The
oblique viewing endoscope with a bridge is ideal for accurate
positioning of the injection needle into the varix.

3

In the emergency situation it is important that varices are confirmed to be the source of the haemorrhage. The prominent tortuous variceal columns (V) are seen to extend proximally from the cardio-oesophageal junction. The extent of the variceal columns should be accurately documented for later assessment of the efficacy of treatment.

3

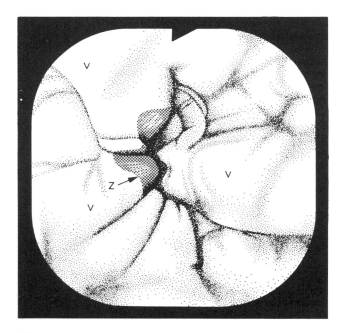

4

4

The varices (V) are followed to the squamocolumnar junction or 'Z' line. The site of injection should be as close as possible to the cardio-oesophageal junction because obliteration of the perforating veins at this level will control the variceal columns.

5

Occasionally, smaller variceal columns (V) may be missed because they sometimes prolapse into the stomach (S).

5

6

6

It is important in the absence of obvious bleeding oesophageal varices, the presence of gastric varices (GV) is excluded by manoeuvring the gastrocope (G) to allow visualization of the cardia from within the stomach (the 'J' manoeuvre).

7

To start sclerotherapy the needle (N) is advanced through the endoscope and introduced *into* the varix (V). *Intravariceal* injection of sclerosant is associated with a much smaller incidence of oesophageal ulceration and stricturing than *perivariceal* injection.

7

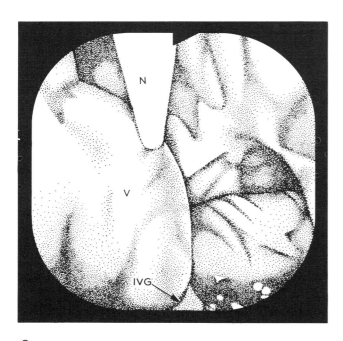

8

8

Successful intravariceal injection is recognized by a gentle distention of the varix (V), without the formation of a submucosal blister or obliteration of the intervariceal groove (IVG). Confirmation of the correct site of injection may be obtained under image-intensifier control, by the addition of contrast medium to the ethanolamine. A total of 2–3 ml of ethanolamine is injected into each varix.

9

Perivariceal injection of sclerosant occasionally occurs. While this probably also obliterates the varices, the higher incidence of complications makes this technique less favourable. Perivariceal injection may be recognized by the raising of a 'bleb' at the site of the injection, pallor of the oesophageal mucosa, obliteration of the intervariceal groove (IVG) and the absence of bleeding on withdrawal of the needle. Repeated perivariceal injection or the use of too much sclerosant will result in oesophageal ulceration and possible stricturing.

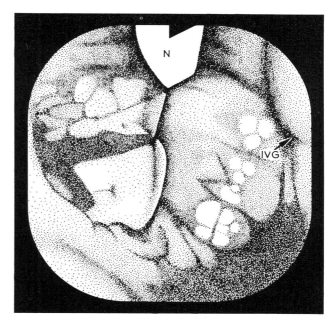

9

Postoperative management

1. The maintenance of balloon tamponade for 8–12 h is advisable after emergency injection of bleeding varices.
2. Small doses of intravenous diazepam are given for sedation and small doses of intravenous pentazocine are given for analgesia as necesary. The use of opiates is avoided. Mucaine is given for the retrosternal discomfort sometimes encountered following injection.
3. Attention must then be focused on all aspects of liver function. Lactulose is given by mouth (or down the Minnesota tube) to prevent encephalopathy after major haemorrhage. Accurate fluid balance with adequate blood replacement and correction of clotting abnormalities with vitamin K and fresh frozen plasma is essential. Ascites is treated as necessary by spironolactone.
4. The patient is entered into a programme of elective sclerotherapy at 3–4 week intervals until all the varices are obliterated.

References

Conn, H. O. (1974). Therapeutic portacaval anastomosis; to shunt or not to shunt. *Gastroenterology* **67**, 1065.

Crafoord, C. and Frenckner, P. (1939). New surgical treatment of varicose veins of the oesophagus. *Acta Oto-Laryngologica* **27**, 422.

MacBeth, D. (1966). Treatment of oesophageal varices in portal hypertension by means of sclerosing injections. *British Medical Journal* **2**, 877.

Palani, C. K., Abuabara, S., Kraft, A. R. and Jonasson, O. (1981). Endoscopic sclerotherapy in acute variceal hemorrhage. *American Journal of Surgery* **141**, 164.

Surgical techniques in the treatment of varicose veins

Sidney S. Rose   MB, ChB, FRCS

Consulting Surgeon, University Hospital of South Manchester, Withington Hospital, Manchester, UK

Introduction

The surgical treatment of varicose veins has in the past produced notoriously bad results, even in experienced hands. It is felt that this is due to the prevalence of the older concept of aetiology, namely that of primary valvular incompetence. This has led to concentration of operative techniques on proximal ligation of main stem superficial veins and/or ligation of incompetent deep perforators. Full-length stripping has had its advocates and been found wanting because of failure to remove varicose bunches. Our concept of the aetiology is somewhat different and has led us to adopt our present techniques.

We believe that the primary lesion is in the muscle and elastic layers of the vein wall where a degenerative fibrosis develops, producing dilatation not only of the vein wall in between the valves but of the valve ring itself where dilatation leads to secondary valvular incompetence because the valve cusps can no longer meet and eventually undergo disuse atrophy. This applies to both the superficial veins and the deep perforators.

The surgical treatment is therefore based on removal of the varicose veins themselves combined if necessary with proximal ligation at the main saphenofemoral or saphenopopliteal junction if incompetence exists at these points. We maintain that meticulous removal of the superficial varices renders it unnecessary to ligate deep perforators as most of the connections to the superficial veins will be interrupted by this procedure, and the veins into which they feed will be eliminated surgically.

Preoperative

Indications for surgery

Relief of symptoms

Varicose veins are often asymptomatic but the sensation of heaviness of the legs and chronic aching in the calves may be so severe as to require treatment. The other symptoms which cause patients to seek advice are night cramps, 'restless' legs, localized pain and tenderness over incompetent perforating veins, even in the absence of phlebitis. Itching and irritation of the overlying skin may occur. Any of these symptoms may be severe enough to require treatment by surgery.

To treat complications

The common complications are haematoma, even after slight trauma, haemorrhage which may be spontaneous or traumatic, eczema which may be local or generalized, recurrent superficial phlebitis, the development of subcutaneous and intradermal induration and varicose ulceration. Deep venous thrombosis may occur although the relationship to varicose veins is not as clear-cut as might be expected. Pulmonary embolism has also been recorded although it is probably related to a subclinical deep venous thrombosis. A history of any of the above complications is an indication for surgery, although an interval of 3 months should be allowed after an attack of superficial thrombophlebitis.

Cosmetic considerations

There is no doubt that varicose veins can be extremely ugly, both from a subjective and objective point of view. The development of a cosmetic procedure which also provides efficient and long-lasting relief justifies operating for cosmetic reasons.

Contraindications

1. Age and general condition. General condition is more important than age in this respect but it is obviously unwise and unnecessary to carry out operative procedures requiring long anaesthetics in the aged.
2. Obesity. This increases the hazards of any surgical procedure, and may produce special difficulties in removing varicose veins. This should be corrected if possible before proceeding.
3. Active superficial thrombophlebitis. This must always be controlled before embarking upon surgery for varicose veins.
4. Subcutaneous induration (lipodermatosclerosis). It is often impossible to remove veins from these areas. The local condition may be improved by support (firm bandaging or pressure-graded elastic stockings), elevation of the legs at night, calf muscle and ankle exercises, and stanozolol in acute cases. The feeding veins may then be dealt with by ligation, sclerotherapy, or a combination of the two.
5. Infected ulceration. The presence of an ulcer alone is not a contraindication to surgery provided it is clean, but infection must be treated first.
6. Pregnancy. It is inadvisable to operate during pregnancy and in any event many of the veins regress within 3 months of termination.
7. Arterial insufficiency. Peripheral pulses must always be recorded.
8. The presence of a large intra-abdominal tumour which may be the cause of venous back pressure and will require primary treatment.

Both the latter conditions will have been excluded by the preliminary examination.

Preoperative preparation

A pubic shave is only necessary where the groin is to be explored. The leg must be shaved, especially in men, and the patients are instructed to do this themselves before admission.

The veins are marked with the patient standing using a black or blue fine-point felt pen, the sites of maximum discomfort being marked with a circle, so that special attention may be given to the underlying vein. If the veins are extensive in one leg, both legs are not operated on unless the contralateral limb is only slightly involved. This is because an extensive procedure on both sides will hinder the postoperative walking ability, essential to avoid phlebitis, and will involve an unjustifiably long anaesthetic.

Anatomy

1

Normal distribution of main superficial veins of the lower limb with common sites of deep perforators (after *Gray's Anatomy*). A similar chart is used to record the distribution of the varicosities at the first examination.

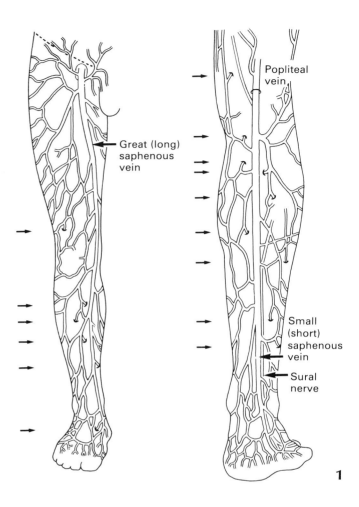

1

2

Normal anatomy of the saphenofemoral junction (after *Gray's Anatomy*). The position of the inguinal ligament is shown dotted, but this is not synonymous with the groin crease. This is usually lower than the inguinal ligament.

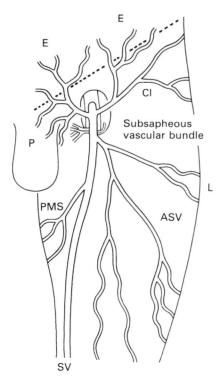

2

SV = long saphenous vein; ASV = anterior saphenous veins; PMS = posterior medial saphenous veins; P = superficial internal pudendal veins; E = superficial epigastric veins; CI = superficial circumflex iliac veins; L =

376

The operation

Position of patient

The patient is positioned on the table with a sandbag under the contralateral buttock to rotate the affected limb outwards to improve access to the groin, and this is further improved by having the knee moderately flexed.

Most aspects of the limb can be reached by judicious rotation but exploration of the saphenopopliteal junction and veins at the back of the thigh must be carried out with the patient in the prone position. If this is necessary, this part of the procedure is carried out first.

3

4

The groin incision

Exploration of the groin is indicated where there is a pronounced cough impulse at the groin on palpation. Reflux may be confirmed by Doppler examination. This may be confined to the immediate vicinity of the saphenofemoral junction or propagated down the leg in more advanced cases. The incision must be placed so that an adequate exposure of the saphenofemoral junction is obtained. Its position and length will be governed by the degree of obesity of the patient since the groin fold only approximates to the inguinal ligament when there is a minimum of subcutaneous fat. It will be appreciably lower in obese patients, in whom the incision needs to be above the groin crease. In any event, the incision is parallel to the inguinal ligament, using the femoral pulse as the lateral landmark, and will be on average 3.5–7 cm long.

3

The saphenous vein and its tributaries are identified by blunt dissection, remembering that it lies much more superficially in the male. The saphenofemoral junction must be clearly visualized before the clamps are applied, since considerable anatomical variation may occur. Two clamps are applied proximally and one distally and the vein is divided between them. It is safer to leave a small proximal stump than to carry out a flush ligation, because if a clamp slips it can be picked up without difficulty. A short stump cannot be the site of significant thrombus formation. The tributaries are divided and ligated as the saphenous vein is mobilized.

4

The saphenous vein is ligated with No. 1 linen thread and the most proximal clamp is removed.

A second ligature of 2/0 linen thread is placed above the second proximal clamp which is then removed.

In cases where there is no downward propagation of the cough impulse, ligation of the distal end with 2/0 linen thread completes the groin operation. The rest of the operation is then completed by multiple removal of the varicosities by the technique described below (*see Illustrations 11–16*).

Where the impulse is propagated down the leg, limited stripping of the long saphenous vein is indicated and is carried out as follows.

Limited stripping of long saphenous vein

5

The stripper is inserted into the distal end of the saphenous vein. Mosquito forceps are applied as shown to make this easier.

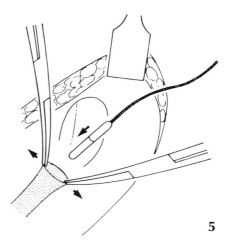

5

6

The vein is tied round the stripper head with 1/0 linen thread, leaving one end of the thread long enough to follow the stripper all the way down to the lowest point of the strip. Alternatively, the acorn of the stripper is drilled and the long end of the thread is tied through the hole. This prevents the stripper angling at the junction with the acorn when it is drawn upwards (*b*). The end of the thread is secured with an arterial clamp.

6

7

The lower end of the stripper is identified by palpation and the vein is dissected out through a small transverse incision using curved mosquito forceps. The vein is doubly clamped and the tip of the stripper is drawn out through a small incision in the vein just above the proximal clamp.

7

8 & 9

The vein is divided between the clamps and the stripper is now pulled gently downwards keeping the proximal retaining thread taut until the head of the stripper is just above the lower incision. The end of the vein is freed by traction on the retaining forceps which is now removed.

10

The vein is then removed by upward traction on the retaining thread so that the head of the stripper is removed through the groin incision, thus avoiding enlarging the incision at the lower end in order to pull the head through.

Firm pressure is applied over the whole length of the stripped channel for a few minutes to prevent haematoma formation. This part of the operation is not completed by removing the lower end of the saphenous vein by firm traction until it breaks in the manner shown in *Illustration 14.* Haemostasis is again secured by firm pressure.

This method of stripping ensures that only the incompetent saphenous vein is removed and incidentally avoids damage to the saphenous nerve at the ankle – a frequent cause of lingering postoperative discomfort.

Routine orthograde stripping has been abandoned in favour of this technique, since not only does that method endanger the saphenous nerve but it often removes long lengths of normal saphenous vein which should be preserved whenever possible.

Multiple excision of varicose veins

11

Multiple tiny (2–3 mm) transverse incisions are made over the previously marked veins, at such intervals that the maximum length of vein can be removed through the minimum number of incisions. The number will be dictated by the size and the fragility of the veins and by familiarity with the technique. Formerly, an 11-blade was used to make the incisions, but a No. 65 Beaver blade and handle have made appreciably smaller incisions possible. Once all the incisions are made, the marking ink is rubbed off with spirit to avoid tatooing of the scars.

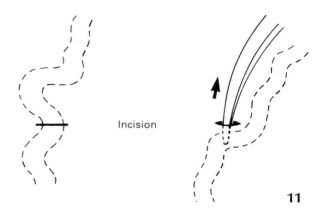

11

12

Using small curved mosquito forceps, a loop of vein is drawn out through the incision.

12

13

The vein is now divided between the forceps and each end is 'winkled out' in turn by firm but gentle traction.

13

14

The vein is always pulled in the direction shown and never across the incision, which would otherwise become enlarged. Heavier curved forceps (Cairns) should be used to apply traction as the broader grip will prevent the vein from breaking prematurely. Sometimes a deep perforator will come into view if traction continues, and it may be grasped and broken by traction in the usual way. No ligatures are required.

14

15

Haemostasis is secured by firm pressure over each incision as before while the next incision is being explored.

Skin sutures are not necessary and the tiny incisions are sealed with Steristrips reinforced with a plastic spray (Rikospray) and a gauze roll is applied from foot to groin with the limb elevated.

Firm pressure is maintained by the application of Gamgee pads to include all the operated areas. The limb is firmly bandaged from foot to groin using 15-cm crêpe bandages.

In patients over 50 years of age, 1 u of Rheomacrodex 40 is given at the end of the operation to minimize the possibility of postoperative venous thrombosis.

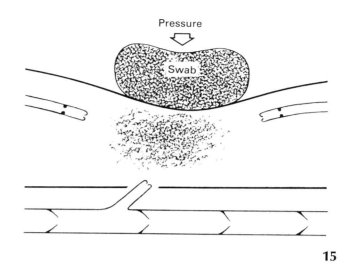

15

Postoperative care

The limb remains elevated for 8 h postoperatively and this is followed by immediate brisk ambulation. The patient may be treated as a day case but if the procedure has been extensive an overnight stay is advisable. The limb is rebandaged firmly before discharge after the Gamgee pads are removed. This encourages freer movement of the leg and allows the patient to undertake brisk walking exercise. They are advised to do this for 10 min at a time, at least six times a day, for the first 2 postoperative weeks. This is preferable to recommending long time-consuming walks of 5–8 km (3–5 miles) and is more likely to be carried out conscientiously.

The patient takes a full bath on the 7th postoperative day and the strips come off with each succeeding bath. A firm tubular bandage support should be worn for a further 4 weeks. The pressure helps to accelerate healing. A postoperative instruction sheet is given to the patient as an *aide-mémoire*. The multiple avulsion technique may be carried out under a local anaesthetic as an out-patient procedure, thus saving hospital beds. The average patient is able to tolerate as many as 15 incisions without difficulty and follows substantially the same postoperative regime.

Operative treatment of varicose veins with tourniquet

John P. Royle   MB BS, BS, FRCS(Ed), FRCS, FRACS, FACS
Director of Vascular Surgery Unit, Austin Hospital, Heidelberg, Australia;
Senior Associate, University of Melbourne, Australia;
Consultant Vascular Surgeon, Fairfield Hospital, Melbourne, Australia

Introduction

1a & b

The preoperative assessment of a patient with varicose veins should include Doppler evaluation of the saphenofemoral and saphenopopliteal junctions. These should not be ligated as a routine, but their ligation is required when reflux is present. Clinical examination, particularly in obese patients, often fails to reveal any abnormality at these sites, but such abnormality is revealed with ease by a Doppler (Chan, Chisholm and Royle, 1983).

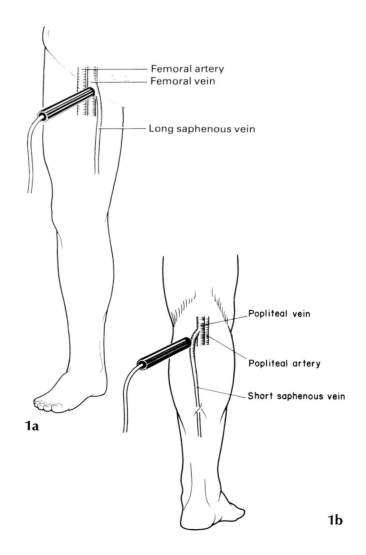

Femoral artery
Femoral vein
Long saphenous vein
Popliteal vein
Popliteal artery
Short saphenous vein

1a

1b

2a & b

Marking the veins

Very careful preoperative marking of the varices is performed with the patient in a standing position in a good light. All visible varices are marked and in particular the most superficial portions of the varices are marked clearly (these will be the sites for subsequent stab avulsion). The obvious normal veins on the dorsum of the foot are not marked for removal, but genuine varices on the dorsum of the foot are so marked.

2a   **2b**

Long saphenous vein

3

Skin incision

The groin incision should be made directly over the saphenofemoral junction, i.e. *above* the groin skin crease. The incision is made in a line parallel to the skin crease centred over a point 1 cm medial to the femoral pulse and 1 cm distal to the line of the pubic tubercle. Except in obese patients, the incision does not need to exceed 4 cm. A small self-retaining retractor is inserted to spread the skin edges apart. The fat separates easily, revealing Scarpa's fascia.

- Femoral artery
- Femoral vein
- Pubic tubercle
- Skin incision
- Long saphenous vein

3

4

Scarpa's fascia

The incision is deepened through Scarpa's fascia and the self-retaining retractor is placed in a deeper plane to spread this layer. At this stage the long saphenous vein is usually visible. The vein is grasped with forceps and gently pulled outwards.

5

7

6

Saphenofemoral junction

The junction of the long saphenous vein with the femoral vein must be clearly identified before the saphenous vein is divided. The junction on the medial side must be carefully inspected, along with the medial aspect of the femoral vein at this point to check for the point of entry of the deep external pudendal vein. This may enter the long saphenous vein itself, the junction of the long saphenous vein and the femoral vein, or the femoral vein itself (as illustrated). It should be ligated and divided (Royle, Eisner and Fell, 1981).

5

Division of tributaries

Thereafter dissection takes place in the immediate perivenous plane. The plane immediately alongside the vein is avascular and consists only of loose areolar tissue. The tributaries of the terminal portion of the long saphenous vein are all identified at the site where they drain into the long saphenous vein and pass across this loose areolar tissue. They are ligated and divided.

Deep external pudendal vein

Femoral vein
Long saphenous vein

6

7

Flush ligation

The long saphenous vein is divided some 2 cm from the junction, and is then transfixed and tied. To provide a flush ligation, the needle of the transfixion suture enters the long saphenous vein one-half of the diameter of the long saphenous vein away from the saphenofemoral junction. The ligature is then tied, looped around the vein and tied again. The transfixion suture will then lie flush with the femoral vein, and constriction of the femoral vein by the suture is avoided.

8

Long saphenous vein removal

When it is intended to remove the long saphenous vein, traction is applied to its cut end, so that the vein can be identified farther down the leg. A small incision is made with a No. 11 blade over the long saphenous vein, the vein is grasped with toothed mosquito forceps and extracted through the wound. The vein is removed down the leg by similar traction, identification, stab incision and extraction (as described below).

Groin wound closure

The orifice left by the removal of the long saphenous vein is closed over. This prevents any haematoma from passing up to the groin wound. The subcutaneous tissue in the groin is approximated with an absorbable deep suture. The skin is closed with a subcuticular absorbable suture. The wound edges are infiltrated with 0.5% Bupivacaine HCl local anaesthetic solution. There is then little discomfort in the leg for some hours (but even when multiple varicose tributaries are also removed through stab incisions as in *Illustrations 9–16*).

8

Varicose tributaries

Thigh veins are approached in the following manner.

9

A small stab incision 3 mm long is made directly over the vein in the long axis of the limb and passing through the dermis only. A pair of toothed mosquito forceps (shown magnified) is passed through the incision and the underlying vein grasped.

9

10

The grasped vein is pulled to the surface and the toothed forceps are replaced by stronger artery forceps.

10

11

The vein is pulled further until it emerges as a loop. A pair of forceps is placed on each limb of the loop.

11

12

Taking one limb of the loop at a time, the vein is pulled gently.

12

13

As it emerges through the skin, the vein is grasped with another pair of forceps near the skin and pulled farther, a new pair of forceps being placed on nearer the skin as every 2 cm or so is extracted.

13

14

This process is continued until the vein breaks off. A new incision is then made farther down the marked vein to pick up the vein again. In this manner the whole of the superficial varicosity is removed.

14

15 & 16

Tourniquet

When sufficient thigh veins have been dealt with so that a tourniquet can be positioned higher than all the remaining veins, an Esmarch's bandage is applied from medial malleolus to thigh. The upper turns are used on the thigh as a tourniquet and the lower turns are then removed. After application of the tourniquet, the remainder of the varices in the leg are removed from the now avascular field through multiple small stab incisions as described above (*see Illustrations 9–14*).

15

16

17

Wound dressings

The incisions are *not sutured*; they are dressed with tulle gras, gauze, cotton wool and a crêpe bandage. The bandage must be firm enough to occlude the surface veins, as no venous connections have been ligated except in the groin incision. The wounds distal to the tourniquet are dressed and bandaged while the tourniquet is still in place. The tourniquet is removed and any thigh wounds are then dressed and bandaged. If any bloody ooze comes through the bandages after removal of the tourniquet, an extra, firmer crêpe bandage is applied over the top of the original bandage.

17

Short saphenous vein

18

Venography

When the Doppler has shown saphenopopliteal incompetence, after induction of anaesthesia, a venogram is taken to locate accurately the saphenopopliteal junction, the position of which is quite variable. The skin crease is marked with a radiopaque marker (a needle will do for this). The venogram will also confirm whether the reflux heard with the Doppler has been from the saphenopopliteal junction or from a communication with the long saphenous vein (when saphenopopliteal ligation would be unnecessary) (Hoare and Royle, 1984).

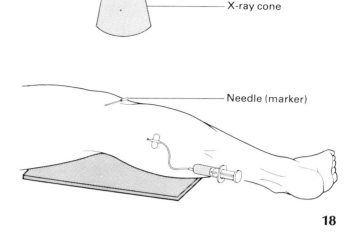

18

Saphenopopliteal ligation

When only the short saphenous vein is abnormal, the patient may be placed in the prone position and an Esmarch's tourniquet applied. When the saphenopopliteal junction is being ligated as part of a more generalized operation on other veins, the flush ligation of the saphenopopliteal junction is usually delayed until after the tourniquet has been applied and all the superficial varices have been removed by stab avulsions as described above (*see Illustrations 9–14*). In these circumstances the patient is turned on his side.

19

19

The skin incision is made transversely at the level indicated by venography and a small self-retaining retractor is inserted to separate the skin. The fat usually parts to reveal the deep fascia.

20

The deep fascia is opened transversely in the line of its fibres. The short saphenous vein can then usually be seen easily.

The short saphenous vein is grasped with forceps and dissection is conducted in the immediate perivenous avascular plane.

The vein that passes upwards from the short saphenous vein to form the posteromedial vein of the thigh is ligated and divided. Gastrocnemius veins joining the incompetent short saphenous vein are ligated and divided. The dissection of the short saphenous vein is continued down to the saphenopopliteal junction.

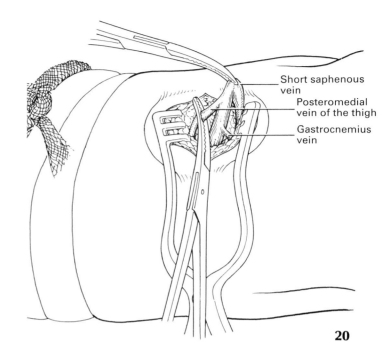

Short saphenous vein

Posteromedial vein of the thigh

Gastrocnemius vein

20

21

21

Flush ligation

A transfixion flush ligation is performed as described for the saphenofemoral junction, with the needle passing through the saphenous vein one-half of the diameter away from the popliteal vein in order to produce a flush ligation without constriction.

Short saphenous vein removal

The short saphenous vein can be removed by putting tension on the vein and locating it at a lower level through small stab incisions as described for long saphenous vein removal (*see Illustration 8*). More often just the ligation and excision of the length of short saphenous vein in the wound itself is performed. This lessens the incidence of sural nerve hyperaesthesia and anaesthesia postoperatively. The fascia is closed with an absorbable deep suture. The skin is closed with a subcuticular absorbable suture. The wound edges are infiltrated with 0.5% Bupivacaine HCl local anaesthetic solution as for a groin wound.

Postoperative management

The patient is returned to the ward with the foot of the bed elevated. Narcotic analgesia is seldom necessary. The patient is ambulated later the same day. If there is any bloody ooze through the bandage, an extra, reinforcing bandage is applied. The patient leaves hospital later the same day or on the following day.

The bandages and dressing are left in place for 5–7 days and then removed. After removal of the dressings, occasionally one or two of the stab wounds may not be quite healed and a small dressing may be used over such wounds for several days.

Because the wounds have not been sutured the scars tend to be more prominent than usual for the first few weeks after surgery. However, the cosmetic result after 6 months is generally better when the wounds have not been sutured than when they have been.

References

Chan, A., Chisholm, I and Royle, J. P. (1983). The use of directional Doppler ultrasound in the assessment of saphenofemoral incompetence. *Australian and New Zealand Journal of Surgery* 53, 399.

Hoare, M. C. and Royle, J. P. (1984). Doppler ultrasound detection of saphenofemoral and saphenopopliteal incompetence and operative venography to ensure precise saphenopopliteal ligation. *Australian and New Zealand Journal of Surgery* 54.

Royle, J. P., Eisner, R. and Fell, G. (1981). The saphenofemoral junction. *Surgery, Gynecology and Obstetrics* 152, 282.

Ligation of perforating veins

F. B. Cockett MS, FRCS

Consulting Surgeon, St Thomas's Hospital, London, UK

Introduction

The perforating veins referred to here are the so-called 'direct' perforators – defined as those veins which perforate the *deep fascia* of the limb to enter directly into a main deep vein (such as the femoral or posterior tibial). These veins are few in number and in definite regular anatomical sites. The termination of the long saphenous vein at the groin and of the short saphenous vein in the popliteal vein behind the knee are the two most well-known perforator sites. There is also the 'Hunterian' or mid-thigh perforator.

This chapter deals with the important direct perforators in the lower half of the leg, which normally drain the venous blood from the subcutaneous tissue and skin of the ankle directly into the posterior tibial and peroneal veins.

1

On the inner side of the limb there are two main direct perforating veins (2) emerging from holes in the deep fascia. They are situated behind the long saphenous vein (1). The upper one is approximately halfway up the leg. The lower one is four fingers' breadth above the medial malleolus. Note that the perforating veins communicate by fine venous arches, and with the long saphenous vein by a large constant posterior arch vein (3) arising at knee level.

On the outer side of the limb there is only one constant large perforator (5) which communicates directly with the short saphenous vein (4). Much less constant is the so-called midcalf perforating vein (6) emerging close to the insertion of the gastrocnemius into the soleus tendon. When present, however, it is often large and important.

1

2

Clinically, these perforators are easily located by the 'hand's breadth' rule. In other words, the perforating veins on the medial aspect are separated by approximately the breadth of a hand as shown.

2

3

In the normal erect exercising limb, very high pressure (about 100 mmHg) develops in the deep calf veins during the contraction phase of the calf muscles. Blood is normally prevented from leaking out into the skin and subcutaneous tissue by the valve in the perforating vein, but when this valve is destroyed or becomes incompetent for any reason, the high pressure is exerted directly on to the fine mesh veins on the inner side of the ankle. These veins dilate rapidly, giving rise to the typical and important sign called 'ankle flare'. This process eventually leads to sclerosis and skin destruction – the lesion we know as a venous ulcer.

Normal   *Perforator leak established*   3

Essential diagnostic points

There are three distinct groups of cases in which incompetent ankle perforators occur. In the first two groups, they are the main cause of the steady deterioration of the ankle skin and subcutaneous tissues which leads eventually to venous ulceration.

4

Group 1: Incompetent ankle perforators occurring as a late complication of primary varicose veins

In many longstanding cases of primary hereditary long saphenous incompetence, as the varicose veins of the posterior arch branch become bigger and more prominent, they connect with and drain into a competent medial ankle perforator. This competent perforator 'drains off into the deep veins', the high pressure coming down the long saphenous system, and thus protects the ankle skin. However, in many cases, as time goes on, the ankle perforator enlarges and its valve is either destroyed or becomes inefficient. When this occurs a massive venous hypertension from the perforator is added to that coming down the saphenous system, and rapid deterioration of the ankle occurs, leading to ulcer (hence the old name, 'varicose ulcer').

These cases are fairly common, and give the best results after long saphenous ligation and stripping, combined with ankle perforator exposure and ligation. In this group, associated varicose veins will be seen and should be marked as they must be dealt with when the perforating veins are tied.

4

5

Group 2: Incompetent ankle perforators occurring late (2–5 years) after an acute venous thrombosis of the peripheral type

In this type, the thrombosis starts deep in the calf, either in the calf sinusoids or in the posterior tibial or peroneal veins. It spreads upwards into popliteal or femoral veins, but rarely higher. Usually, the clot spreads into the perforator up to its valve. During the recanalization phase the valve is destroyed and a 'perforator leak' is established. This causes swelling, venular dilatation, sclerosis and pigmentation of the ankle (the classic post-thrombotic syndrome), eventually leading to ulcer.

Often, in these cases, there is a remarkable degree of recanalization of the main deep veins in the post-thrombic phase. Also in the profunda vein and its branches there is usually an efficient collateral channel from the lower leg, so that there is often very minimal deep vein obstruction after a peripheral type of thrombosis, leaving the incompetent perforator as the main lesion responsible for the ankle ulcer. It is essential to discover any past history of possible deep vein thrombosis in order to recognize this state of affairs, because it implies that the only surgery required is ligation of these perforating veins.

Acute thrombosis　　　*Post-thrombotic phase (2–5 years later)*　**5**

6

Group 3: Incompetent ankle perforators occurring after a patient has had a proximal or iliofemoral type of thrombosis

In these cases the thrombosis starts in the iliac vein segment; usually, patients are young and have the developmental anomaly known as the 'iliac compression syndrome'. The left iliac vein is partly (or sometimes wholly) obstructed by the right common artery passing over it and compressing it against the promontory of the sacrum. When this partly obstructed left iliac vein thromboses, the thrombosis usually spreads down to the groin. After this resolves and attempts recanalization, the patient is left with an obstructed iliac vein, but a *normal* calf pump and perforators.

Occasionally, the thrombus extends peripherally right back into the calf, producing a very severe clinical picture (phlegmasia caerulae dolens). When this resolves and recanalizes, there may be extensive deep vein obstruction *plus* incompetent ankle perforators. These patients develop the worst and most intractable ulcers and even though incompetent perforating veins are detected, ligation in this situation gives poor results, because the venous hypertension due to obstructed deep veins is unrelieved. More frequently, venous reconstructive surgery is required.

Acute iliofemoral thrombosis

Possible incompetent perforator

Post-thrombotic phase

6

Preoperative preparation

If there is an open ulcer, active eczema or swelling, this should be first brought under control by a period of rest with elevation of the leg. This means the ankle must be above the level of the heart, so that 'sitting up in bed' is not allowed. With this simple antigravity treatment all ulcers and eczemas rapidly improve and start healing. If there is a chronic open ulcer or infected eczema, a culture should be taken and the patient put on a potent oral antistaphylococcal antibiotic (erythromycin stearate 0.5 g four times a day is the author's choice). If the *Staphylococcus* is resistant, flucloxacillin may be needed.

Ideally, this ulcer or eczema may be simply cleaned with saline and then dried and left open to the air, or lightly covered with a layer of plain unmedicated gauze. On no account should local lotions, creams or antibiotic ointments or any medicated type of paraffin gauze be used in the vicinity of the ulcer, as these can produce or perpetuate contact allergic eczema.

After 2 or 3 days of this treatment the operation may be done even in the presence of an open ulcer, provided it is in the healing phase.

The operation

The operation, which may be either extrafascial or subfascial, is performed in a cool operating theatre. The foot of the table is elevated and the patient is placed on his back and the knee slightly flexed. Halothane anaesthesia is best avoided because it causes vasodilatation and unnecessary profuse bleeding.

The extrafascial operation

7

When the subcutaneous tissues are in good condition, freely mobile and contain obviously palpable masses of veins, the extrafascial approach is used. The incision for full exploration is a straight line from about halfway up the leg to a point just *above* and *behind* the medial malleolus. This is the direct line of emergence of the medial ankle perforators from their holes in the deep fascia.

7

8

The knife is carried cleanly down to the deep fascia and if necessary any ulcer is excised.

8

9

The subcutaneous tissues are swept aside laterally by gauze pledget dissection *right down on the deep fascia*. This layer is important, because if sharp lateral dissection is carried out in the subcutaneous plane, the arterial supply of the skin flaps is impaired and skin necrosis may occur.

The middle and upper medial ankle perforators are ligated with fine plain catgut just at their emergence from the foramina in the fascia. All large varicose veins in the subcutaneous tissue in their vicinity are then also pulled out causing as little trauma to the subcutaneous tissues as possible.

Under the anterior flap the long saphenous vein can be identified and this may be stripped also from the groin if it is enlarged and incompetent as described in the chapter on 'Surgical techniques in the treatment of varicose veins'.

9

The subfascial operation

This approach, first described by Linton (1953), is preferred in the more advanced stage of the post-thrombotic syndrome, when the subcutaneous tissues of the leg are indurated and fibrotic.

10

The incision may be the same as for the extrafascial operation, or it may be slightly posterior to avoid an ulcerated area. Sometimes it is best to excise an ulcerated area altogether, down to the deep fascia. This is then later grafted with a split-skin graft.

10

11

11

The knife is carried straight down through the deep fascia to expose the muscle beneath. The deep fascia of the anterior flap is lifted up with artery forceps and the perforating veins are sought as they pass straight from the posterior tibial veins to the hole on the deep surface of the fascia. The perforators are ligated in this plane with fine plain catgut. Non-absorbable sutures such as silk or linen should never be used as they cause sinuses. In the deep subfascial plane, wide lateral and medial dissection and exploration can be done without jeopardizing the blood supply of the skin.

12

Closure

In the extrafascial operation there is seldom any difficulty. The author uses fine silk sutures for the skin only. It is extremely important not to tie these sutures too tightly (just tightly enough for skin apposition and no more) because this part of the ankle is susceptible to skin necrosis if there is incorrect and rough manipulation of subcutaneous tissues and the use of tight skin sutures with wide bites.

There is often more difficulty in closing the skin after a subfascial operation on an indurated ankle. Here, a few fine catgut sutures may be placed in the fascial layer to aid apposition, and fine silk stitches, without tension, used for the skin.

12

13

13

If the skin cannot be closed without tension, it is best to leave the whole wound open. This relieves the tourniquet effect of the tight fibrous tissue round the ankle. A dressing and bandage are applied, and after about 5 days when granulation tissue is forming a long split-skin 'gusset' graft is laid on the wound. The leg is again dressed and a firm circumflex crêpe bandage applied. After about 10 days to 2 weeks in elevation the graft will be firm and graduated walking with good supporting bandages can be started. The late results of this sort of case are extremely gratifying!

Lateral perforating veins

When they are prominent and there is evidence of their incompetence (distended veins and venules on the back and *lateral* side of the ankle, often in communication with an incompetent *short* saphenous vein), the lateral and mid-calf perforators may be approached and ligated by short vertical incisions over them. Incompetence is much less common in the lateral perforating veins than in the medial ankle perforators.

Variants of the subfascial operation

14

Mid-calf 'stocking seam' incision

This incision goes straight down through the deep fascia and allows wide dissection on both sides of the flap. Both lateral and medial perforators can be reached with some difficulty through this incision.

However, the scar is long and rather prominent on the back of the calf, and therefore not very popular in female patients.

14

15

15

Use of the Edwards' blunt dissector or 'phlebotome' (Edwards, 1976)

The instrument is inserted through a small horizontal incision just below the knee and pushed down deep to the deep fascia to sheer off the perforators blindly. The advantage of this method is that no incision near the poor skin of the ankle is needed. However, it tends to miss the upper medial ankle perforator, and often there is 'profuse bleeding'.

Postoperative care

A dry gauze dressing is placed over the wound, and a firm circumflex crêpe pressure bandage from toes to just above the knee is applied. For about a week the patient should rest with the foot of the bed elevated and no more than two or three pillows (so that the leg is just above heart level). During this time the patient should be up for active walking periods three or four times a day, and even in bed should be encouraged to move the ankle and knee frequently. Stitches are removed on about the 7th–9th day, according to the magnitude of the operation.

After about a week the patient should be fully ambulatory at home but should wear strong elastic webbing supporting bandages all the time he is up, for at least a month.

After this, bandages can be discarded altogether or a below-knee firm elastic stocking substituted. Permanent firm support is particularly needed in the group 3 cases mentioned previously.

References

Cockett, F. B. (1955). Surgery of venous ulcers. *British Journal of Surgery* **43**, 179.

Cockett, F. B. and Jones, D. E. (1953). Ankle blow-out syndrome. *Lancet* **1**, 17.

Cockett, F. B., Lea Thomas, M. and Negus, D. (1967). Iliac vein compression – its relation to iliofemoral thrombosis and the post-thrombotic syndrome. *British Medical Journal* **2,** 14.

Dodd, H., and Cockett, F. B. (1976). *Pathology and Surgery of the Veins of the Lower Limb*, 2nd ed. Edinburgh: Churchill-Livingstone

Edwards, J. M. (1976). Sherry operation for incompetent perforating veins. *British Journal of Surgery* **63**, 885.

Linton, R. R. (1953). *Annals of Surgery* **138**, 415

Negus, D. and Friedgood, A. (1983). Effective management of venous ulceration. *British Journal of Surgery* **70**, 623.

Venous reconstructive surgery

John J. Bergan MD
Clinical Professor of Surgery, University of California, San Diego, California, USA;
Magerstadt Professor Emeritus of Surgery, Northwestern University Medical School, Chicago, Illinois, USA

James S. T. Yao MD, PhD
Professor of Surgery and Director, Blood Flow Laboratory, Northwestern University Medical School, Chicago, Illinois, USA

Introduction

Direct surgery of veins has lagged behind direct arterialization of the extremities and viscera partly because surgeons have been more fascinated with the drama of cardiac and arterial surgery and partly because of the genuine difficulties which attend venous reconstruction and anastomosis. The standard operations with expected good results are bypasses of venous obstruction. Kistner has been successful with valveplasty (Ferris and Kistner, 1982), but others have found it to be a technically difficult procedure (Sottiurai, 1988). Kistner's technique of segment transfer is less demanding and enables venous flow to be directed through competent valves; unfortunately, it is applicable to a very small number of patients. The procedure championed by Taheri, Lazar and Alias (1982) of transplantation of valve-containing venous segments must await long-term evaluation before it is considered acceptable. Free-segment venous transfer must also be regarded as experimental. This chapter presents our current techniques of direct venous reconstruction.

Femorofemoral cross-over grafts

1 & 2

In this procedure, the saphenous vein is used as a conduit to bypass contralateral common and external iliac venous occlusion. Exposure is gained through vertical incisions over the femoral veins; one-third of the incision extends above the inguinal ligament. The saphenous vein is removed from the thigh under direct vision, through multiple, discontinuous incisions. Preparation of the graft must be meticulous to avoid venous trauma. As much adventitia as possible is carefully removed to allow maximum venous dilation. All tributary veins are ligated and divided at least 2 mm from the main trunk, in order to avoid constriction of the trunk during dilation. The graft is gently distended with heparinized saline solution to check for inadvertent tears or leaks. Localized varicosities, if present, must be dealt with either by resection or external support using normal vein tissue as recommended by Palma (1976).

The junction of the saphenous vein with the femoral vein is left intact. The superficial epigastric and external pudendal tributaries must be maintained so that angulation of the saphenofemoral junction is prevented.

The tunnel is made deeply, but subcutaneously, in the suprapubic region by digital dissection. The saphenous vein is passed through the tunnel using a long vascular clamp. Twisting of the vessel must be avoided. If possible, the graft should gradually curve into Scarpa's triangle on the affected side, and if necessary the vein can be stitched to the deep fascia using adventitial stitches.

The anastomosis should be 2–3 cm in length. It can be made to the saphenous vein on the affected side, but is best made to the common femoral vein, if possible. The venous intima should not be traumatized.

1

2

3a & b

Illustration 3(a) shows the orientation of the structures after mobilization. Atraumatic clamps, as shown here, or siliconized rubber slings can be used for venous occlusion. *Illustration 3(b)* indicates the anastomotic technique, with careful atraumatic eversion of the venous edges and approximation with 6/0 or 7/0 monofilament suture.

The wounds are closed in several layers to obliterate dead space. On our service, the arteriovenous fistula has been abandoned; instead, intermittent calf compression boots are applied using a 15-second on-cycle and 45-second off-cycle. Anticoagulants are not used.

Late results of the procedure are comparatively good. Harris *et al.* (1988), reporting from Sydney, Australia, described a 17-year experience, ending in 1982, involving 40 cross-saphenous bypasses. The cross-over bypass graft managed symptoms in all patients, except two who required some distal reconstructive or ablative surgery. There were five late deaths, all unrelated to venous disease; three patients were lost to follow-up. The 5-year cumulative patency rate was 83%, but this was based on clinical judgement only. It is known that 8 of the 41 grafts have occluded. In this study, 11 patients had surgical interruption of perforating veins or removal of distal varicosities, either concomitantly (8) or following the bypass (3). The remaining 28 patients constituted a follow-up group: 11 have normal legs, 9 confirmed by photoplethysmography (PPG), and 9 have residual calf symptoms controlled with stocking support. Only one patient has had recurrent ulcerations. The eight patients with occluded grafts continue to have swelling, pigmentation and ulceration of the affected limb.

Saphenopopliteal bypass

When deep venous thrombosis of the superficial femoral vein is poorly recanalized, severe distal venous stasis may appear. When wearing of supportive bandages or well-fitted elastic stockings does not relieve stasis symptoms, direct surgical bypass of the obstruction is required. The calf muscle pump is relatively ineffective when working below an obstruction, and the long saphenous vein is inefficient because it is not connected to the muscle pump mechanism. Therefore, the objective of the operation is to provide a conduit to connect the deep venous system of the calf with a patent proximal venous pool.

In the United States, first Warren (Warren and Thayer, 1954), and then Husni (1970) performed saphenopopliteal bypass. May (1979), in Innsbruck, also advocated this procedure. In 50% of Warren's patients, the saphenous vein was transplanted deep to the sartorius muscle.

As time has passed, we have become increasingly disappointed with this procedure.

For this procedure the poorly recanalized venous segment must be confined to the superficial femoral vein, the iliac system being spared, and the saphenous vein must be of good calibre preferably with functioning valves and no varicosities.

Careful ascending venography should show at least the distal half of the popliteal vein to be completely patent. There should be no evidence of smouldering, sub-acute venous thrombosis, as this will cause the procedure to fail.

3a

3b

Operative procedure

4

The patient lies supine on the operating table, with the leg slightly externally rotated and the knee moderately flexed. An incision is made parallel to the tibia, distal to its crest. The vein is marked prior to the operation, so that the skin incision can be made directly over it. The saphenous vein is mobilized and transected 2–3 cm distal to the distal end of the operative incision. The deep fasica is divided. The medial head of the gastrocnemius muscle is retracted medially. The soleus is exposed. The popliteal vein may be doubled, but the larger portion will lie posterior to the artery, with the anterior tibial veins crossing that structure.

Additional exposure can be gained by cutting the semitendinosus and semimembranosus muscles. These do not have to be repaired.

Once an adequate segment of vein for anastomosis has been mobilized, attention is turned to the anteromedial aspect of the thigh. A 6-cm incision is made at the junction of the middle and distal thirds of the thigh and is carried through the deep fascia, displacing the sartorius posteriorly and incising the fascia over the popliteal space. A tunnel is made between the thigh and calf wounds, so that the mobilized saphenous vein can be inserted parallel to the popliteal vessels from above downward and thus lie in a gentle curve in the thigh, without tension behind the knee joint.

The leg is extended to make sure that the saphenous vein is of adequate length, and a site is chosen for the distal anastomosis. Thin, siliconized vessel loops are used to encircle the popliteal vein. A venotomy is created, and the venotomy and the distal end of the saphenous vein are irrigated with heparinized saline solution. The distal end of the saphenous vein is fishmouthed to conform exactly to the venotomy in the popliteal vein. A long anastomosis, 1.5 cm in length, is then made using 6/0 or 7/0 monofilament polypropylene suture.

Following the attainment of haemostasis, the wounds are closed, leaving the fascia open, both in the calf and in the thigh. The skin is approximated with synthetic, absorbable intradermal suture. Suction drainage may be used, but an arteriovenous fistula is not created.

Postoperatively, the patient is not anticoagulated but may receive 500 ml of 10% Rheomacrodex each day for the first 5 days. An intermittent compression pump is applied to the calf, with a cycle of 15 seconds on, 45 seconds off.

The patency of the anastomosis is monitored by the transcutaneous Doppler technique.

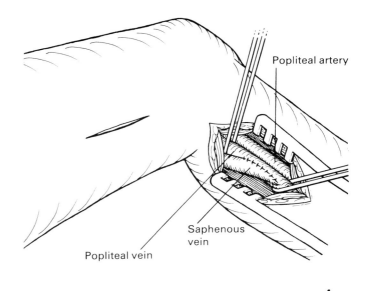

4

Prostheses in venous reconstruction

Anecdotal reports have been received about the use of polytetrafluoroethylene (PTFE) grafts in the cross-over femorofemoral position. None of these has been successful below the femoral vein.

Investigators using prosthetic grafts have been encouraged by experimental models which have used short-segment venous interposition grafts in the portal and vena caval systems, yet the clinical application of PTFE has been limited. There are reports of successful cross-over grafts (Clowes, 1980), but these are few, and the operation should be applied with great caution.

As externally reinforced grafts have become available, they have been used clinically although, admittedly, in situations of great difficulty. A 1983 report from Japan (Takaba et al., 1983) included a follow-up of 3–15 months in five patients requiring such femorofemoral cross-over grafts. The grafts used were 16, 12, 8 and 6 mm, the last two being externally reinforced.

Direct venous valve surgery

Operations to correct valvular incompetence include direct valvuloplasty, transposition of the venous stream through a competent valve system, and valve transplantation.

Valvuloplasty, as invented by Kistner (Ferris and Kistner, 1982), can be a technically difficult operation. It is performed under magnification, using a 7/0 to 9/0 sutures. It is used in patients who have demonstrated a grossly incompetent superficial femoral valve, through which retrograde flow is visualized on descending venography.

5a, b & c

The femoral vein is exposed through a linear incision extending from the inguinal ligament. After complete mobilization of the superficial femoral vein, the anterior aspect is studied carefully, so that the incision in the vein can be made from below upward exactly through the valve commissure. It is very easy to carry the incision through a valve cusp and destroy the valvuloplasty operation.

6a, b & c

It is essential not to tear the valve cusp while sutures are being placed, and the reefing sutures must be placed precisely, in order to shorten the valve cusp but not excessively.

The venotomy may be closed from above downward to test the competence of the valve under direct vision. A dental mirror may be inserted into the venotomy to check the status of the reconstruction further or, alternatively, as the venotomy is being created from below upward, to assist in placing the venotomy precisely through the valve commissure (Samuels, P., 1983, personal communication).

5a

5b

5c

6a

6b

6c

Transposition of the venous stream

7a, b & c

Kistner made a second major contribution to direct venous surgery by inventing the procedure of transposition of the venous stream through a demonstrably competent valve. He has called this redirection of venous flow through competent proximal valves the 'segment transfer operation'.

In this procedure, competent valves are identified in the profunda femoris vein, the saphenous vein or the superficial femoral vein by means of descending phlebography. After a competent valve is identified, an adjacent deep vein is transected and anastomosed to the venous segment containing the competent valve. An example of this is transection of the superficial femoral vein, which contains only incompetent valves, and anastomosis of this to the saphenous vein, which contains a competent saphenofemoral valve (*a*). Another example is anastomosis of the divided superficial femoral vein to a profunda femoris vein which contains a competent valve (*b*). Otherwise, the superficial femoral vein can be ligated and the saphenous vein anastomosed end-to-side below the ligature (*c*).

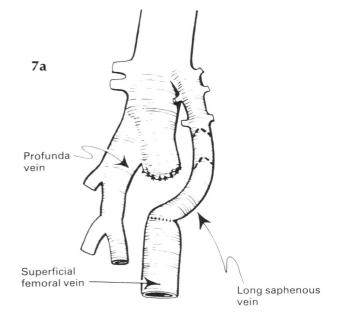

7a

Profunda vein

Superficial femoral vein

Long saphenous vein

7b

7c

The femoral venous confluence is approached through a linear incision made directly over the veins. One-third of the incision should be above the inguinal ligament, and two-thirds below. The saphenous vein and its tributaries are isolated, the common vein is skeletonized, and the profunda and superficial femoral veins are mobilized for a distance of 3–6 cm. The patient is systematically heparinized prior to the application of atraumatic clamps or occlusion of the major veins with siliconized rubber slings. Anastomosis is done with 7/0 polypropylene suture, ensuring that there is no tension between the structures to be anastomosed. Continuous stitching is utilized.

Competence of the valve is checked by emptying the distal vein through the valve and observing the distal vein for refilling. Wound closure is done in layers to avoid dead space. The skin edges are approximated using intradermal sutures of synthetic absorbable material, such as polyglycolic acid. Suction drainage may be used, but anticoagulants have been abandoned on our service.

Intermittent calf compression can be applied to maintain venous velocity through the reconstructed segment.

Kistner's late 1982 report (Ferris and Kistner, 1982) included 53 venous reconstructions in 46 patients, performed over a 14-year period. Seven of these reconstructions were excluded from evaluation. In two of these, superficial femoral vein ligation was required because of haemorrhage. In two others, superficial femoral vein ligation was required because of valve injury during repair or irreparable valve due to postphlebitic state. In another case, external plication rather than valve repair was done. Two patients had lymphoedema but underwent repair of a leaking superficial femoral vein valve; their symptoms of lymphoedema persisted.

In the remaining 46 extremities, there were 32 valve repairs and 14 venous segment transpositions. The results were good-to-excellent in 80% of both groups. Patients with stasis and ulceration had better results than those with pain and oedema. Interestingly, descending postoperative venography was performed in 41 of 46 cases, and thrombosis of the reconstructed segment has not occurred in any patient. Improvement of venous competence was demonstrated in 39 of the 41 cases.

It should be noted that incompetent perforators have been treated in conjunction with femoral vein reconstruction in this series. In another series (Queral et al., 1980), in which incompetent perforators were not treated, good results were only achieved in 11 of 16 patients, and excellent results in only 1 patient. This experience is similar to ours.

Valve transplantation

Taheri has had the greatest experience with valve transplantation. In the original procedure described by him the superficial femoral vein was exposed through a longitudinal incision below the inguinal ligament. Later, he implanted the new segment in the above-knee popliteal vein. The brachial vein is approached through a longitudinal incision 5 cm below the axilla. A 2-cm segment of brachial vein, including valve, is tested for competence and removed. A segment of popliteal vein is excised, and the brachial vein, including the valve, is sutured to the popliteal vein with 7/0 or 8/0 polypropylene suture, using a continuous, everting or interrupted technique.

Taheri uses continuous heparin administration and suction drainage of both the arm and the thigh wound. Oral anticoagulation is used for 3 months.

Taheri, Lazar and Alias (1982) described 38 patients having valve transplantation. Postoperative venography (16 ascending, 12 descending) showed 13 patients with normal venous systems and 3 patients with thrombosis of the superficial femoral system.

The only other large experience with valve transplantation is that of Raju (1983), who reported 20 valvuloplasties, 22 vein valve transplantations and 3 Kistner segment transfer operations. Thrombosis of a valve repair was only found in 1 of 17 patients who had venographic examination of the repair after operation. The valve transplant operation seemed quite satisfactory, with resolution of the primary symptom in 13 limbs (9 ulcers, 2 oedema, 2 chronic pain). Of this group, 10 limbs showed improvement in the venous haemodynamics, as measured in the laboratory, and in 3 limbs, despite subjective improvement, the laboratory parameters remained unchanged. Eight patients were surgical failures: there was a technical problem in one small axillary vein; in the other seven patients there was recurrence of reflux through the transplanted axillary vein segment, proved by venography/venous testing.

Superior vena cava bypass

8

Superior vena cava obstruction may have a variety of causes, including granulomatous mediastinitis, tuberculosis and malignant tumour. When cerebral insufficiency syndromes occur, consideration may be given to the performance of a bypass of the superior vena cava (Chiu, Terzis and MacRae, 1974; Wright and Doty, 1980). A suitable graft for such bypass may be obtained by removing the long saphenous vein, ligating all of its branches, distending the vein with heparinized saline solution under gentle hydrostatic pressure, and splitting the vein longitudinally throughout its length. The open vein is then wrapped around a previously chosen stent of appropriate size (No. 40 chest tube). The continuous anastomosis can be made utilizing 6/0 or 7/0 polypropylene suture.

A median sternotomy incision is made, and the innominate vein exposed and mobilized throughout its length. The pericardium is then opened through a vertical incision,

retracted laterally and held in place with stay sutures. Biopsy of the upper mediastinum can be obtained at this time. The distance between the innominate vein and atrial appendage is measured. The distal anastomosis can be made end-to-end, as preferred by Doty and Wright, or end-of-graft to side-of-innominate vein. Meticulous performance of the anastomosis is eased by use of loop magnification. The suture material is 6/0 polypropylene.

The anastomosis to the right atrial appendage can be done using a partial occlusion clamp. The trabeculated portion of the atrial appendage is excised and the anastomosis constructed with 6/0 polypropylene. The clamps are removed, and the blood flow through the graft is checked. As in all venous surgery, meticulous technique must be utilized for construction of the spiral graft and both of the anastomoses. Fibrous adventitial strings must not be allowed to cross the suture lines; neither should purse-stringing of either anastomosis be allowed to occur.

The pericardium is not closed, but the median sternotomy is closed by peristernal wire, in order to immobilize the sternum entirely. Drainage tubes are left in the mediastinum, but anticoagulation is unnecessary.

8

Acknowledgements

Supported in part by the Conrad Jobst Foundation, the Seabury Foundation and the Northwestern Vascular Research Foundation.

Illustrations 5 and 6 are from Kistner and Ferris (1980, pp. 293 and 295). *Illustration 7* is from Queral (1980, p. 304).

References

Chiu, C. J., Terzis, J. and MacRae, M. L. (1974). Replacement of superior vena cava with the spiral composite vein graft. *Annals of Thoracic Surgery* **17**, 555.

Clowes, A. W. (1980). Extra-anatomical bypass of iliac vein obstruction. *Archives of Surgery* **115**, 767.

Ferris, E. B. and Kistner, R. L. (1982). Femoral vein reconstruction in management of chronic venous insufficiency. *Archives of Surgery* **117**, 1571.

Harris, J. P., Kidd, J., Burnett, A. and Halliday, P. (1988). Patency of femorofemoral venous crossover grafts assessed by duplex scanning and phlebography. *Journal of Vascular Surgery* **8**, 679.

Husni, E. A. (1970). *In situ* sapheno-popliteal bypass grafts for incompetence of femoral and popliteal veins. *Surgery, Gynecology and Obstetrics* **130**, 279.

Kistner, R. L. and Ferris, E. B. (1980). Technique of surgical reconstruction of femoral vein valves. In *Operative Techniques in Vascular Surgery*. Bergan, J. J., Yao, J. S. T., eds. London and San Diego: Grune and Stratton.

May, R. (1979). *Surgery of the Veins of the Leg and Pelvis*. London and Philadelphia: W. B. Saunders, p. 150.

Palma, E. C. (1976). Vein grafts for treatment of post-phlebitic syndrome. In: *Vascular Surgery: Principles and Techniques*. Haimovici, H., ed. New York: McGraw Hill, p. 857.

Queral, L. A. (1980). Correction of deep venous insufficiency by valvular transposition. In *Operative Techniques in Vascular Surgery*. Bergan, J. J., Yao, J. S. T., eds. London and San Diego: Grune and Stratton.

Queral, L. A., Whitehouse, W. M. Jr, Flinn, W. R. *et al*. (1980). Surgical correction of chronic deep venous insufficiency by valvular transposition. *Surgery* **87**, 688.

Raju, S. (1983). Venous insufficiency of the lower limb and stasis ulceration. *Annals of Surgery* **197**, 688.

Sottiurai, V. S. (1988). Techniques in venous valvuloplasty. *Journal of Vascular Surgery* **8**, 646.

Taheri, S. A., Lazar, L. and Alias, S. (1982). Status of vein valve transplant after 12 months. *Archives of Surgery* **117**, 1313.

Takaba, T., Yamamoto, N., Fumami, M., *et al*. (1983). Reconstruction with expanded polytetrafluoroethylene (EPTFE) for iliac venous obstruction (abstract). *Journal of Cardiovascular Surgery* **24**, 422.

Warren, C.B. and Thayer, T. P. (1954). Transplantation of the saphenous vein for post-phlebitic stasis. *Surgery* **35**, 867.

Wright, C. B. and Doty, D. B. (1980). Spiral vein grafting: the technique. In: *Operative Techniques in Vascular Surgery*. Bergan, J. J., Yao, J. S. T., eds. London and San Diego: Grune and Stratton, pp. 307–310.

Repair of venous valves using silicone cuffs

Rodney J. Lane   MS, FRCS, FRCSE, DDU, FRACS

Visiting Vascular Surgeon, The Royal North Shore Hospital, St Leonards, New South Wales, Australia;
Visiting Vascular Surgeon, North Harbour Private Hospital, Harbord, New South Wales, Australia

Introduction

The present indications for the use of silicone valve cuffs are to correct chronic deep venous insufficiency usually associated with ulceration unresponsive to other forms of therapy. Similar silicone cuffs may be used for varicose veins. The underlying aetiology of lower limb venous insufficiency is first determined using non-invasive testing. If deep venous incompetence is thought to be the problem it is confirmed by venography. Grades of III or IV (Kistner) of reflux must be demonstrated and the best results are obtained when the whole venous system is uniformly dilated with multiple valves. These must be clearly demonstrated by venography, particularly by descending venography. Both cusps must be seen to be present and the attachment of the cusps on to the wall must be symmetrical. Radio-opaque markers are essential during all forms of venography in order to allow accurate location of the valves at the time of operation.

There are reservations about this technique in patients with extensive deep venous thrombosis and associated inflammatory changes with destruction of valve cusps. However, patients who have venographically intact valve cusps either above or below a previous thrombosis do not necessarily have to be excluded. At present, at least three valves in more than one area (i.e. popliteal or femoral level) should be corrected. The distal repairs are always performed initially, because one of the operative tests for valve function requires maximal hydrostatic pressure with anaesthetic-induced val-

salva. Additional back pressure is created by elevating the head as much as possible and clearly this is best achieved without having interposing competent valves. Main axial valves are selected in order to minimize distal alternate retrograde flow. In patients where the function of a particular valve cannot be totally corrected (but a good pressure gradient can be maintained), additional valves should be repaired. It is essential that all valves are tested at operation usually via the 'milking' and the 'proximal occlusion' techniques to check competence visually. Typically, complete competence is obtained with reduction of the lumen by apparently one-third.

Preoperative precautions

Microbiological examination of swabs from the ulcer is used to determine the presence of pathogens and patients are covered with the appropriate antibiotics during the anaesthetic induction. Heparin is also given. Our practice is to give 5000 u subcutaneously and 2000 u intravenously. The level of the valve is marked on the skin with an indelible pencil based on preoperative venogram with magnification taken into account.

The operation

1

The popliteal fossa or thigh is prepared and draped in the usual manner and the skin covered with a suitable plastic drape. The incision is curved to minimize contracture at the skin fold.

2

The incision is carried through the deep fascia and the vein is located adjacent to the artery. Minimal dissection is required in order to obviate or minimize lymphatic interruption. The segment of vein above and below the valve is isolated and minor tributaries are ligated and divided. If there are major tributaries then these are slung.

3

During the dissection the valve is located and appears as an oblique curvilinear line of attachment joining in a proximal apex. There is commonly a bulge just proximal to the valve cusp and it may be necessary to refer to the venogram and remeasure the actual site of the valve from a bony prominence.

If the valve cannot be identified by these means, intraoperative B-mode imaging may be used. Occasionally, to decide finally on the presence or absence of a valve, the vein is narrowed to see if competence is achieved. Very gentle dissection is essential as spasm of the valve may occur and cause temporary competence interfering with testing. This can always be overcome, however, by proximal occlusion and digital pressure between the occlusive loop and the valve.

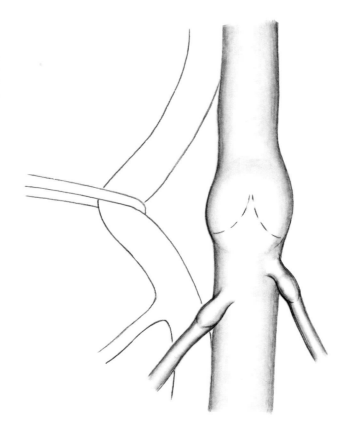

4

Having identified the valve and dissected at least 3 cm distally and 1 cm proximally, silastic vessel loops are placed around the vein in order to control inflow and outflow.

4

5

The silicone cuff used is called the 'Venocuff'. A right-angle forceps is used to pass one end of the 'Venocuff' around the vein. The other end of the 'Venocuff' is already attached to its applicator. Sometimes the end of the 'Venocuff' may impinge upon the vein wall and great care should be taken.

6

The free end of the 'Venocuff' is engaged into the applicator 'Venocuff' slot. The 'Venocuff' is now wrapped around the vein and is positioned at the valve site. The buckle action is similar to a car seat belt. At this stage, irrigation solution containing antibiotics in saline is used to irrigate the wound to maintain asepsis. The 'Venocuff' should not be allowed to touch the patient's skin.

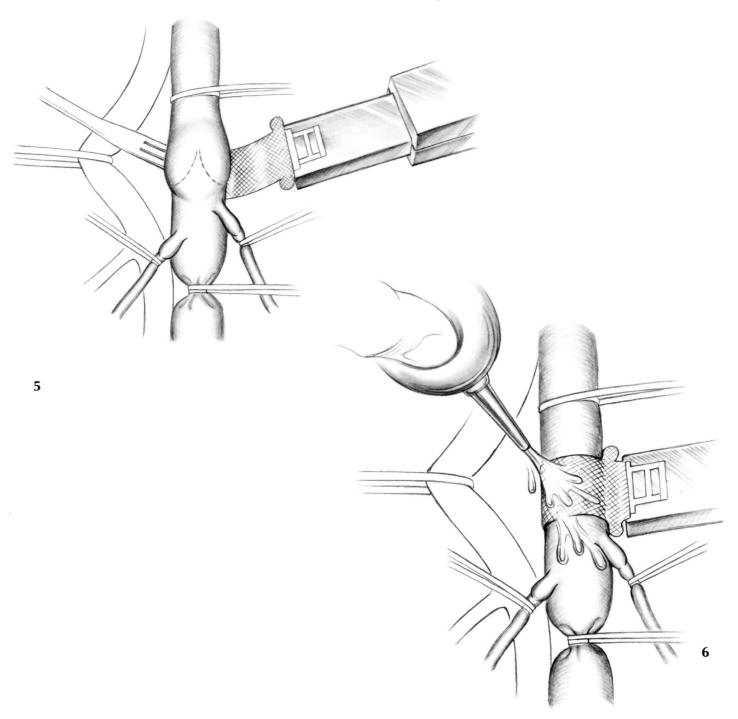

5

6

7

The applicator tensioning bar is then activated to decrease the valve ring circumference and so bring valve cusps closer together to produce competence. This is checked frequently during the tightening using the 'milking technique'. The inflow is first occluded with the distal silastic slings and the segment up to the valve ring is milked free of blood with the finger and thumb. Maximum 'head up' of the patient on the operating table is required during this testing. A 'valsalva manoeuvre' is performed by the anaesthetist to obstruct venous return and further stress the valve being tested. It becomes clear if the valve withstands the downward force of venous pressure if the distal vein segment stays collapsed. The distal silastic loop is now released to fill the distal segment and again the test is repeated.

7

8

The proximal compression test or close segment compression test is then performed by obstructing the proximal sling, cranial to the valve being tested and allowing the segment between to fill. Digital pressure then compresses this segment and a competent valve generates a high pressure. This can be compared with the pressure in the distal vein. This test is useful when access to the more distal parts of the vein are not possible because of tributaries or inadequate dissection. If a valve seems to be incompetent following 'Venocuff' application on repeated testing, an unsighted tributary should be sought. In many cases, competence is demonstrated when this hidden tributary is controlled. If the valve is not completely competent under high pressure but clearly maintains a gradient, the 'Venocuff' is left in place.

8

414

9

When valve function has been corrected or, at least, improved, the staple trigger on the applicator is fired and the staple automatically fastens the 'Venocuff' at the appropriate diameter and cuts off excess strapping. Occasionally, the operator may place excessive downward pressure on the actual vein, so that when the applicator has been removed, the valve subsequently becomes incompetent again. Therefore, both testing manoeuvres should be repeated after fastening the 'Venocuff'. The diameter of the 'Venocuff' should always be noted using the graduations on the applicator. Hence, if incompetence occurs, a new 'Venocuff' is applied and the diameter is further decreased, which usually imparts competence.

9

10

10

Occasionally, the ends of the 'Venocuff' require a metal vessel clip at the join of the two straps. These may be inserted at either end above or below.

11

There are two fixation tags on the 'Venocuff' which are then used to suture the 'Venocuff' to surrounding tissue. A 5/0 polypropylene suture is used to do this. Two further sutures are used to fasten the 'Venocuff' directly to the adventitia of the vein as shown. Sometimes when checking for competence it becomes necessary to cut the distal fixation tag off, and this direct extra suturing to the vein is then mandatory.

11

12

In cases of a valve being very close to a tributary, a 'Venocuff' with a V-notch (Venocuff S) can be chosen to allow adequate and suitable reduction of the circumference of the valve. There are two notched 'Venocuffs', the left and right (Venocuff SL and SR), to suit the situation.

It should be emphasized that the corners of the notch must be sutured directly to the adventitia, preferably anteriorly and posteriorly in order to maintain the diameter and tension of the 'Venocuff'.

12

13

Closure is completed in layers and sterility maintained by again irrigating with an antibiotic solution. A suction drain is used routinely and careful haemostasis is essential. Mobilization should begin as soon as possible, preferably the next day, and subcutaneous heparin is administered until ambulation is complete. Intravenous antibiotics are continued for 24 h. The patient is usually discharged at 4 days and ulcer care is continued.

13

Deep venous thrombectomy

O. Wagner MD

Professor of Surgery, University of Vienna, Vienna, Austria

Introduction

Intervention for the removal of acute thrombosis of the iliac and femoral veins consists of thrombolysis or venous thrombectomy. The aim of these procedures is the prevention of lethal pulmonary embolism as well as the immediate restoration of venous blood-flow, thereby also preserving the valvular system and preventing a post-thrombotic syndrome. The advantages of these procedures over elevation and heparin therapy are the immediate relief of the compromised venous drainage, lowered and shortened morbidity, venous valve preservation and prevention of the postphlebitic syndrome in a large percentage of these patients. Success of surgical thrombectomy can only be expected in cases of very recent thrombosis, which means that surgery should be performed within the first few days of occurrence. If thrombectomy is performed after a longer interval, adherence of the thrombus to the vessel wall makes removal of the clot increasingly more difficult and enhances the chance of rethrombosis. Surgery performed after a period of 6 days shows results similar to those after conservative treatment; thrombolysis, however, may be successful up to 15 days (Minar *et al.*, 1983).

Preoperative

Indications
Surgery is indicated for thrombosis of the deep femoral and iliac veins with a history of onset up to 5 days. However, floating thrombus or segmental femoral or iliac thrombosis can be operated on successfully up to 4 weeks.

Contraindications
Surgery is contraindicated in patients with a short life expectancy (such as those with inoperable tumour) or when postoperative heparin or anticoagulant therapy is inadvisable.

Preoperative assessment
The clinical course with sudden onset of swelling and pain is characteristic. A reliable diagnosis depends on clinical findings only and can be supplemented by ultrasound examinations. Venography is not obligatory but provides helpful information on the extent of the thrombosis. The blood group should be determined and 2 u of blood prepared in case of extensive blood loss.

The operation

This operation was first described in 1937 by Läwen, Professor of Surgery in Königsberg, Germany and followed up by Mahorner, Castleberry and Coleman in 1957.

The operation is performed under general anaesthesia. Systemic heparinization is attained by administration of 5000 i.u. of heparin i.v.

1 & 2

A transverse inguinal incision is made just above the groin crease, and the femoral vein, saphenous vein, deep femoral vein and superficial femoral vein are controlled by Silastic slings.

After heparinization a longitudinal incision of 2–3 cm is made at the entrance of the saphenous vein. First the local thrombus is removed; then each orifice is explored for clots which are removed by forceps and Fogarty catheters. The same procedure is performed on the deep femoral veins. The veins are then controlled by bulldog clamps (Fogarty and Kreppoehne, 1965). Proximal clots are removed by passing Fogarty catheters into the iliac venous system. During this procedure the pressure in the intra-abdominal vena cava is increased by hyperbaric respiration to prevent pulmonary embolism. (A blocking catheter from the collateral side should not be used since this would constitute an added trauma to the normal collateral vein without providing absolute security against embolization.)

Intraoperative phlebography of the iliac veins is helpful when additional information on the completeness of thrombectomy is necessary. In some patients repeated attempts at thrombectomy are necessary before normal venograms can be obtained.

Intraoperative endoscopy is another possibility for checking completeness of clot removal and to demonstrate residual disease in the iliac veins (Loeprecht, Weber and Monnig, 1985).

1

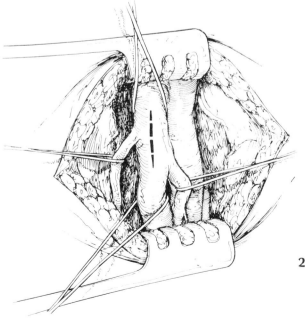

2

3

If a chronic thrombus in the iliac vein cannot be removed with the Fogarty catheter despite successful catheterization, the Fogarty catheter can be guided through the hole of a ringstripper and used to block the entrance of the common iliac vein. Following this procedure, the ringstripper can be used to remove the thrombotic material with gentle force from the vessel wall. When the clots are loosened they can then be removed by retracting the Fogarty catheter.

3

4

Finally, the distal clot is removed. When the thrombus is of recent origin and not yet firmly attached to the vessel wall, it can be removed by circumferential manual pressure which is exerted at the calf and gradually advanced upward. In cases of fresh thrombosis, sudden compression of the calf and thigh muscles by hand or with an Esmarch bandage results in complete removal of a thrombus throughout the whole deep venous sytem. The thrombus is then flushed out *in toto* by the bloodstream.

4

5

When the thrombus is adherent and compression does not work, a Fogarty catheter is used. In most cases introduction of this catheter is not possible over a longer distance because of competent valves. In such cases the catheter is attached to a small ringstripper and guided downward through the superficial femoral vein. If this procedure is not successful, because of patent venous valves, an additional incision at the proximal or distal popliteal vein might be helpful. A soft catheter can be brought up from the distal incision, the Fogarty catheter inserted into the lumen of the catheter, moved distally without problems, and the thrombus material can then be removed without interference from the valves.

After satisfactory thrombectomy, the incision(s) is (are) closed with a continuous 6/0 polypropylene suture, a suction drain is inserted and the wound is closed in layers. Postoperative continuous heparin therapy is administered (1000 i.u./h i.v.).

The patient is mobilized on the third postoperative day and anticoagulation with warfarin is started as a longer-term therapy. Anticoagulation treatment should be continued lifelong, because the rate of recurrent thrombosis in the diseased leg is very high (50%) among those patients who stopped anticoagulation even some years after their operation (Polterauer *et al.*, 1988).

Ligation of veins is never performed. If the thrombus cannot be removed during the operation because of its adherence, there is also no danger of pulmonary embolism.

The chances of developing a postphlebitic syndrome are the same as in non-operated cases. The recanalization in coming months or years is probably not adversely influenced by the surgical exploration (Wagner, 1986).

5

422

Problems

6

Venous spur

In 20–25% of cases a circumscribed stenosis at the entrance of the common iliac vein into the vena cava is found which in many of these cases might be the major cause of thrombosis. This stenosis was described by May and Thurner (1957) and is probably caused by the pulsating irritation of the crossing right iliac artery. It is nearly always possible to pass the stenosis with the balloon catheter and to dilate the spur with the inflated balloon using moderate force. Direct exploration of this area and surgical resection of the spur is not advisable as this results in a rather extensive operation. The danger of postoperative haematoma or haemorrhage as a consequence of vigorous interference and heparin therapy is high.

6

7

7

Impaction in an ascending lumbar vein

Occasionally, the Fogarty catheter, in spite of careful manipulation, repeatedly enters the lumbar ascending vein. In this case the tip of the catheter should be curved (inset). This catheter is introduced for the first few centimetres with the curve backwards and then with the curve towards the medial side of the vein in order to enter the vena cava.

Thrombus of longer duration

Even with a history of recent thrombosis, organized clots may be found during the operation, because old thrombi in the major deep veins are sometimes silent. However, acute symptoms follow sudden propagation, and occlusion of small segments (particularly the common femoral vein) as well as of small collateral branches with obstruction of venous drainage may occur. Therefore, even though the indication for venous thrombectomy is restricted to patients with a history of onset up to 5 days, an old thrombosis may be found unexpectedly during operation in the iliac and/or femoral veins in up to 50% of patients. Since the success of clot removal is directly related to intraoperatively determined thrombus age (which may not necessarily correspond to the patient's history), there are definitely two groups of patients with an entirely different prognosis. The most favourable prognosis can be made for patients with a short history of

thrombosis and when recent thrombosis is found intraoperatively. The success rate is much lower in patients with a history of over a week or when a chronic thrombosis is found during surgery.

Surgical possibilities

Chronic thrombosis of the superficial femoral vein in combination with fresh iliac vein thrombosis Thrombectomy of the acute thrombus is performed on the iliac vein, thus returning the patient to the preoperative asymptomatic condition. Partial thrombectomy is also beneficial if the venous drainage from the deep femoral veins in iliac veins and vena cava can be preserved.

8

Chronic thrombosis of the iliac vein combined with acute thrombosis of the superficial femoral vein In addition to thrombectomy of the acute thrombosis of the superficial femoral vein, thrombectomy of a chronic thrombosis of the iliac vein is often possible. In many of these cases the iliac vein stays patent. If the inflow from the femoral vein is poor, the formation of an arteriovenous fistula at the inguinal level is advisable. This arteriovenous fistula is also indicated when only the deep vein circulation can be obtained. The technique recommended is to mobilize a suitable branch of the long saphenous vein as shown and anastomose its end to the side of the femoral artery.

8

Additional technical factors

An obstruction in the thigh caused by a doubled superficial femoral vein makes the removal even of a recent thrombus difficult   In these cases distal incisions in the proximal or distal popliteal vein are sometimes helpful. The decision can depend on the preoperatively obtained venogram.

9

If the thrombus is adherent but removable, a distal arteriovenous fistula on a branch of the artery or the vein keeps the thrombectomized vein open in a sufficient number of cases. These fistulae might be located at the level of the proximal or distal popliteal artery, or even at the ankle (between the long saphenous vein and the posterior tibial artery). Arteriovenous fistulae are marked with a silk suture and should be closed after 2–3 months. The closure of an iatrogenic arteriovenous fistula in many cases presents a difficult technical problem.

Obstruction of the iliac veins by tumour, pregnancy or chronic fibrosis of the thrombus   When a thrombectomy of the femoral vein can be performed but the iliac vein cannot be cleared of thrombosis, distal thrombectomy should be combined with a femoral cross-over saphenous vein bypass (Palma and Esperon, 1960). This procedure was successful in a series of cases of primary undiagnosed pelvic tumour and in cases where pregnancy was the cause of the iliac vein thrombosis (Wagner, Piza and Müller Hartburg, 1973).

Arterio-venous fistula above the knee

Arterio-venous fistula below the knee

9

Complications

Intraoperative lethal pulmonary embolism is rare (around 0.5%) when appropriate caution is taken. There are some deaths in the postoperative period in patients where peripheral pulmonary embolisms of longer duration are found, but it is difficult to decide whether this embolization occurred before, during or after surgery. It is well established, however, that the pulmonary embolism rate in patients with iliac vein thrombosis is around 75%. The older patient group also shows an additional low mortality in myocardial infarctions. A rare complication is the loss of a transplanted kidney when the unsuspected intubation of the renal vein with the Fogarty catheter and the subsequent inflation results in an arteriovenous fistula and an untreatable haematuria leading to the removal of the otherwise well-functioning kidney transplant.

Rethrombosis is observed in a variable number of cases. In a few of those, restoration of blood flow can be obtained with a second operation and repeated thrombectomy with and without an arteriovenous fistula. In many cases it is advisable to accept the spontaneous course with rethrombosis and not insist on repeated and sophisticated operations.

References

Fogarty, T. J. and Kreppoehne, W. W. (1965). Catheter technique for venous thrombectomy. *Surgery, Gynecology and Obstetrics* **121**, 362.

Läwen, A. (1937). Über Thrombektomie bei Venethrombose und Arteriospasmus. *Zentralblatt für Chirurgie* **64**, 961.

Loeprecht, H., Weber, H. and Monnig, J. (1985). Vascular endoscopy. In *Diagnostic Techniques and Assessment Procedures in Vascular Surgery*. Greenhalgh, R. M., ed. London and San Diego: Grune and Stratton.

Mahorner, H., Castleberry, S. W. and Coleman, W. O. (1957). Attempts to restore functions in major veins which are the site of massive thrombosis. *Annals of Surgery* **146**, 510.

May, R. and Thurner, J. (1957). The cause of the predominantly sinistral occurrence of thrombosis of the pelvic veins. *Angiology* **8**, 419.

Minar, E., Ehringer, H., Marosi, L., Piza, F., Wagner, O. and Czembirek, H. (1983). Klinische, funktionelle und morphologische Spätergebnisse nach venöser Thrombektomie. *VASA* **12**, 346.

Palma, E. and Esperon, R. (1960). Vein transplants and grafts in the surgical treatment of the postphlebitic syndrome. *Journal of Cardiovascular Surgery* **1**, 94.

Polterauer, P., Holzenbein, Th., Huk, I., Kretschmer, G. and Wagner, O. (1988). Die akute tiefe Bëin-Beckenvenenthrombose: Retrospektive Analyse chirurgischen Therapie ergebuisse. *Chirurg.*

Wagner, O. (1986). Chirurgischen Thrombektomie. In *Angiologie 86*. Widmer, L. K. and Zemp, E., eds. Bern: Hans Huber.

Wagner, O., Piza, F. and Müller-Hartburg, W. (1973). Zur chirurgischen Therapie der Beckenvenenthrombose in der Schwangerschaft. *Wiener Klinische Wochenschrift* **85**, 17.

Transvenous insertion of the inferior vena caval filter

Lazar J. Greenfield   MD
Professor and Chairman, Department of Surgery, University of Michigan, Ann Arbor, Michigan, USA

Introduction

Most patients with deep vein thrombosis or pulmonary embolism can be managed by anticoagulation alone; however, it is essential to provide timely mechanical protection from thromboembolism for those patients who have a contra-indication to anticoagulation, who have a complication of anticoagulation forcing it to be discontinued or who fail anti-coagulation and sustain recurrent embolism. Patients who have a propagating tail on a thrombus in a major vein, who have required pulmonary embolectomy or who sustain recurrent embolism after another device within, or ligation of the inferior vena cava, will also benefit from a vena caval filter. In some high-risk patients with serious underlying cardiac or pulmonary disease, filter insertion may be considered as an adjunct to anticoagulation which itself provides 90% protection against recurrent thromboembolism. This is particularly appropriate in the presence of a free-floating proximal thrombus where anticoagulation is less effective. This situation can be identified either by retrograde veno-graphy or by duplex echographic or MRI imaging of the proximal thrombus. When a thrombus has propagated to the level of the renal veins or when there is pelvic or ovarian vein thrombosis, the filter should be placed above the level of the renal veins at T12–L1. This suprarenal location is also appropriate for pregnant patients and young women anticipat-ing pregnancy, since placement in the standard infrarenal location may subject the filter to compression from the gravid uterus. On rare occasions, the filter has been inserted in the superior vena cava in an inverted position for subclavian vein thrombosis.

Methods

There are two techniques for insertion of the Greenfield vena caval filter, which is the only device available approved by the FDA. Earlier unfavourable experiences with the Mobin-Uddin umbrella and the Hunter balloon has led to the withdrawal of these devices.

1

The standard Greenfield filter (SGF) is fashioned from stainless steel (*left*) and designed to be inserted operatively from either the right jugular or right femoral vein. Alternative sites include the left jugular or left axillary vein as well as intraoperative insertion via the right atrium. Interventional radiologists have reported their experience with percutaneous insertion of the SGF using the Seldinger technique for progressive dilatation to a Fr 24 sheath, usually from the femoral vein. This, however, has been associated with a 40% incidence of post-insertion femoral vein thrombosis. A new titanium Greenfield filter (TGF, *right*) is available with the same design as the SGF but with the ability to be placed in a Fr 12 carrier.

1

2

The smaller TGF carrier (*below*) is safer for percutaneous insertion and also allows intraoperative insertion directly into the inferior vena cava. Carrier systems are available to allow either filter to be inserted from either vein. The SGF in the femoral insertion carrier is shown here (*above*).

2

Operative technique

The technique of operative insertion of the SGF via the jugular vein will be described, then the technique of percutaneous insertion of the TGF via the femoral vein. The open procedure is usually performed in the operating room on a table which allows portable fluoroscopy over the chest and abdomen. Local anaesthesia is preferred to a general anaesthetic if the patient is cooperative, but it is essential to control the open jugular vein during inspiration to prevent air embolism.

The patient is positioned supine with the table slightly head-up. Placing a small roll under the shoulders and turning the head to the left facilitate exposure of the base of the neck. If the patient is heparinized, it is usually discontinued 6 h prior to the procedure and resumed postoperatively. Full heparinization is not a contraindication to filter insertion, but will lead to a higher incidence of wound haematomas.

3

A transverse incision is made one finger breadth above the clavicle overlying the sternal and clavicular heads of the sternocleidomastoid muscle. Separation of the heads of the muscle allows ready access to the internal jugular vein which is freed for a distance of at least 3 cm. After loops are passed around the vein, a vascular clamp is applied distally, taking care to avoid injury to the vagus nerve. Twill tape is preferred for proximal control to allow repeated clamping by a haemostat.

3

4

A 0.038-inch flexible tip Teflon-coated guide-wire is passed through a No. 14 plastic sheath needle puncture of the jugular vein and threaded under fluoroscopy to the level of the bifurcation of the inferior vena cava. Torque manipulation is usually required in order to pass the eustachian valve at the atriocaval junction. Once the guide-wire is in position, the external end is threaded retrograde through the carrier system of the SGF and a clamp applied to it when it emerges from the proximal catheter. The venotomy is enlarged at the point of guide-wire entry by incision and clamp dilation after which the carrier is threaded over the guide-wire to the desired level of filter discharge. This would be the L3 level for infrarenal discharge and the T12–L1 level for suprarenal discharge.

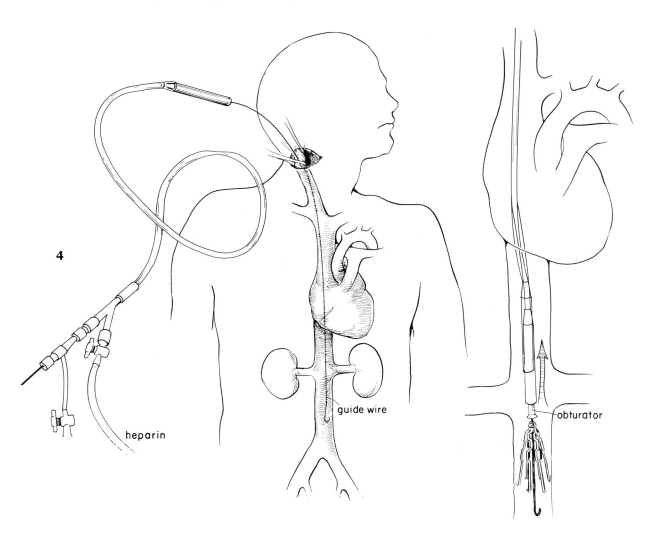

4

heparin

guide wire

obturator

5

The locking hub is unscrewed to release the stylet and the main catheter is drawn backward holding the Y connector which uncovers the filter, allowing it to spring open and attach itself to the wall of the inferior vena cava.

5

6

6

The carrier system and guide-wire are withdrawn and the jugular venotomy is repaired using continuous 5/0 polypropylene. Meticulous haemostasis is obtained and the wound is closed without drainage, usually with subcuticular closure. A compression dressing is applied with elastic adhesive tape.

Percutaneous technique

The procedure is usually performed in the radiology suite, often after a catheter has already been introduced into the right femoral vein for venous or pulmonary angiography. The presence of iliofemoral venous thrombosis is a contra-indication to the use of that side for percutaneous filter insertion. Although the left common iliac vein is usually flattened by the cross-over of the right common iliac artery, the smaller size of the TGF carrier system allows it to be inserted from either the right or left common femoral vein.

7

Percutaneous needle aspiration of the common femoral vein allows insertion of a guide-wire through an attached plastic cannula once the needle is withdrawn. Following this, a small skin incision is made in order to allow passage of the dilator and sheath over the guide-wire. (Reprinted with permission from *Atlas of Bedside Procedures*, 2nd ed., Little, Brown & Co., 1988.)

7

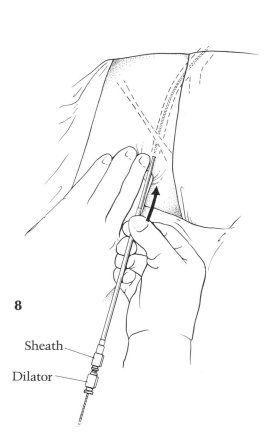

8

Sheath

Dilator

8

The dilator with attached sheath is passed under fluoroscopy over the guide-wire into the inferior vena cava. Angulation between the iliac vein and inferior vena cava over the brim of the pelvis may require advancement of the dilator and guide-wire together. Once the dilator and sheath are in position in the vena cava, the dilator and guide-wire are withdrawn, leaving the sheath in place. (Reprinted with permission from *Atlas of Bedside Procedures*, 2nd ed., Little, Brown & Co., 1988.)

9

The filter carrier is then introduced into the sheath and, again if there is difficulty negotiating the angle over the brim of the pelvis, the guide-wire and sheath should be advanced together. Prior to insertion of the carrier system, the sheath should be flushed with heparinized saline. Digital occlusion of the luerlock will avoid excessive blood loss. (Reprinted with permission from *Atlas of Bedside Procedures*, 2nd ed., Little, Brown & Co., 1988.)

9

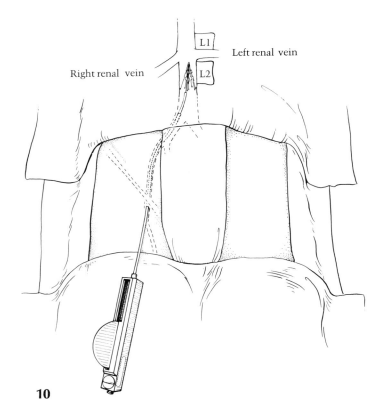

L1

L2

Right renal vein

Left renal vein

10

10

It is important to advance the carrier through the sheath until the sheath hub contacts the control handle in order to prevent accidental release of the filter into the sheath. The carrier should be positioned under fluoroscopy at the level of L3 and then the locking mechanism on the control handle can be released by moving the control tab to the unlock position. The control tab is then pulled backward in order to uncover the filter which will be discharged within the vena cava. Once the filter has been discharged, no attempt should be made to alter its position. The carrier and sheath are then withdrawn and pressure applied to the puncture site for at least 5 min. A firm bolus dressing should be applied and an abdominal radiograph obtained to document filter position. (Reprinted with permission from *Atlas of Bedside Procedures*, 2nd ed., Little, Brown & Co., 1988.)

11

Predictable patency rate of the Greenfield filter in excess of 95% is due to its geometry. The cone shape of the filter allows it to be filled to 70% of its depth (above) without interfering with flow. Preservation of flow allows for spontaneous resolution of entrapped thrombi, with or without systemic anti-coagulation. Anticoagulation should always be used to control the underlying thrombotic disorder, but is not necessary for long-term patency of the filter. Filter design also enhances entrapment of smaller thrombi, since axial flow is directed into the apex of the filter. (Reprinted with permission, Meditech, Inc., Watertown, Pennsylvania, USA.)

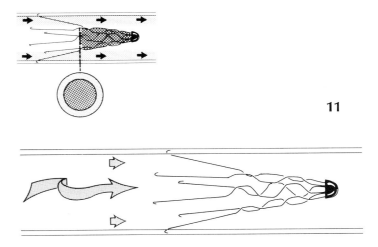

11

Complications

It is advisable to have a vena cavogram prior to filter insertion in order to document the proximal extent of the thrombus and to reveal any congenital anomalies such as duplication of the vena cava. Prior to insertion, the span of the filter should be checked for all limbs at 30 mm for the SGF. The TGF comes preloaded and should not be discharged for test purposes since it cannot be reloaded. Premature discharge of the SGF can occur if the locking nut is not secure, but other misplacement is rare if a guide-wire is used. Flushing the catheter system with heparinized saline prevents thrombus from forming within the carrier which can tether the limbs of the filter, preventing its opening and fixation to the cava. After fixation to the wall of the cava, the filter will not migrate proximally but can be deformed and the limbs extruded from the cava by external forces at the time of laparotomy or through the flaccid abdominal wall of the quadriplegic during a 'quad cough'.

References

Greenfield, L. J. (1979). Technical considerations for insertion of vena caval filters. *Surgery, Gynecology and Obstetrics* **148**, 422.

Greenfield, L. J. and Michna, B. A. (1988). Twelve year clinical experience with the Greenfield vena caval filter. *Surgery* **104**(4), 706.

Greenfield, L. J., Zocco, J., Wilk, J. D., Schroeder, M. D. and Elkins, R. C. (1977). Clinical experience with the Kim-Ray Greenfield vena caval filter. *Annals of Surgery* **185**(6), 692.

Greenfield, L. J., Peyton, R., Crute, S. and Branes, R. (1981). Greenfield vena caval filter experience: Late results in 156 patients. *Archives of Surgery* **116**, 1451.

Greenfield, L. J., Stewart, J. R. and Crute, S. (1983). Improved technique for Greenfield vena caval filter insertion. *Surgery, Gynecology and Obstetrics* **156**(2), 217.

Jones, T. K., Barnes, R. W. and Greenfield, L. J. (1986). Greenfield vena caval filter rationale and current indications. *Annals of Thoracic Surgery* **42**, S48.

Stewart, J. R., Peyton, J. W. R., Crute, S. L. and Greenfield, L. J. (1982). Clinical results of suprarenal placement of the Greenfield vena caval filter. *Surgery* **92**(1), 1.